SBAs and EMQs in
CLINICAL
PATHOLOGY

SBAs and EMQs in
CLINICAL
PATHOLOGY

Sukhpreet Singh Dubb MBBS Bsc (Hons) FY1 Doctor,
Imperial College London, UK

Neeral Patel MBBS BSc (Hons) Academic FY1 Doctor,
West Midlands Deanery, Imperial College London, UK

Nishma Manek MBBS BSc (Hons) Oxford Deanery,
Imperial College London, UK

Dhruv Panchal MBBS Bsc (Hons) FY1 Doctor, Oxford Deanery,
Imperial College London, UK

Shams Shamoon BSc (Hons) Final Year Medical Student,
Imperial College London, UK

Editorial Advisor:
Karim Meeran, Professor of Endocrinology, Imperial College London, UK

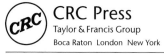

CRC Press
Taylor & Francis Group
Boca Raton London New York

CRC Press is an imprint of the
Taylor & Francis Group, an **informa** business

CRC Press
Taylor & Francis Group
6000 Broken Sound Parkway NW, Suite 300
Boca Raton, FL 33487-2742

© 2013 by Taylor & Francis Group, LLC
CRC Press is an imprint of Taylor & Francis Group, an Informa business

No claim to original U.S. Government works

Printed and bound by CPI Group (UK) Ltd, Croydon, CR0 4YY
Version Date: 20121105

International Standard Book Number: 978-1-4441-6730-6 (Paperback)

Library of Congress Cataloging-in-Publication Data

Dubb, Sukhpreet Singh.
  Single best answers and EMQs in clinical pathology / Sukhpreet Dubb ... [et al.].
    p. ; cm.
  Single best answers and emergency medicine questions in clinical pathology
  Includes index.
  ISBN 978-1-4441-6730-6 (alk. paper)
  I. Title. II. Title: Single best answers and emergency medicine questions in clinical pathology.
    [DNLM: 1. Emergency Medicine--Examination Questions. 2. Pathology, Clinical--methods--Examination Questions. QY 18.2]

616.02'5076--dc23   2012043460

Visit the Taylor & Francis Web site at
http://www.taylorandfrancis.com

and the CRC Press Web site at
http://www.crcpress.com

Dedication

To my parents and brother, who during the darkest of nights have forever remained the brightest stars

Sukhpreet Singh Dubb

To my parents, family, and friends – thank you for your invaluable support

Neeral Patel

To my parents, brother, and late aunty Usha- I wouldn't be where I am without you. And a special thank you to all the inspiring teachers I came across at Imperial.

Nishma Manek

SECTION 9 – HISTOPATHOLOGY EMQs

SECTION 10 – HISTOPATHOLOGY SBAs

Preface

There has been a transition in the method used by medical schools to test the knowledge base and clinical acumen of medical students with the adoption of extending matching questions (EMQs) and more recently the single best answers (SBAs) question format. EMQs and SBAs overcome the ambiguity that occurs in multiple choice question (MCQ) exams as well as being able to provide more clinical question stems reflecting real life situations. The SBA format is highly favoured in examinations at both the undergraduate and postgraduate levels since students must not only demonstrate their clinical knowledge and understanding but also make sound judgments that are more congruent with clinical practice.

Although there are multiple sources for clinical medicine, there is a shortfall in the resources available for explaining the pathology behind all clinical diseases and processes. *Single Best Answers and EMQs in Clinical Pathology* provides a comprehensive and unique examination of the medical undergraduate curriculum and focuses on the pathology and science behind clinical diseases. Each question not only provides an opportunity to apply clinical knowledge and correctly identify the single best answer to a question but also to learn why the other answers are wrong, greatly increasing the reader's learning opportunity. This book aims to provide medical students with a useful source for exam revision as well as supplementing their knowledge such that they may enter their clinical years with a sound scientific basis.

Dr. Sukhpreet Singh Dubb
Professor Karim Meeran

Acknowledgements

We would like to thank Dr. Joanna Koster and Stephen Clausard and the rest of the Hodder Arnold team, as well as Judith Simon of Taylor & Francis, whose support and advice have made this project possible.

Reference intervals

Investigation/Test	Range	Units
Alanine Transaminase ALT	0–31	IU/L
Albumin	33–47	g/L
Alkaline Phosphatase ALP	30–130	IU/L
Amylase	70–400	U/L
APTT	22.0–29.0	secs
Aspartate Transaminase AST	0–31	IU/L
Bicarbonate	22–29	mmol/L
Bilirubin	0–17	umol/L
Calcium	2.15–2.65	mmol/L
Chloride	95–108	mmol/L
Cholesterol	<5	mmol/L
Cholesterol HDL Ratio	0–5.00	
C-Reactive Protein	0–10	mg/L
Creatinine	60–110	umol/L
Eosinophils	0.0–0.4	x10
Ferritin	10–120	ug/L
Free T4	9.0–26.0	pmol/L
Gamma GT	2.0–30	IU/L
Glucose Fasting	3.0–6.0	mmol/L
Glucose Random	3.0–8.0	mmol/L
Haemoglobin AIC	4.3–6.1	%
HDL Cholesterol	1.00–2.20	mmol/L
Hgb	11.4–15.0	g/dl
Insulin	3.0–17.0	mU/L
Iron	7.0–27	umol/L
LDL Cholesterol	2.0–5.0	mmol/L
Lymphocytes	1.0–3.5	xl0
MCH	26.7–32.9	pg
MCV	83.0–101.0	fl
Monocytes	0.3–1.0	x10
MPV	8.0–12.0	fl
Neutrophils	2.0–7.5	x10
Osmolality Serum	275–295	mOsm/kg
Osmolality Urine	50–1200	mmol/kg
PaCO2:	4.7–6	Kpa
PaCO2:	35–45	mmHg
PaO2:	>10.6	Kpa
PaO2:	75–100	mmHg
PH	7.35–7.45	
Phosphate	0.80–1.40	mmol/kg

(Continued)

Investigation/Test	Range	Units
Platelets	120–400	10^9/L
Potassium	3.8–5.5	mmol/kg
Prolactin Female	0–750	mU/L
Prolactin Male	150–500	mU/L
Prothrombin Time	9.0–12.0	secs
RBC	3.74–4.99	x10
Serum Vitamin B12	160–800	ng/L
Sodium	135–145	mmol/L
Total Iron Binding Capacity	49–78	umol/L
Total Protein	64–83	g/L
Transferrin Sat	20–45	%
Triglycerides	0.00–1.80	mmol/L
TSH	0.3–4.2	mU/L
Urea	2.5–7.0	mmol/L
WBC	4.0–11.0	10^9/L

SECTION 1: CHEMICAL PATHOLOGY EMQs

Questions

Answers

QUESTIONS

1. Sodium handling

A	Ethanol	F	Diarrhoea
B	SIADH	G	Congestive cardiac failure
C	Frusemide	H	Addison's disease
D	Chronic kidney disease	I	Hyperlipidaemia
E	Conn's syndrome		

For each scenario below, choose the most appropriate answer from the list above. Each option may be used once, more than once or not at all.

1 A 50-year-old woman with known diabetes has a routine blood test which demonstrates the following:

Na 130 (135–145 mmol/L)
K 4.1 (3.5–5.0 mmol/L)
Urea 4.2 (3.0–7.0 mmol/L)
Glucose 3.1 (2.2–5.5 mmol/L)
Osmolality 283 (275–295 mOsm/kg)

2 A 45-year-old man is seen by his specialist. His last blood and urine tests demonstrated the following:

Na 129 (135–145 mmol/L)
K 5.5 (3.5–5.0 mmol/L)
Urea 8.2 (3.0–7.0 mmol/L)
Glucose 4.2 (2.2–5.5 mmol/L)
Osmolality 265 (275–295 mOsm/kg) dilute
Urine osmolality 26 mOsm/kg dilute

3 A 30-year-old woman visits her GP due to pigmentation of her palmar creases. Two weeks later the following blood and urine tests are received:

Na 128 (135–145 mmol/L)
K 5.9 (3.5–5.0 mmol/L)
Urea 5.2 (3.0–7.0 mmol/L)
Glucose 1.8 (2.2–5.5 mmol/L)
Osmolality 264 (275–295 mOsm/kg)
Urine osmolality 24 mOsm/kg

4 A 30-year old woman is seen by her GP after a 5-day episode of productive cough and lethargy. The GP notes dullness on percussion of the patient's left lower lung. Blood and urine tests reveal the following:

↓ Na 128 (135–145 mmol/L)
K 4.1 (3.5–5.0 mmol/L)
Urea 3.5 (3.0–7.0 mmol/L)
Glucose 3.2 (2.2–5.5 mmol/L)
↓ Osmolality 265 (275–295 mOsm/kg)
— Urine osmolality 285 mOsm/kg

5   A 63-year-old man with chronic obstructive pulmonary disease (COPD) sees his
     GP due to oedematous ankles. His blood and urine tests show the following:

Na 130 (135–145 mmol/L)
K 4.4 (3.5–5.0 mmol/L)
Urea 4.2 (3.0–7.0 mmol/L)
Glucose 3.1 (2.2–5.5 mmol/L)
Osmolality 268 (275–295 mOsm/kg)
Urine osmolality 16–mmol/LmOsm/kg

2. Potassium handling

A   Spurious sample   F   Bartter syndrome
B   Anorexia   G   Frusemide
C   Diarrhoea   H   Renal failure
D   Renal tubular acidosis   I   ACE inhibitors
E   Insulin overdose

For each scenario below, choose the most appropriate answer from the list
above. Each option may be used once, more than once or not at all.

1   A 15-year-old boy presents to accident and emergency with loss of
     consciousness. His blood sugars are found to be extremely low. Blood tests
     demonstrate the following:

Na 138 (135–145 mmol/L)
K 3.0 (3.5–5.0 mmol/L)
Urea 4.2 (3.0–7.0 mmol/L)
Creatinine 74 (60–120 mmol/L)
pH 7.48 (7.35–7.45)
HCO_3 31 (22–28 mmol/L)

2   A 64-year-old man who is an inpatient on the Care of the Elderly ward is found
     to have the following blood results:

Na 136 (135–145 mmol/L)
K 5.5 (3.5–5.0 mmol/L)
Urea 14.4 (3.0–7.0 mmol/L)
Creatinine 165 (60–120 mmol/L)
pH 7.44 (7.35–7.45)
HCO_3 27 (22–28 mmol/L)

3   A 16-day-old baby girl is found to have low blood pressure. Urinary calcium levels are found to be elevated. Blood tests demonstrate the following results:

Na 138 (135–145 mmol/L)
K 2.8 (3.5–5.0 mmol/L)
Urea 3.4 (3.0–7.0 mmol/L)
Creatinine 62 (60–120 mmol/L)
pH 7.51 (7.35–7.45)
HCO_3 33 (22–28mmol/L)

4   A 32-year-old man presents to his GP for a check-up. His serum aldosterone is found to be low. Blood tests reveal the following:

Na 140 (135–145 mmol/L)
K 5.6 (3.5–5.0 mmol/L)
Urea 5.3 (3.0–7.0 mmol/L)
Creatinine 92 (60–120 mmol/L)
pH 7.38 (7.35–7.45)
HCO_3 24 (22–28 mmol/L)

5   A 68-year-old woman on the Care of the Elderly ward is found to have the following blood results:

Na 138 (135–145 mmol/L)
K 3.0 (3.5–5.0 mmol/L)
Urea 4.2 (3.0–7.0 mmol/L)
Creatinine 74 (60–120 mmol/L)
pH 7.31 (7.35–7.45)
HCO_3 28 (22–28 mmol/L)

3. Acid–base balance

A	Metabolic acidosis	F	Respiratory acidosis with metabolic compensation
B	Metabolic acidosis with respiratory compensation	G	Respiratory alkalosis
C	Metabolic alkalosis	H	Respiratory alkalosis with metabolic compensation
D	Metabolic alkalosis with respiratory compensation	I	Mixed metabolic and respiratory acidosis
E	Respiratory acidosis		

For each scenario below, choose the most appropriate answer from the list above. Each option may be used once, more than once or not at all.

1 pH 7.31 (7.35–7.45)
pO$_2$ 7.6 (10.6–13 kPa)
pCO$_2$ 8.2 (4.7–6.0 kPa)
HCO$_3$ 26 (22–28 mmol/L)

2 pH 7.36 (7.35–7.45)
pO$_2$ 14.2 (10.6–13 kPa)
pCO$_2$ 4.1 (4.7–6.0 kPa)
HCO$_3$ 14 (22–28 mmol/L)

3 pH 7.45 (7.35–7.45)
pO$_2$ 10.2 (10.6–13 kPa)
pCO$_2$ 7.2 (4.7–6.0 kPa)
HCO$_3$ 32 (22–28 mmol/L)

4 pH 7.30 (7.35–7.45)
pO$_2$ 8.2 (10.6–13 kPa)
pCO$_2$ 7.2 (4.7–6.0 kPa)
HCO$_3$ 19 (22–28 mmol/L)

5 pH 7.49 (7.35–7.45)
pO$_2$ 13.6 (10.6–13 kPa)
pCO$_2$ 4.1 (4.7–6.0 kPa)
HCO$_3$ 23 (22–28 mmol/L)

4. Liver function tests

A Alcohol abuse
B Gilbert's syndrome
C Gallstones
D Dublin–Johnson syndrome
E Non-alcoholic fatty liver disease
F Crigler–Najjar syndrome
G Alcoholic liver disease
H Paracetamol poisoning
I Hepatocellular carcinoma

For each scenario below, choose the most appropriate answer from the list above. Each option may be used once, more than once or not at all.

1 AST 65 (3–35 IU/L)
ALT 72 (3–35 IU/L)
GGT 82 (11–51 IU/L)
ALP 829 (35–51 IU/L)
Total bilirubin 234 (3–17 μmol/L)
Conjugated bilirubin 63 (1.0–5.1 μmol/L)

2 AST 32 (3–35 IU/L)
ALT 29 (3–35 IU/L)
GGT 34 (11–51 IU/L)
ALP 53 (35–51 IU/L)
Total bilirubin 36 (3–17 μmol/L)
Conjugated bilirubin 3.4 (1.0–5.1 μmol/L)

3   AST 1259 (3–35 IU/L)
     ALT 1563 (3–35 IU/L)
     GGT 73 (11–51 IU/L)
     ALP 46 (35–51 IU/L)
     Total bilirubin 15.2 (3–17 μmol/L)
     Conjugated bilirubin 4.2 (1.0–5.1 μmol/L)

4   AST 2321 (3–35 IU/L)
     ALT 2562 (3–35 IU/L)
     GGT 62 (11–51 IU/L)
     ALP 182 (35–51 IU/L)
     Total bilirubin 14 (3–17 μmol/L)
     Conjugated bilirubin 3.4 (1.0–5.1 μmol/L)

5   AST 34 (3–35 IU/L)
     ALT 32 (3–35 IU/L)
     GGT 134 (11–51 IU/L)
     ALP 123 (35–51 IU/L)
     Total bilirubin (3–17 μmol/L)
     Conjugated bilirubin (1.0–5.1 μmol/L)

5. Endocrine chemical pathology

A   Prolactinoma   F   Conn's syndrome
B   Grave's disease   G   Kallman's syndrome
C   Addison's disease   H   Secondary hypoaldosteronism
D   Schmidst's syndrome   I   De Quervain's thyroiditis
E   Acromegaly

For each scenario below, choose the most appropriate answer from the list above. Each option may be used once, more than once or not at all.

1   A 38-year-old woman is referred by her GP to the Endocrine Clinic for further tests after experiencing fatigue and orthostatic hypotension. After a positive short synACTHen test, a long synACTHen test reveals a cortisol of 750 nmol/L after 24 hours.

2   A 48-year-old man visits his GP complaining of muscle pain and weakness. He is found to have raised blood pressure. Blood tests reveal Na 149 (135–145 mmol/L) and K 3.1 (3.5–5.0 mmol/L).

3   A 39-year-old woman sees an endocrinologist due to recent onset galactorrhoea. She denies recent child birth. Thyroid function tests are found to be normal.

4   A 46-year-old man is seen by his GP after experiencing tremors, heat intolerance and weight loss. His wife complained that his eyes were bulging. Blood tests reveal T_3 (1.2–3.0 nmol/L), T_4 (70–140 nmol/L), TSH (0.5–5.7 mIU/L).

5   A 45-year-old woman is referred to an endocrinologist due to the appearance of enlarged hands and feet as well as a protruding jaw. After conducting an oral glucose tolerance test, growth hormone levels are found to be 5 mU/L (<2 mU/L).

6. Calcium handling

A   Primary hyperparathyroidism
B   Secondary hyperparathyroidism
C   Tertiary hyperparathyroidism
D   Pseudohypoparathyroidism
E   Primary hypoparathyroidism
F   Osteoporosis
G   Osteomalacia
H   Paget's disease
I   Familial benign hypercalcaemia

For each scenario below, choose the most appropriate answer from the list above. Each option may be used once, more than once or not at all.

1   Ca 2.4 (2.2–2.6 mmol/L)
    PTH 4.2 (0.8–8.5 pmol/L)
    ALP 250 (30–150 u/L)
    PO_4 1.1 (0.8–1.2 mmol/L)
    Vitamin D 76 (60–105 nmol/L)

2   Ca 3.1 (2.2–2.6 mmol/L)
    PTH 10.5 (0.8–8.5 pmol/L)
    ALP 165 (30–150 u/L)
    PO_4 0.6 (0.8–1.2 mmol/L)
    Vitamin D 78 (60–105 nmol/L)

3   Ca 2.1 (2.2–2.6 mmol/L)
    PTH 10.4 (0.8–8.5 pmol/L)
    ALP 190 (30–150 u/L)
    PO_4 0.69 (0.8–1.2 mmol/L)
    Vitamin D 41 (60–105 nmol/L)

4   Ca 1.8 (2.2–2.6 mmol/L)
    PTH 9.6 (0.8–8.5 pmol/L)
    ALP 50 (30–150 u/L)
    PO_4 1.9 (0.8–1.2 mmol/L)
    Vitamin D 82 (60–105 nmol/L)

5   Ca 1.8 (2.2–2.6 mmol/L)
    PTH 0.69 (0.8–8.5 pmol/L)
    ALP 89 (30–150 u/L)
    PO_4 1.5 (0.8–1.2 mmol/L)
    Vitamin D 76 (60–105 nmol/L)

7. Plasma proteins

A	Bence–Jones protein	F	Ferritin
B	Carcino-embryonic antigen	G	α-Fetoprotein
C	Caeruloplasmin	H	Albumin
D	Fibrinogen	I	CA125
E	Amylase		

For each scenario below, choose the most appropriate answer from the list above. Each option may be used once, more than once or not at all.

1   A 13-year-old boy presents to his GP with parotitis with pain in his testes. His previous history reveals an incomplete childhood vaccination record.

2   A 50-year-old patient who has a 4-week history of tiredness undergoes a colonoscopy. Bleeding is noted in the large intestine.

3   A 62-year-old smoker with a history of ulcerative colitis presents to his GP with weight loss and tiredness. The patient admits noticing fresh blood mixed in with the stool.

4   A 42-year-old woman presents to her GP with weight loss and abdominal pain. Bimanual examination reveals a mass in the left adnexa.

5   A 15-year-old boy is brought in by his mother who has noted a change in his behaviour as well as a tremor. On slit lamp examination, Keiser–Fleischer rings are noted around the iris.

8. Vitamin deficiencies

A	Vitamin A	F	Vitamin C
B	Vitamin B_1	G	Vitamin D
C	Vitamin B_2	H	Vitamin E
D	Vitamin B_6	I	Vitamin K
E	Vitamin B_{12}		

For each scenario below, choose the most appropriate answer from the list above. Each option may be used once, more than once or not at all.

1   A 40-year-old patient with a history of Graves' disease presents with bilateral weakness of her legs. On examination she is Babinski sign positive and blood tests reveal a megaloblastic anaemia.

2   A 26-year-old man presents to his GP with a 5-month history of bleeding gums. Petechiae are also observed on the patient's feet. The man admits he has had to visit his dentist recently due to poor dentition.

3   A 5-year-old girl who is a known cystic fibrosis sufferer is noted by her mother to have developed poor coordination of her hands and on examination her reflexes are absent. Blood tests also reveal anaemia.

4   A 35-year-old man who is being treated for tuberculosis develops a rash on his trunk. Blood tests also reveal anaemia.

5   A 40-year-old known alcoholic develops confusion and an unsteady gait. On examination bilateral lateral rectus palsy is noted.

9. Inborn errors of metabolism

A   Phenylketonuria (PKU)
B   Peroxisomal disorders
C   Maple syrup urine disease
D   Short-chain acyl-coenzyme A dehydrogenase (SCAD) deficiency

E   Von Gierke's disease
F   Fabry's disease
G   Urea cycle disorder
H   Homocystinuria
I   Galactosaemia

For each scenario below, choose the most appropriate answer from the list above. Each option may be used once, more than once or not at all.

1   An 18-month-old girl is seen by the GP. Her mother is concerned by the child's brittle hair and inability to walk. The mother reports her daughter has had two previous convulsions.

2   A fair haired 8-month-old baby, born in Syria, is seen together with his mother in the paediatric outpatient clinic. He is found to have developmental delay and a musty smell is being given off by the baby.

3   A 9-month-old baby is seen in accident and emergency as her mother has reported that she has become 'floppy'. The baby is found to be hypoglycaemic and on examination an enlarged liver and kidneys are noted.

4   A 14-day-old girl of Jewish descent presents with lethargy, poor feeding and hypotonia. The paediatrician examining the child also notices excessively sweaty feet.

5   A 5-month-old boy is seen by the community paediatrician due to concerns of developmental delay. On examination dysmorphic features are noted, as well as a 'cherry-red spot' on the baby's trunk.

10. Therapeutic drug monitoring

A   Procainamide
B   Lithium
C   Methotrexate
D   Theophylline
E   Gentamicin

F   Carbamazepine
G   Cyclosporine
H   Phenytoin
I   Digoxin

For each scenario below, choose the most appropriate answer from the list above. Each option may be used once, more than once or not at all.

1 A 35-year-old man presents to accident and emergency with feelings of lightheadedness and slurred speech. His wife mentions that the patient has been walking around 'like a drunk'. The man's blood pressure is found to be low.

2 A 45-year-old woman is told she may be demonstrating signs of toxicity, 12 hours after being given an initial dose of medication. She has a coarse tremor and complains of feeling nauseous.

3 A 65-year-old man being treated as an inpatient develops sudden onset 'ringing in his ears' as well as difficulty hearing.

4 A 45-year-old woman is seen by her GP for a routine medications review. The patient complains of recent onset abdominal pain and tiredness. An electrocardiogram (ECG) reveals prolonged PR interval.

5 A 45-year-old man presents to his GP for a routine medications review. The patient complains of recent diarrhoea and headaches. The GP notes the patient was treated with erythromycin for a community acquired pneumonia 1 week previous to the consultation.

ANSWERS

1. Sodium handling

ANSWERS: 1) I 2) D 3) H 4) B 5) G

Pseudo-hyponatraemia can occur in patients with hyperlipidaemia (I) or hyperproteinaemia. In such states, lipids and proteins will occupy a high proportion of the total serum volume. Although the sodium concentration in serum water is in fact normal, a lower sodium concentration will be detected due to dilution by increased lipids and protein molecules. As a consequence, there is an apparent hyponatraemia. A spurious result due to the sample being taken from the drip arm can also cause pseudo-hyponatraemia.

A true hyponatraemic state occurs when the osmolality is simultaneously low. Chronic kidney disease (CKD; D) results in urinary protein loss and hence oedema. A reduced circulating volume causes activation of the renin–angiotensin system, thereby raising blood sodium levels. This in turn causes release of antidiuretic hormone (ADH) from the posterior pituitary leading to water retention and hypervolaemic hyponatraemia. Water reabsorption in the renal tubules increases urine osmolality (>20 mmol/L indicates a renal cause of hyponatraemia). CKD is also associated with hyperkalaemia and azotaemia.

Addison's disease (H) is also known as primary adrenal insufficiency (reduced aldosterone and cortisol); consequently there is a rise in the production of adrenocorticotropic hormone (ACTH). An impaired synthesis of aldosterone reduces reabsorption of sodium and increases excretion of potassium in the distal convoluted tubule and collecting ducts of the kidney; this leads to a simultaneous hyponatraemia and hyperkalaemia. Reduced cortisol production causes hypoglycaemia due to impaired gluconeogenesis. Clinical features of Addison's disease include hyperpigmentation, postural hypotension and weight loss.

The syndrome of inappropriate ADH secretion (B; SIADH) results from the excess release of ADH. In this case the clinical features suggest pneumonia is the cause, but the aetiologies of SIADH are numerous, including malignancy, meningitis and drugs (carbamazepine). Criteria to diagnose SIADH include the following:

- Hyponatraemia <135 mmol/L
- Plasma osmolality <270 mmol/L
- Urine osmolality >100 mmol/L
- High urine sodium >20 mmol/L
- Euvolaemia
- No adrenal, renal or thyroid dysfunction

Characteristically the urine osmolality is inappropriately high; in normal circumstances if the plasma osmolality is low, the urine osmolality will stop rising as reduced ADH secretion prevents water retention. As a rule of thumb in SIADH, urine osmolality is greater than plasma osmolality.

Congestive cardiac failure (G) may present with shortness of breath, pitting peripheral oedema and/or raised jugular venous pulse (JVP). In this scenario, shortness of breath may be masked by the patient's COPD. The clinical picture together with the blood result demonstrating a low sodium and low osmolality suggest a hypervolaemic hyponatraemia. This scenario can be differentiated from hypervolaemia as a result of CKD (D) by the urine osmolality, which is less than 20 mmol/L in this instance, thereby suggesting a non-renal cause for the hyponatraemia.

Ethanol (A) may cause hyponatraemia in the context of a raised plasma osmolality (>295 mmol/L). Other low molecular weight solutes that can cause hyponatraemia (when osmolality is raised) include mannitol and glucose.

Frusemide (C) and other diuretics cause a hypovolaemic hyponatraemia. As well as a low plasma sodium and osmolality, the urine osmolality will be greater than 20 mmol/L, signifying a renal cause of hyponatraemia.

Conn's syndrome (E), also known as primary aldosteronism, results from an aldosterone-producing adenoma producing excess aldosterone. Biochemical (and concurrent clinical) features include hypernatraemia (hypertension) and hypokalaemia (paraesthesia, tetany and weakness).

Diarrhoea (F) leads to a hypovolaemic hyponatraemia (as does vomiting). Plasma sodium and osmolality will be low and urine osmolality will be lower than 20 mmol/L indicating an extra-renal cause of hyponatraemia.

2. Potassium handling

ANSWERS: 1) E 2) H 3) F 4) I 5) D

Insulin overdose (E) in a diabetic patient will cause a redistributive hypokalaemia and concurrent metabolic alkalosis. Insulin causes a shift of potassium ions from the extracellular space to the intracellular space, thereby lowering blood potassium levels. Metabolic alkalosis can also cause a redistributive hypokalaemia; a reduced hydrogen ion concentration in the blood causes increased intracellular hydrogen ion loss to increase extracellular levels via Na^+/H^+ ATPase; potassium ions therefore diffuse intracellularly to maintain the electrochemical potential. Adrenaline and re-feeding syndrome also cause redistributive hypokalaemia.

Renal failure (H) can lead to hyperkalaemia secondary to reduced distal renal delivery of sodium ions. As a consequence, there is reduced exchange of potassium ions via the Na/K ATPase pump in the collecting duct, which thereby leads to accumulation of potassium ions in the blood and hence hyperkalaemia. An increase in aldosterone release will initially cause a compensatory loss of potassium ions; as renal failure progresses, this homeostatic mechanism will become decompensated and hyperkalaemia will result. Renal failure will also be reflected in the deranged urea and creatinine levels due to reduced excretion.

Bartter syndrome (F) is an autosomal recessive condition due to a defect in the thick ascending limb of the loop of Henle. It is characterized by hypokalaemia, alkalosis and hypotension. The condition may also lead to increased calcium loss via the urine (hypercalcuria) and the kidneys (nephrocalcinosis). Various genetic defects have been discovered; neonatal Bartter syndrome is due to mutations in either the NKCC2 or ROMK genes. In the associated milder Gitelman syndrome, the potassium transporting defect is in the distal convoluted tubule of the kidney.

ACE inhibitors (I) will lead to hyperkalaemia due to reduced potassium excretion. ACE inhibitors antagonize the effect of angiotensin converting enzyme, the enzyme which catalyzes the production of angiotensin II from angiotensin I. A decreased level of angiotensin II reduces the production of aldosterone in the adrenal glands, a key hormone causing the excretion of potassium. Other causes of reduced excretion of potassium include Addison's disease, renal failure and potassium sparing diuretics.

Renal tubular acidosis (D) occurs when there is a defect in hydrogen ion secretion into the renal tubules. Potassium secretion into the renal tubules therefore increases to balance sodium reabsorption. This results in hypokalaemia with acidosis. Renal tubular acidosis is classified according to the location of the defect: type 1 (distal tubule), type 2 (proximal tubule), type 3 (both distal and proximal tubules). Type 4 results from a defect in the adrenal glands and is included in the classification as it results in a metabolic acidosis and hyperkalaemia.

Spurious sampling (A) of blood results in hyperkalaemia. Excessive vacuuming of blood or using too fine a needle can cause haemolysis, leading to a raised potassium.

Anorexia (B) will result in reduced potassium intake and hence hypokalaemia. Other causes of reduced potassium intake include dental problems, alcoholism and total parental nutrition deficient in potassium.

Diarrhoea (C) results in hypokalaemia due to increased gastrointestinal losses of potassium. Other causes of increased gastrointestinal loss of potassium include villous adenoma and VIPoma.

Frusemide (G) intake leads to hypokalaemia secondary to increased renal loss of potassium. This occurs due to increased collecting duct permeability and hence potassium loss.

3. Acid–base balance

ANSWERS: 1) E 2) B 3) D 4) I 5) G

Respiratory acidosis (E) is defined by a low pH (acidosis) together with a high pCO_2, due to carbon dioxide retention secondary to a pulmonary, neuromuscular or physical causes. There is no metabolic compensation in this case, suggesting this is an acute pathology; a compensatory metabolic rise in HCO_3 from the kidneys can take hours or days. This patient is also hypoxic with a low pO_2. Causes of an acute respiratory acidosis include an acute exacerbation of asthma, foreign body obstruction and cardiac arrest.

Metabolic acidosis with respiratory compensation (B) occurs when pH is low (acidosis) and HCO_3 is low with concurrent respiratory compensation by decreasing pCO_2. The anion gap can differentiate between causes of metabolic acidosis (anion gap = $[Na^+ + K^+] - [Cl^- + HCO_3^-]$; normal range between 10 and 18 mmol/L). Causes of a raised anion gap can be remembered by the mnemonic MUDPILES: methanol/metformin, uraemia, diabetic ketoacidosis, paraldehyde, iron, lactate, ethanol and salicylates. Causes of a normal anion gap include diarrhoea, Addison's disease and renal tubular acidosis.

Metabolic alkalosis with respiratory compensation (D) occurs when pH is high (alkalosis) and HCO_3 is high with a compensatory reduction in respiratory effort that increases pCO_2. As respiratory effort is reduced there is the possibility of the patient becoming hypoxic. Causes of metabolic alkalosis include vomiting, potassium depletion secondary to diuretic use, burns and sodium bicarbonate ingestion. Respiratory compensation increase serum CO_2 concentration, which reduces pH back towards normal.

Mixed metabolic and respiratory acidosis (I) occurs when there is a low pH and a simultaneous high pCO_2 and low HCO_3. In the case of a mixed metabolic and respiratory acidosis, the metabolic acidosis component may be due to conditions such as uraemia, ketones produced as a result of diabetes mellitus or renal tubular acidosis. The respiratory acidosis component may be due to any cause of respiratory failure. Hence, this mixed picture may occur in a COPD patient with concurrent diabetes mellitus.

Respiratory alkalosis (G) is biochemically defined by a raised pH (alkalosis) and reduced pCO_2. As previously mentioned, metabolic compensation can take hours or days to occur. The primary pathology causing respiratory alkalosis is hyperventilation which causes increased CO_2 to be lost via the lungs. Causes of hyperventilation may be due to central nervous system disease, for example stroke. Other causes of hyperventilation include anxiety (panic attack), pulmonary embolism and drugs (salicylates).

Metabolic acidosis (A) occurs when pH is reduced due to low HCO_3. If there is no respiratory compensation, pCO_2 will be normal or elevated.

Metabolic alkalosis (C) occurs when pH is increased as a result of raised HCO_3. If there is no respiratory compensation, pCO_2 will be normal or low.

Respiratory acidosis with metabolic compensation (F) is defined as a low pH as a consequence of high pCO_2. There is a raised HCO_3 concentration in order to raise pH back towards normal.

Respiratory alkalosis with metabolic compensation (H) is defined as a high pH due to low pCO_2. There is a reduced HCO_3 concentration in order to lower pH back towards normal.

4. Liver function tests

ANSWERS: 1) C 2) B 3) E 4) H 5) A

Gallstones (C) may be composed of cholesterol, bilirubin or mixed in nature. The major complication of gallstones is cholestasis, whereby the flow of bile is blocked from the liver to the duodenum. This results in right upper quadrant abdominal pain, nausea and vomiting. Other causes of cholestasis include primary biliary cirrhosis, primary sclerosing cholangitis and abdominal masses compressing the biliary tree. Biochemically, cholestasis is defined by rises in GGT and ALP (obstructive picture) that are greater than the rises in AST and ALT.

Gilbert's syndrome (B) is an autosomal dominant condition in which there is a mutation in the enzyme UDP glucuronosyl transferase which reduces conjugation of bilirubin in the liver. As a consequence patients experience mild, intermittent jaundice. Jaundice in patients with Gilbert's syndrome may be precipitated by infection or starved states. Biochemistry will reveal that all liver function tests are normal apart from an isolated raised unconjugated bilirubin level, while conjugated bilirubin is within the normal range.

Non-alcoholic fatty liver disease (NAFLD; E) is due to fatty deposits in the liver (steatosis), but where the underlying cause is not due to alcohol. In such circumstances, aetiological factors include obesity, diabetes, parenteral feeding and inherited metabolic disorders (glycogen storage disease type 1). NAFLD may present with right upper quadrant pain or may be asymptomatic. Liver function tests will reveal raised AST and ALT levels (AST:ALT ratio <1) and increased GGT. Bilirubin and albumin levels are normal.

Paracetamol poisoning (H) is a common cause of acute liver failure. The clinical features of acute liver failure reflect the diminished synthetic and metabolic functioning of the liver. Characteristics include reduced blood sugar level, metabolic acidosis, increased tendency to bleed and hepatic encephalopathy. Biochemical tests will reveal AST and ALT levels greater than 1000 IU/L. AST and ALT levels will be greater than GGT and ALP levels, reflecting the hepatic rather than obstructive picture of the pathology.

Alcohol abuse (A) can lead to deranged liver function tests. In the absence of underlying liver disease, biochemical investigation may demonstrate an isolated rise in GGT. There may also be mild elevations in AST and ALT, reflecting mild hepatic damage. Haematology results will show a macrocytic picture due to toxic effects of alcohol on the bone marrow. Isolated raised GGT levels may also occur due to the consumption of enzyme-inducing drugs such as phenytoin, carbamazepine and phenobarbitone.

Dublin–Johnson syndrome (D) is an autosomal recessive disorder that results in a raised conjugated bilirubin level due to reduced secretion of conjugated bilirubin into the bile. AST and ALT levels are normal.

Crigler–Najjar syndrome (F) is a hereditary disease resulting in either complete (type 1) or partial (type 2) reduction in the conjugating enzyme UDP glucuronosyl transferase causing an unconjugated hyperbilirubinaemia.

Alcoholic liver disease (ALD; G) occurs in three stages: alcoholic steatosis, alcoholic hepatitis and eventually cirrhosis. GGT, AST and ALT will be markedly elevated (AST:ALT ratio >2).

Hepatocellular carcinoma (HCC; I) occurs as a result of underlying cirrhosis. Raised α-fetoprotein levels can be indicative of HCC. Deranged liver function tests will reflect the underlying pathology.

5. Endocrine chemical pathology

ANSWERS: 1) C 2) F 3) A 4) B 5) E

Addison's disease (C) is caused by primary adrenal insufficiency resulting in a reduced production of cortisol and aldosterone. It is diagnosed using the synACTHen test. In the short synACTHen test, baseline plasma cortisol is measured at 0 minutes, the patient is given 250 μg of synthetic ACTH at 30 minutes and plasma cortisol is rechecked at 60 minutes; if the final plasma cortisol is <550 nmol/L, a defect in cortisol production exists. The long synACTHen test distinguishes between primary and secondary adrenal insufficiency. A 1 mg dose of synthetic ACTH is administered; after 24 hours, a cortisol level of <900 nmol/L signifies a primary defect. Due to reduced mineralocorticoid production, blood tests will also reveal a hyponatraemia and hyperkalaemia.

Conn's syndrome (F) is defined as primary hyperaldosteronism second-ary to an aldosterone-producing adrenal adenoma. As a result of the high aldosterone levels produced there will be an increased excretion of potassium and reabsorption of sodium, leading to hypokalaemia and hypernatraemia. The increased delivery of sodium to the juxtaglomeru-lar apparatus causes renin levels to be reduced. Plasma aldosterone will either be raised or inappropriately normal (as ACTH is suppressed, aldosterone should physiologically be reduced).

A prolactinoma (A) is a prolactin-producing tumour and is the most prevalent pituitary tumour. Prolactinomas are classified according to size: microprolactinoma <10 mm diameter and macroprolactinoma >10 mm diameter. The clinical consequences of prolactinoma are divided into, first, those that occur as a result of increased prolactin production and, second, effects due to the mass effect of the tumour. Hormonal effects of prolactin include amenorrhoea, galactorrhoea and gynaeco-mastia in males. Mass effects of the tumour can lead to compression of pituitary cells producing other hormones such as thyroid stimulating hormone, growth hormone and ACTH.

Grave's disease (B) is an autoimmune condition resulting in the produc-tion of TSH-receptor antibodies, leading to elevated levels of T_3 and T_4. TSH levels will therefore be suppressed as a result of negative feedback. Clinical features will include exophthalmos, pretibial myxoedema, diffuse thyroid enlargement as well as other systemic features of hyper-thyroiditis (tremor, excess sweating, heat intolerance and unintentional weight loss). There is a strong association with other autoimmune con-ditions such as vitiligo and type 1 diabetes mellitus.

Acromegaly (E) is caused by the increased secretion of growth hormone as a result of a pituitary adenoma (rarely there may be ectopic production). Serum growth hormone levels are not a useful marker of acromegaly due to its pulsatile release from the pituitary. The diagnostic test for acromegaly is the oral glucose tolerance test with synchronous growth hormone measurement: 75 mg of glucose is administered to the patient; if growth hormone levels are not suppressed to below 2 mU/L, a diagnosis of acromegaly is made.

Schmidst's syndrome (D), also known as autoimmune polyendocrine syndrome type 2, is associated with Addison's disease, hypothyroidism and type 1 diabetes mellitus.

Kallman's syndrome (G) is a genetic disorder that results in hypogon-adotropic hypogonadism. As a consequence there is reduced production of LH and FSH in the pituitary. Anosmia is an associated feature.

Secondary hypoaldosteronism (H) is defined by a defect in the pituitary gland which results in reduced ACTH production, and hence reduced cortisol and aldosterone. The long synACTHen test will reveal a cortisol of >900 nmol/L as there is a delayed rise in production in the adrenal glands.

De Quervain's thyroiditis (I) is a post virus induced thyroiditis which initially presents as hyperthyroidism because thyroxine from colloid enters the circulation. Hypothyroidism then ensues for a period as thyroxine stores are depleted.

6. Calcium handling

ANSWERS: 1) H 2) A 3) G 4) I 5) E

Paget's disease (H) is a condition associated with impaired bone remodelling. New bone is larger but weak and prone to fracture. The pathogenesis has been postulated to be linked to paramyxovirus. All calcium blood studies will be normal apart from ALP, which will be raised. Paget's disease is associated with extreme bone pain, bowing and chalk-stick fractures. Bossing of the skull may lead to an eighth cranial nerve palsy and hence hearing loss. X-ray findings include lytic and sclerotic lesions.

Primary hyperparathyroidism (A) is caused by a parathyroid adenoma or parathyroid chief cell hyperplasia that leads to increased PTH production. Primary hyperparathyroidism leads to hypercalcaemia due to a raised PTH level. PTH achieves this by activating osteoclastic bone resorption (increasing blood ALP), stimulating calcium reabsorption in the kidney (with concurrent excretion of phosphate) and potentiating the action of the enzyme 1α hydroxylase in the kidney. 1α Hydroxylase acts on 25-hydroxyvitamin D_3 to produce 1,25-dihydroxyvitamin D_3 (calcitriol), which increases gut absorption of calcium.

Osteomalacia (G; rickets in children) results from insufficient bone mineralization, secondary to vitamin D or phosphate deficiency. Low vitamin D causes hypocalcaemia, due to reduced 1,25-dihydoxyvitamin D_3 production, and hence reduced reabsorption of calcium from the gut. Low blood calcium levels cause an increase in production of PTH in an attempt to normalize calcium. Therefore, calcium levels will either be low or inappropriately normal. Increased bone resorption will cause ALP levels to rise.

Familial benign hypercalcaemia (I) is a genetic condition leading to raised blood calcium levels. The disease results from a mutation in the calcium receptor located on the parathyroid glands and kidneys. This receptor defect therefore leads to underestimation of calcium, causing an increased production of PTH, despite the raised calcium levels. It is important to distinguish these patients from hyperparathyroid patients as the management of these conditions differs. Receptor failure in the kidneys reduces calcium excretion, leading to a hypocalcuric state.

Primary hypoparathyroidism (E) is defined as dysfunction of the parathyroid glands leading to reduced production of PTH. As a result, the actions of PTH are blunted leading to reduced bone resorption as well as renal and gut calcium reabsorption. As a consequence there is hypocalcaemia and hyperphosphataemia. Other causes of hypocalcaemia include pseudoparathyroidism, vitamin D deficiency, renal disease (unable to make 1,25-dihydroxyvitamin D_3), magnesium deficiency (magnesium required for PTH rise) and post-surgical (neck surgery may damage parathyroid glands).

Secondary hyperparathyroidism (B) is defined as the release of PTH as a consequence of hypocalcaemia that arises due to non-parathyroid pathology. The most common cause is chronic renal failure.

Tertiary hyperparathyroidism (C) results from hyperplasia of the parathyroid glands after a long period of secondary hyperparathyroidism. Autonomous production of PTH causes hypercalcaemia.

Pseudohypoparathyroidism (D) is a genetic condition in which there is resistance to PTH. As a result patients have high PTH and phosphate levels but are hypocalcaemic.

Osteoporosis (F) results in reduced bone density and all calcium studies are normal. Menopause, alcohol and drugs such as goserelin and steroids are risk factors.

7. Plasma proteins

ANSWERS: 1) E 2) F 3) A 4) I 5) C

Amylase (E) is an enzyme that breaks down starch into maltose. Serum amylase levels are often elevated during inflammation involving the parotid glands (parotitis) as occurs in mumps. Amylase is produced in the salivary glands, the parotid gland being the largest producer of the enzyme. Inflammation of the parotid glands cause a release of amylase into the blood stream, hence elevating levels. Raised serum amylase levels are also used in the diagnosis of pancreatitis; the pancreas is another amylase producing site.

Ferritin (F) is an intracellular protein responsible for the safe storage of iron, as free iron can be toxic to cells. Gastrointestinal bleeding may cause iron deficiency anaemia (microcytic anaemia), characterized haematologically by a reduced serum iron, raised total iron binding capacity and reduced ferritin. Ferritin levels will distinguish between other causes of microcytic anaemia: anaemia of chronic disease (raised ferritin) and thalassaemia (normal ferritin). As ferritin is an acute-phase protein, it will also be raised secondary to inflammation.

Bence–Jones proteins (A) are monoclonal globular proteins that are a diagnostic feature of multiple myeloma. Multiple myeloma is defined as the proliferation of plasma cells in the bone marrow and is commonly associated with the elderly population. Malignant plasma cells produce monoclonal antibodies and/or κ or λ light chains (paraproteins). The light chains appear in the urine and can be detected by electrophoresis of a urine sample as a monoclonal band. Bence–Jones proteins are also a feature of Waldenstrom's macroglobulinaemia and amyloid light chain amyloidosis.

CA-125 (cancer antigen 125; I) is a protein encoded by the *MUC16* gene that may suggest the presence of ovarian cancer. Its low sensitivity and specificity prevents it from being a diagnostic marker but it is useful when used in conjunction with imaging modalities for the diagnosis of ovarian cancer. Many ovarian cancers are coelomic epithelial carcinomas and hence will express CA-125, which is a coelomic epithelium-related glycoprotein. CA-125 may be associated with endometrial, pancreatic and breast carcinomas but plasma levels are most elevated in ovarian cancer.

Caeruloplasmin (C) is a copper carrying protein encoded by the *CP* gene. Low plasma caeruloplasmin levels are associated with Wilson's disease, an autosomal recessive condition in which there is an accumulation of copper within organs due to a defect in the copper transporter ATP7B (linking copper to caeruloplasmin). As a result caeruloplasmin is degraded in the blood stream. Clinical manifestations include neurological and psychiatric symptoms, and copper accumulation within the iris of the eyes leading to Keiser–Fleischer rings is pathognomonic.

Carcino-embryonic antigen (CEA; B) is a glycoprotein that is raised primarily in gastrointestinal cancers such as colorectal carcinoma, gastric carcinoma and pancreatic carcinoma.

Fibrinogen (D) is a glycoprotein synthesized in the liver. It has an essential role in the coagulation cascade, being converted to fibrin in the presence of thrombin, an essential process during clot formation.

α-Fetoprotein (G) is a tumour marker especially raised in hepatocellular carcinoma and germ cell tumours. α-Fetoprotein is also used antenatally to screen for neural tube defects and Down syndrome.

Albumin (H) is synthesized in the liver. Low plasma albumin levels result in oedema (liver disease, nephrotic syndrome and malabsorption). Raised plasma albumin levels are associated with dehydration.

8. Vitamin deficiencies

ANSWERS: 1) E 2) F 3) H 4) D 5) B

Vitamin B$_{12}$ (cobalamin; E) deficiency may result from pathologies affecting the stomach or ileum, as well as pernicious anaemia. In pernicious anaemia, autoantibodies exist against intrinsic factor. Pernicious anaemia is also commonly associated with other autoimmune conditions, such as Graves' disease. Anaemia is a common manifestation of vitamin B$_{12}$ deficiency, with raised mean cell volume and hypersegmented neutrophils evident. Subacute combined degeneration of the cord can also result, causing ataxia and progressive weakness in limbs and trunk; Babinski sign may be positive.

Vitamin C (F) is a water soluble vitamin, essential for the hydroxylation of collagen. When deficiency of vitamin C is present, collagen is unable to form a helical structure and hence cannot produce cross-links. As a consequence, damaged vessels and wounds are slow to heal. Vitamin C deficiency results in scurvy, which describes both bleeding (gums, skin and joints) and bone weakness (microfractures and brittle bones) tendencies. Gum disease is also a characteristic feature.

Vitamin E (tocopherol; H) is an important anti-oxidant which acts to scavenge free radicals in the blood stream. Deficiency leads to haemolytic anaemia as red blood cells encounter oxidative damage and are consequently broken down in the spleen. Spino-cerebellar neuropathy is also a manifestation, which is characterized by ataxia and areflexia. Vitamin E deficiency has also been suggested to increase the risk of ischaemic heart disease in later life, as low-density lipoproteins become oxidized perpetuating the atherosclerotic process.

Vitamin B$_{6}$ (pyridoxine; D) is an essential co-factor in a number of metabolic pathways including the synthesis of amino acids and neurotransmitters. Common causes of deficiency include reduced dietary intake and isoniazid use for the treatment of tuberculosis. Vitamin B$_{6}$ deficiency causes blood and skin abnormalities. Haematologically, vitamin B$_{6}$ deficiency causes sideroblastic anaemia; dermatologically seborrhoeic dermatitis can occur. Diagnosis is made by determining erythrocyte levels of aspartate aminotransferase.

Vitamin B$_{1}$ (thiamine; B) deficiency most commonly occurs in cases of alcoholism. The acute presentation of vitamin B$_{1}$ deficiency is Wernicke's encephalopathy, characterized by the triad of confusion, ophthalmoplegia and ataxia. Chronic alcoholism can lead to Korsakoff's syndrome (amnesia and confabulation) and peripheral neuropathy. Beriberi can also occur, classified into wet and dry beriberi. Wet beriberi presents in a similar manner to heart failure, with cardiomegaly, oedema and dyspnoea. Dry beriberi involves an ascending impairment of nervous function involving both sensory (paraesthesia) and motor (foot drop, wrist drop and paralysis) components.

Vitamin A (A) deficiency primarily impairs the production of rods and hence causes night blindness; ocular epithelial changes also cause conjunctival Bitot's spots. Deficiency may cause predisposition to measles and diarrhoeal illnesses.

Vitamin B_2 (riboflavin; C) deficiency leads to mucosal damage and hence presents with angular stomatitis, glossitis and/or corneal ulceration.

Vitamin D (G) deficiency results from reduced dietary intake as well as inadequate sunlight exposure. Deficiency leads to bone pathology, including rickets in children and osteomalacia in adults.

Vitamin K (I) deficiency may result from reduced intestinal uptake or dietary deficiency. Presenting features may include ecchymosis, petechiae, haematomas and slow healing at wound sites.

9. Inborn errors of metabolism

ANSWERS: 1) H 2) A 3) E 4) C 5) F

Homocystinuria (H) is an amino acid disorder in which there is a deficiency in the enzyme cystathionine synthetase. This metabolic disorder presents in childhood with characteristic features such as very fair skin and brittle hair. The condition will usually lead to developmental delay or progressive learning difficulties. Convulsions, skeletal abnormalities and thrombotic episodes have also been reported. Management options include supplementing with vitamin B_6 (pyridoxine) or maintaining the child on a low-methionine diet.

Phenylketonuria (PKU; A) is also an amino acid disorder. Children classically lack the enzyme phenylalanine hydroxylase, but other co-factors may be aberrant. Since the 1960s PKU has been diagnosed at birth using the Guthrie test but in some countries the test may not be available. The child will be fair-haired and present with developmental delay between 6 and 12 months of age. Later in life, the child's IQ will be severely impaired. Eczema and seizures have also been implicated in the disease process.

Von Gierke's disease (E) is one of nine glycogen storage disorders, in which a defect in the enzyme glucose-6-phosphate results in a failure of mobilization of glucose from glycogen. The metabolic disease presents in infancy with hypoglycaemia. The liver is usually significantly enlarged and kidney enlargement can also occur. Other glycogen storage disorders (and enzyme defects) include Pompe's (lysosomal α-glucosidase), Cori's (amylo-1,6-glucosidase) and McArdle's (phosphorylase); each disorder presents with varying degrees of liver and muscle dysfunction.

Maple syrup urine disease (C) is an organic aciduria, a group of disorders that represent impaired metabolism of leucine, isoleucine and valine. As a result, toxic compounds accumulate causing toxic encephalopathy which manifests as lethargy, poor feeding, hypotonia and/or seizures. Characteristic of maple syrup urine disease are a sweet odour and sweaty feet. The gold standard diagnostic test is gas chromatography with mass spectrometry. Management involves the avoidance of the causative amino acids.

Fabry's disease (F) is a lysosomal storage disorder in which there is deficiency in α-galactosidase. Presentation is almost always a child with developmental delay together with dysmorphia. Other findings may involve movement abnormalities, seizures, deafness and/or blindness. On examination, hepatosplenomegaly, pulmonary and cardiac problems may be noted. The pathognomonic feature of lysosomal storage disorders is the presence of a 'cherry-red spot'.

Peroxisomal disorders (A) result in disordered β-oxidation of very-long-chain fatty acids (VLCFA); these accumulate in the blood stream. In neonates, such disorders lead to seizures, dysmorphic features, severe muscular hypotonia and jaundice.

Short-chain acyl-coenzyme A dehydrogenase (SCAD) deficiency (D) is one of the four fatty acid oxidation disorders, which is unique in its neonatal presentation with failure to thrive, hypotonia, metabolic acidosis and hyperglycaemia.

Urea cycle disorders (G) arise due to deficiency in one of the six enzymes in the urea cycle, resulting in hyperammonaemia. Enzyme deficiency occurs in an autosomal recessive fashion. Symptoms depend on age of presentation, but overall encephalopathy ensues with primarily neurological features.

Galactosaemia (I) results from the deficiency in the enzyme galactose-1-phosphate uridyl transferase (Gal-1-PUT). Symptoms occur in the infant after milk ingestion, usually poor feeding, vomiting, jaundice and hepatomegaly. A galactose-free diet is the primary management option.

10. Therapeutic drug monitoring

ANSWERS: 1) H 2) B 3) E 4) I 5) D

Phenytoin (H) is a commonly used anti-epileptic agent. Serum levels of phenytoin must be monitored due to its narrow therapeutic range (10–20 µg/mL). Phenytoin also exhibits saturation kinetics; a small rise in dose may lead to saturation of metabolism by CYP enzymes in the liver, hence producing a large increase in drug concentration in the blood as well as associated toxic effects. Phenytoin toxicity can lead to hypotension, heart block, ventricular arrhythmias and ataxia.

Lithium (B) is a therapeutic agent used in the treatment of bipolar disorder. Drug monitoring is essential (12 hours post dose) due to its low therapeutic index as well as the potential life-threatening effects of toxicity. Lithium is excreted via the kidneys and therefore serum drug levels may increase (with potential toxicity) in states of low glomerular filtration rate, sodium depletion and diuretic use. Features of lithium toxicity include diarrhoea, vomiting, dysarthria and coarse tremor. Severe toxicity may cause convulsions, renal failure and possibly death.

Gentamicin (E) is an aminoglycoside antibiotic, particularly useful against Gram-negative bacteria. It exhibits a low therapeutic index. Factors that may potentiate toxicity include dosage, kidney function (gentamicin is excreted through the kidneys) and other medications such as vancomycin. Gentamicin is an ototoxic and nephrotoxic agent and hence toxicity can lead to deafness and renal failure. Toxic effects on the ear are not limited to hearing, as the vestibular system is also affected, which may cause problems with balance and vision.

Digoxin (I) is an anti-arrhythmic agent used in the treatment of atrial fibrillation and atrial flutter. Symptoms of under-treatment and toxicity are similar. Toxicity commonly arises due to the narrow therapeutic index of the agent. Non-specific symptoms of toxicity include tiredness, blurred vision, nausea, abdominal pain and confusion. ECG changes may include a prolonged PR interval and bradycardia. As digoxin is excreted via the kidneys, renal failure may cause accumulation of digoxin.

Theophylline (D) is a drug used in the treatment of asthma and COPD. A low therapeutic index and wide variation in metabolism between patients lead to requirement for drug monitoring. Toxicity may manifest in a number of ways including nausea, diarrhoea, tachycardia, arrhythmias and headaches. Severe toxicity may lead to seizures. The toxic effects of theophylline are potentiated by erythromycin and ciprofloxacin. Without monitoring, many patients would be under-treated.

Procainamide (A) is an anti-arrhythmic agent. Toxicity may lead to rash, fever and agranulocytosis. Drug induced lupus erythematosus may result from toxic levels.

Methotrexate (C) is an anti-folate drug used in the treatment of cancers and autoimmune conditions. Toxicity may lead to ulcerative stomatitis, leukocytopenia and rarely pulmonary fibrosis.

Carbamazepine (F) is an anti-convulsant medication. Toxic levels may commonly result in headaches, ataxia and abdominal pain. Toxicity may also cause SIADH and, rarely, aplastic anaemia.

Cyclosporine (G) is an immunosuppressant. Toxicity is associated with acute renal failure. Calcium channel antagonists and certain antibiotics such as erythromycin predispose to nephrotoxicity, whereas anti-convulsants such as phenytoin reduce blood levels of the drug.

SECTION 2: CHEMICAL PATHOLOGY SBAs

Questions

18. Vitamin D deficiency
19. Raised alkaline phosphatase
20. Nutritional deficiency
21. Therapeutic drug monitoring
22. Hypoglycaemia
23. Acute pancreatitis
24. Treatment of hyperkalaemia
25. Myocardial infarction

Answers

QUESTIONS

1. Arterial blood gas sample

A 67-year-old woman presents to accident and emergency after having a fall. She is diagnosed with a fractured neck of femur which is fixed with a hemi-arthroplasty. She also suffers from metastatic breast cancer. Four days postoperatively, she develops shortness of breath with an increased respiratory rate of 24 breaths per minute. The doctor on call takes an arterial blood gas sample which shows the following results:

pH 7.48
PaO_2 15.4 kPa on 2 L of oxygen
pCO_2 2.6 kPa
Base excess +1
Saturations 99 per cent

What does the blood gas show?

A   Metabolic alkalosis with respiratory compensation
B   Metabolic alkalosis
C   Respiratory alkalosis with metabolic compensation
D   Respiratory alkalosis
E   None of the above

2. Paradoxical aciduria

A 19-year-old female student presents to the GP with low mood, lethargy and muscle weakness. She is anxious that she is putting on weight and admits to purging after meals to keep her weight under control for several months. She has a past history of depression and is taking citalopram. On examination, her body mass index is 18, she is clinically dehydrated with signs of anaemia including conjunctival pallor. She has bilateral parotidomegaly and the GP also notices erosions of the incisors. He orders some blood tests which reveal the following:

Hb 9.5
White cells 7.8
Platelets 345
Na 143
K 3.1
Urea 8.5
Creatinine 64
Arterial pH 7.49

Urinalysis is normal except for acidic urine. The cause of this patient's acidic urine is:

A   Acute renal failure
B   Renal tubular acidosis
C   Citalopram
D   Anaemia
E   Physiological

3. Hyponatraemia

A 55-year-old man with severe learning difficulties presents with shortness of breath on exertion, fever and a productive cough of rusty red sputum. On examination, there is increased bronchial breathing in the lower right zone with inspiratory crackles. The patient is clinically euvolaemic, and urine dipstick is normal. A chest X-ray demonstrates right lower zone consolidation with the presence of air bronchograms. He is on carbemezepine for epilepsy and risperidone. Blood tests reveal the following:

Hb 13.4
White cell count 12.8
C reactive protein 23
Na 123
K 4.7
Urea 6
Creatinine 62

What is the most likely cause of hyponatraemia?

A   Pneumonia
B   Carbamezepine
C   Risperidone
D   Syndrome of inappropriate antidiuretic hormone (SIADH)
E   Cerebral salt wasting syndrome

4. Hypercalcaemia

A patient with end stage renal failure presents with depression. He is on haemodialysis three times a week but feels it is not working anymore and is getting more tired lately. He says he has lost his appetite and consequently feels rather constipated too. He feels his mind is deteriorating and there is little worth in attending dialysis anymore. His doctor wants to exclude a reversible cause of his depression and orders some blood tests. The doctor finds the patient has a raised corrected calcium, normal phosphate levels and high parathyroid hormone levels. What is the diagnosis?

A   Primary hyperparathyroidism
B   Secondary hyperparathyroidism
C   Tertiary hyperparathyroidism
D   Pseudohypoparathyroidism
E   Pseudopseudohypoparathyroidism

5. Vitamin deficiency tests

A 59-year-old man presents with a fall and haematemesis after a heavy night drinking at the local pub. This is his third admission in a month with alcohol-related problems. He has stopped vomiting, and on examination he is haemodynamically stable. He has digital clubbing, spider naevi and gynaecomastia. He is admitted for neurological observations overnight as he hit his head. The doctors notice the patient suffers from complex ophthalmoplegia, confusion and ataxia. Given his neurological symptoms which test would confirm the associated vitamin deficiency?

A   Red cell folate
B   Red blood cell transketolase
C   Red blood cell glutathione reductase
D   Red blood cell aspartate aminotransferase activity
E   Carbohydrate deficient transferrin

6. Hyperkalaemia

A 75-year-old man presents with acute onset abdominal pain. The patient has not passed stools for 3 days and looks unwell. His past medical history includes bowel cancer which was treated with an abdominoperineal resection and chemotherapy 6 years ago. On examination, there is a large parastomal mass which is tender and irreducible. An arterial blood gas shows metabolic acidosis with a rasied lactate. The on-call doctor immediately starts normal saline fluids and prepares the patient for theatre. A strangulated hernia is diagnosed by the registrar and an emergency laparotomy is performed to resect the ischaemic bowel. One day postoperatively the patient has the following blood results:

Hb 13.2
WCC 10.9
Platelets 234
Na 145
K 6.3
pH 7.38
Urea and creatinine normal

What is the most likely cause of hyperkalaemia?

A   Acute kidney injury
B   Tissue injury
C   Resolving metabolic acidosis
D   Adrenal failure from metastases
E   Overhydration from intravenous fluids

7. Hypernatraemia

A 54 year old with a background of hypertension, presents to the GP with a 2-week history of diarrhoea. He has been travelling in South East Asia recently and developed symptoms of diarrhoea 3 weeks ago. He went to the local doctor whilst in China who prescribed tetracycline, but his symptoms have persisted and only improved slightly. His past medical history includes an undisplaced parietal skull fracture he sustained when he was 10. He takes no other medications. The GP orders blood tests which show the following:

Na 148
K 4.8
Urea 13
Creatinine 112

What is the most likely cause of his hypernatraemia?

A   Conn's syndrome
B   Nephrogenic diabetes insipidus
C   Cranial diabetes insipidus
D   Tetracycline
E   Dehydration

8. Water deprivation test

A 42-year-old woman with persistent polyuria and polydipsia is admitted for a water deprivation test. At the beginning of the test her weight, urine volume and osmolality and serum osmolality are measured and hourly thereafter for 8 hours. After 8 hours, she is given intramuscular desmopressin but drinks 3 L of water before going to bed. Her blood is taken again the next morning (16 hours after beginning the test) and the results are as follows:

	Start	**8 hours**	**16 hours**
Weight	70 kg	67.8 kg	66.8 kg
Urine volume (total)	0 mL	2200 mL	4000 mL
Urine osmolality	278 mosmol/kg	872 mosmol/kg	980 mosmol/kg

What is the most likely diagnosis?

A   Nephrogenic diabetes insipidus
B   Craniogenic diabetes insipidus
C   Psychogenic polydipsia
D   Invalid test
E   Normal

9. Acute abdominal pain

A 24-year-old previously fit and well woman presents with sudden onset
abdominal pain the night after a party where she drank five units of alcohol. She
complains of central abdominal pain, with nausea and vomiting. She also finds
it difficult to control her bladder. On examination, she is tachycardic, hypertensive and is beginning to become confused. On looking back at her previous
admissions, the doctor notices she has had similar episodes after drinking. This
was also true for when she started the oral contraceptive pill and when she had
tuberculosis which was treated with standard antibiotic treatments. She is also
seeing a neurologist for peripheral neuropathy of unknown cause. The admitting
doctor, an Imperial college graduate, suggests the possibility of acute intermittent
porphyria. What enzyme deficiency is responsible for this disease?

A   Porphobilinogen deaminase
B   Uroporphyrinogen synthase
C   Coproporphyrinogen oxidase
D   Protoporphyrinogen oxidase
E   Uroporphyrinogen decarboxylase

10. Exacerbating factors for gout

A patient presents with an acutely painful, inflamed elbow. He has decreased range
of movement passively and actively and the joint is tender, erythematous and warm.
His past medical history includes hypertension, chronic lower back pain for which
he takes aspirin, lymphoma for which he has just completed a course of chemotherapy and psoriasis which is well controlled. He is also a heavy drinker. A joint aspirate shows weakly negative birefringent crystals confirming the diagnosis of acute
gout. Which factor in this patient is the least likely to contribute to this attack?

A   Bendroflumethiazide
B   Chemotherapy
C   Alcohol
D   Psoriasis
E   Aspirin

11. Anion gap

A patient has the following blood results; calculate the anion gap:

Na 143 mmol/L
K 4 mmol/L
Cl 107 mmol/L
HCO_3 25 mmol/L
PO_4 1 mmol/L
Glucose 8 mmol/L
Urea 7 mmol/L

A   14 mmol/L
B   15 mmol/L
C   16 mmol/L
D   17 mmol/L
E   Not enough information

12. Estimated plasma osmolarity

A patient has the following blood results:

Na 143 mmol/L
K 4 mmol/L
Cl 107 mmol/L
HCO_3 25 mmol/L
PO_4 1 mmol/L
Glucose 8 mmol/L
Urea 7 mmol/L

What is the estimated plasma osmolarity?

A   309
B   279
C   426
D   294
E   Not enough information

13. Biochemical abnormalities in chronic renal failure

A 67-year-old man with chronic renal failure presents with fatigue. He has been on haemodialysis three times per week for a decade. His past medical history includes diabetes mellitus, hypertension and gout. He has been increasingly tired the last few weeks although he cannot explain why. He has been attending his dialysis appointments and is compliant with his medications. The GP takes some bloods to investigate. Which of the following is NOT a common association with chronic renal failure?

A   Acidosis
B   Anaemia
C   Hyperkalaemia
D   Hypocalcaemia
E   Hypophosphataemia

14. Thyroid function tests

A 45-year-old woman presents feeling tired all of the time. She has been investigated for anaemia which reveals macrocytosis. She denies drinking excessively. She has recently moved house and the GP notices she has a croaky voice, peaches and cream complexion and a slowed reaction to his questions. He examines her and elicits slow relaxing ankle reflexes. He suspects hypothyroidism and orders some thyroid function tests. Which of the following results are consistent with primary hypothyroidism?

A   Low TSH, raised free T_4 and T_3
B   Low or normal TSH with low free T_4 and T_3
C   Raised TSH with normal free T_4 and T_3
D   Normal or raised TSH with raised T_4 and T_3
E   None of the above

15. Biochemical abnormalities of metabolic bone disease

An 86-year-old woman presents to accident and emergency after a fall. She is a frequent faller but was unable to weight bear after the most recent incident. She has a history of rheumatoid arthritis which is controlled with low dose prednisolone. On examination her right leg is clinically shortened and externally rotated and a pelvic X-ray confirms the presence of a fractured neck of femur. The patient's hip is fixed the next day. Her day one postoperative bloods show the following:

Corrected calcium normal
Phosphate normal
Alkaline phosphatase raised
Parathyroid hormone level normal
Vitamin D level low

What is the most likely diagnosis?

A   Normal
B   Osteoporosis
C   Paget's disease
D   Osteomalacia
E   Malignancy

16. Inherited metabolic disorders

A 42-year-old woman presents to maternity in labour. It is her first child and she delivers a baby boy at 42 weeks gestation. During the neonatal period, the child develops feeding difficulty with hypotonia and jaundice. On examination there is a conjugated hyperbilirubinaemia. The mother thinks this has started shortly after she has started feeding the child with milk. After a few months, the child develops cataracts. On testing the urine, there is positive Fehling's and Benedict's reagent tests with a negative glucose oxidase strip test. The milk is eliminated from the child's diet and immediately some of the symptoms improve. What is the diagnosis?

A   Fructose intolerance
B   Galactosaemia
C   Galactokinase deficiency
D   Urea cycle disorder
E   Tyrosinaemia

17. Neonatal jaundice

A 2-week-old neonate born at term with no gestational complications develops uncongutated jaundice. This was following a difficult birth where instrumentation was required after excessive delay in the second stage of labour. On examination, the neonate looks well in a normal flexed position with visible jaundice most noticeable in the soft palate. There are no abnormal facies but there is a visible large caput succedaneum with bruising. Urine dipstick is normal with no markers of infection present in the blood. What is the most likely cause of the jaundice?

A   Urinary tract infection
B   Bruising
C   Haemolysis
D   Crigler–Najjar syndrome
E   Gilbert's disease

18. Vitamin D deficiency

A 54-year-old man with a past history of alcohol abuse, recurrent severe epigastric pain with flatulence and steatorrhoea presents after a fall whilst out drinking with his friends. He had fallen onto his hip, has severe pain and inability to weight bear. On examination, his right lower limb is shortened and externally rotated. His liver function tests were normal apart from a raised alkaline phosphatase. A fractured neck of femur is diagnosed and is fixed that night. As part of a routine follow up, the fracture liaison nurse suspects vitamin D deficiency and orders a full set of vitamin D levels. What set of results would you expect in this man given his history?

A   Low 25-hydroxycholecalciferol, low 1,25-dihydroxycholecalciferol, low parathyroid hormone

B   Low 25-hydroxycholecalciferol, high 1,25-dihydroxycholecalciferol, high parathyroid hormone

C   High 25-hydroxycholecalciferol, low 1,25-dihydroxycholecalciferol, high parathyroid hormone

D   High 25-hydroxycholecalciferol, high 1,25-dihydroxycholecalciferol, high parathyroid hormone

E   High 25-hydroxycholecalciferol, low 1,25-dihydroxycholecalciferol, low parathyroid hormone

19. Raised alkaline phosphatase

Which of the following is not a cause of raised alkaline phosphatase levels?

A   Pregnancy
B   Paget's
C   Congestive heart failure
D   Obstructive jaundice
E   Myeloma

20. Nutritional deficiency

A 44-year-old African man is seen by a volunteer doctor in his village with skin changes around the neck. There are erythematous and pigmented areas around the neck in a necklace-like distribution. His family is also complaining of him becoming more forgetful and unable to perform normal daily tasks. This is made particularly distressing given his increase in bowel movements, although he cannot remember how many times he goes. He and his family, like many of the villagers, eat almost exclusively maize, and the doctor has treated several cases of kwashiorkor in the local area. What is the nutritional deficiency most likely to explain his symptoms?

A   Tocopherol
B   Riboflavin
C   Retinol
D   Vitamin B_3
E   Ascorbate

21. Therapeutic drug monitoring

A 51-year-woman with epilepsy is admitted after suffering a seizure following non-compliance with her phenytoin. She admits to having problems at home and was finding it difficult to continue to take her medication regularly. She is restarted on phenytoin. How many half lives does it normally take for a drug to reach its steady state?

A   1–2 half lives
B   3–5 half lives
C   10–11 half lives
D   50–60 half lives
E   100–150 half lives

22. Hypoglycaemia

A 67-year-old Indian man presents with irritability, sweating and tremor which progresses to stupor. The admitting doctor sends for a laboratory glucose which comes back at 2.2 mmol/L. The patient is resuscitated and given intravenous glucose. A history reveals that he does not suffer from diabetes, and his past medical history is remarkable only for vitiligo. On direct questioning he admits to feeling increasingly more tired, particularly after returning recently from India. His family arrive after which the doctor notices the patient's unusually darker tan compared with his children. Further investigations reveal the patient has low insulin and low C peptide concentrations. What is the most likely diagnosis?

A   Pituitary failure
B   Addison's disease
C   Alcohol induced
D   Glycogen storage disease
E   Medium chain acyl-CoA dehydrogenase deficiency (MCADD)

23. Acute pancreatitis

A 56-year-old presents with sudden onset, severe epigastric pain which radiates through to the back. The pain is relieved only partly by sitting forward and is associated with nausea. The admitting doctor suspects pancreatitis and sends for a serum amylase which is greatly raised. A diagnosis of acute pancreatitis is made. The following results come back following a blood test:

Haemoglobin 14.5 g/dL
White cells 14.2
Na 148
K 4.6
Urea 14
Creatinine 123
Calcium 2.98 (corrected)
Cholesterol 5.5
Albumin 35 g/L
Glucose 8.8 mmol/L

Which biochemical abnormality is not likely to be a consequence of acute pancreatitis?

A Raised white cells
B Raised sodium
C Raised urea and creatinine
D Raised calcium
E Raised glucose

24. Treatment of hyperkalaemia

A 76-year-old man presents following a fall and is diagnosed with a pubic ramus fracture which is treated conservatively. He has a background of chronic renal failure and over the weekend starts to feel palpitations and lightheadedness. An electrocardiograph is performed which shows tenting of the T waves, suggestive of hyperkalaemia. A blood test is performed which confirms the diagnosis. Which of the following treatments does not lower plasma potassium levels?

A Calcium resonium
B Sodium bicarbonate
C Calcium gluconate
D Insulin
E Salbutamol

25. Myocardial infarction

A 54-year-old man is admitted for an elective shoulder repair. The day before his surgery he develops acute onset central crushing chest pain radiating to his left arm and up the jaw. He is also sweaty and feels nauseous. He has a past medical history of coronary artery bypass grafting and angina, and his father died from a heart attack aged 46. An electrocardiogram is performed which shows acute ST elevation in the inferior leads. He is diagnosed with acute coronary syndrome and treated appropriately. His surgery is delayed, but he presents with the same symptoms 2 days later with further ST changes in the lateral leads. Which cardiac enzyme is most useful to confirm re-infarction?

A Troponin I
B Troponin T
C Aspartate transaminase
D Creatine kinase muscle brain (MB)
E Lactate dehydrogenase

ANSWERS

Arterial blood gas sample

1   D   This lady has most likely suffered a pulmonary embolism manifesting as an acute onset of shortness of breath. Acid–base questions are best approached in three steps: first, decide if the pH shows an alkalosis or an acidosis. Next look at the $PaCO_2$ and decide if it is high or low. Carbon dioxide dissolves in water to form carbonic acid, a weak acid. Therefore, if the concentration of carbon dioxide is high, it will lower the pH. You must then decide if the $PaCO_2$ is compounding or helping the patient's pH – in other words, is it worsening an acidotic patient or compensating for an alkalotic patient? Finally, look at the base excess. A greater positive base excess implies a higher concentration of bicarbonate, which is a base. Unlike carbon dioxide, therefore, high levels of bicarbonate will raise the pH. In this scenario, the pH is 7.48 meaning the patient is alkalotic with a low $PaCO_2$, implying a respiratory cause. There is no compensation as the base excess of +1 is within normal limits. Unlike respiratory compensation, metabolic compensation takes several days. Below is a table of common causes of the different acid–base abnormalities with the likely carbon dioxide and base excess values.

Blood gas picture	pH	$PaCO_2$	Base excess	Common causes
Metabolic acidosis	<7.35	Low	More positive	Diabetic ketoacidosis, fistula
Metabolic acidosis with respiratory compensation	Normal	Low	More positive	Any of the above for more than a few days
Metabolic alkalosis	>7.45	High	More negative	Vomiting, hypokalaemia, bicarbonate ingestion
Metabolic alkalosis with respiratory compensation	Normal	High	More negative	Any of the above for more than a few days
Respiratory acidosis	<7.35	High	Normal	Decreased ventilation, poor lung perfusion, impaired gas exchange
Respiratory acidosis with metabolic compensation	Normal	High	More negative	Any of the above for more than a few days
Respiratory alkalosis	>7.45	Low	Normal	Voluntary, tachypnoea for other reasons, artificial ventilation, stimulation of respiratory centres
Respiratory alkalosis with metabolic compensation	Normal	Low	More negative	Any of the above for more than a few days

Another way to tackle acid–base problems is to look at the Flenley Acid–Base normogram which depicts the likely metabolic abnormality given the pH and the arterial PCO_2:

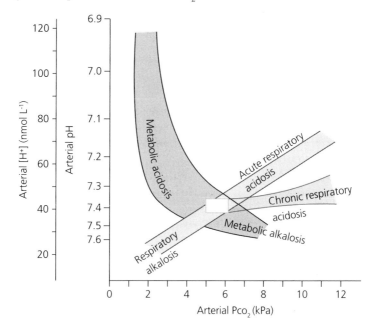

Note the non-linear relationship of metabolic acidosis and alkalosis, in contrast with the linear relationship of the respiratory based acid–base abnormality. This is because ventilation is limited at both ends of the spectrum – too low and you risk hypoxia, too high and you cannot inhale a sufficient tidal volume for meaningful gas exchange!

Paradoxical aciduria

2   E   This is a difficult question but the answer can be deduced with a basic knowledge of electrolyte physiology. This patient suffers from bulimia nervosa as characterized by the use of characteristic purging after meals to keep her weight under control. The main abnormalities in the investigations reveal a hypokalaemia with arterial alkalosis and paradoxical aciduria. The alkalosis is likely to be due to excessive purging leading to a loss of hydrogen ions. The hypokalaemia is secondary to the metabolic alkalosis as potassium and hydrogen are transported across cell membranes by the same transporter. The reduction of plasma hydrogen ions leads to increased potassium uptake leading to hypokalaemia. As part of a normal homeostatic mechanism, potassium is exchanged for

hydrogen ions in the distal convoluted tubule of the nephron, resulting in an apparent paradoxical aciduria.

Acute renal failure (A) tends to give hyperkalaemia and metabolic acidosis. This is due to the failure of homeostatic mechanism, the causes of which are classically defined as pre-renal, renal or post-renal. Pre-renal failure is caused by a reduction in glomerular filtration rate. This may be due to reduced blood flow or reduced perfusion pressure. Common causes include hypovolaemia or hypotension from shock. Intrinsic renal failure has a wide aetiology including drugs, inflammation and infection. Post-renal failure is caused by obstruction anywhere from the collecting ducts distally. This classically presents in elderly men with prostatic disease with urinary retention relieved by catheterization.

Citalopram (C) is a selective serotonin reuptake inhibitor (SSRI) used in the treatment of depression. Some SSRIs cause hyponatraemia, but not usually hypokalaemia. Renal tubular acidosis (B) generally causes a lack of ability to acidify urine and hyperkalaemia. The exception is type II renal tubular acidosis with a bicarbonate leak in the proximal convoluted tubule where hypokalaemia is common but the urine is only acidified during systemic metabolic acidosis. This is not the case in this patient. Finally anaemia (D) does not usually cause electrolyte abnormalities.

Hyponatraemia

3 B This patient's hyponatraemia is most likely secondary to Carbamezepine therapy (B), a well documented side effect of this anti-epileptic medication. Carbamezepine stimulates the production of vaso-pressin, the mechanism of action of which will be discussed shortly. It is also one of the 'terrible 3 Cs' which cause aplastic anaemia, the other two being carbimazole and chloramphenicol. Any patient with signs of infection or bleeding must be taken very seriously as fulminant sepsis may ensue without prompt treatment. This patient, however, has mounted a white cell response with a normal platelet count therefore making aplastic anaemia unlikely.

Pneumonia (A) does not normally cause a sodium abnormality on its own. Less commonly, Legionnaire's disease caused by the bacterium *Legionella pneumophilia* can have extrapulmonary features including hyponatraemia, deranged liver function tests and lymphopenia. This is unlikely to be the case as this organism often colonizes water tanks in places with air conditioning and has a prodromal phase of *dry* cough with flu-like symptoms. The alternative indirect pulmonary cause of hyponatraemia is lung cancer producing a SIADH; the tumour pre-disposes the patient to pneumonia by obstructing the normal ciliary clearance of the bronchi. It is unlikely in this patient given the lack of smoking history or cachexia.

Risperidone (C) is an atypical antipsychotic and only very rarely causes hyponatraemia. More common side effects include gastrointestinal disturbance and dry mouth. SIADH (D) is the excessive production of anti-diuretic hormone (also called vasopressin) from the posterior pituitary. Its release is stimulated physiologically by osmoreceptors responding to an increased plasma osmolality, as well as baroreceptors responding to decreased intravascular volume. Vasopressin activates vasopressin 2 receptors in the renal collecting duct principal cells, which in turn activate adenylate cyclase to increase intracellular cyclic AMP levels. This is turn increases aquaporin 2 gene transcription and the protein inserts into the apical membrane of the cells allowing free water influx to normalize increased plasma osmolality. SIADH occurs when there is excessive production of vasopressin leading to a euvolaemic hyponatraemia. It is a diagnosis of exclusion and requires two criteria in the blood, two criteria in the urine and three exclusion criteria and can be remembered as 'two low in the blood, two high in the urine, three exclusions everywhere else'.

1   Two low in the blood – hyponatraemia and hypo-osmolality

2   Two high in the urine – high urinary sodium >20 mmol/L and high urinary osmolality

3   Three exclusions – NO renal/adrenal/thyroid/cardiac disease, NO hypovolaemia, NO contributing drugs.

Cerebral salt wasting (CSW) syndrome (E) occurs after head injury or neurosurgical procedures where a natriuretic substance produced in the brain leads to sodium and chloride loss in the kidneys, reducing intravascular volume and leading to water retention. There is therefore a baroreceptor-mediated stimulus to vasopressin production. It resembles SIADH in that both are hyponatraemic disorders seen after head injury with high urinary sodium, urinary osmalility and vasopressin levels. The difference is the *primary* event in CSW is high renal sodium chloride loss, not high vasopressin release.

Hypercalcaemia

4   C   This patient has tertiary hyperparathyroidism (C) given the presence of elevated calcium levels with high parathyroid levels in the presence of chronic renal failure. Plasma calcium levels are controlled via parathyroid hormone (PTH) which is produced in the parathyroid glands situated within the thyroid gland. Reduced ionized calcium concentration is detected by the parathyroid glands leading to a release of PTH which circulates in the blood stream. PTH increases calcium resorption from

the kidneys whilst increasing phosphate excretion. PTH also stimulates 1-alpha hydroxylation of 25-vitamin D to make 1,25-vitamin D. Finally, PTH increases bone resorption of calcium via osteoclast activation. The sum effects of increased PTH levels are to increase plasma calcium concentration and to reduce phosphate concentration. PTH has an indirect, but very important, mechanism via 1,25-vitamin D which acts to increase gut absorption of calcium.

Tertiary hyperparathyroidism (C) is seen in the setting of chronic renal failure and chronic secondary hyperparathyroidism leads to hyperplastic or adenomatous change in the parathyroid glands resulting in autonomous PTH secretion. The causes of calcium homeostasis dysregulation are multifactorial including tubular dysfunction leading to calcium leak, inability to excrete phosphate leading to increased PTH levels and parenchymal loss resulting in lower activated vitamin D levels. As a result tertiary hyperparathyroidism gives a raised calcium with a very raised PTH, with normal or low phosphate. Serum alkaline phosphatase is also raised due to the osteoblast and osteoclast activity (note, osteoblasts produce alkaline phosphatase. This is why there is a normal alkaline phosphatase in myeloma, as it directly stimulates the osteoclasts). Treatment of tertiary hyperparathyroidism is subtotal parathyroidectomy. Tertiary hyperparathyroidism is differentiated from primary hyperparathyroidism (A) by the presence of chronic renal failure but is otherwise difficult to distinguish biochemically. Primary hyperparathyroidism is most commonly caused by a solitary adenoma in the parathyroid gland. Surgeons sometimes use sestamibi technetium scintigraphy to locate the offending adenoma prior to surgical removal.

Secondary hyperparathyroidism (B) occurs where there is an appropriately increased PTH level responding to low calcium levels. This is commonly due to chronic renal failure or vitamin D deficiency but can be seen in any pathology resulting in reduced calcium or vitamin D absorption or hyperphosphataemia.

Pseudohypoparathyroidism (also known as Albright's osteodystrophy) results from a PTH receptor insensitivity in the proximal convoluted tubule of the nephron. As a result, calcium resorption and phosphate excretion fail despite high PTH levels. Furthermore, other physical signs associated with this condition include short height, short 4th and 5th metacarpals, reduced intelligence, basal ganglia calcification, and endocrinopathies including diabetes mellitus, obesity, hypogonadism and hypothyroidism. Type 1 pseudohypoparathyroidism is inherited in an autosomal dominant manner where the renal adenylate cyclase G protein S alpha subunit is deficient, thus halting the intracellular messaging system activated by PTH. Patients with pseudopseudohypoparathyroidism (E) have similar physical features to pseudohypoparathyroidism but with no biochemical abnormalities of calcium present. This condition is a result of genetic imprinting where the phenotype expressed is dependent on not just what mutation is inherited but also from *whom*. In other words, inheriting the pseudo-hypoparathyroidism mutation from one's mother leads to pseudohypo-parathyroidism, but inheriting it from one's father leads to pseudo-pseudohypoparathyroidism. At the molecular level, this is signalled by differential methylation of genes thus providing a molecular off switch controlling its expression. Another example of genetic imprint-ing occurs in Prade–Willi syndrome and Angelman's syndrome, caused by a microdeletion on chromosome 15.

Vitamin deficiency tests

5 B   This patient suffers from chronic alcohol abuse with signs of chronic liver disease. He also exhibits the classical triad of Wernicke's encepha-lopathy caused by a thiamine (vitamin B_1) deficiency. The test for this is measuring red blood cell transketolase activity (B). Red cell transke-tolase is a thiamine pyrophosphate requiring enzyme which catalyzes reactions in the pentose phosphate pathway essential for regenerating NADPH in erythrocytes. The test measures enzyme activity by adding thiamine pyrophosphate to a sample of haemolyzed red blood cells and measuring the effluent substances. By calculating the amount of product made and substrates consumed, one is able to calculate the increase of enzyme activity after thiamine addition. A marked increase in activity implies a thiamine deficiency as the other substrate (ribose 5 phosphate) is supplied in excess. Thiamine deficiency has a number of clinical sequelae including Wernicke's encephalopathy, a reversible neurological manifestation characterized pathologically by haemor-rhage in the mammillary bodies. If left untreated, this may progress to Korsakoff's syndrome, an irreversible neurological disease character-ized by severe memory loss, confabulation, lack of insight and apathy. Thiamine deficiency can also lead to wet beriberi syndrome leading to a high output cardiac failure.

Folate (vitamin B_9) is required for cell reproduction and DNA and RNA synthesis. It is particularly important in infancy and pregnancy where cell turnover is high and provides the rationale behind folate supplementation of pregnant women up to 12 weeks' gestation where organogenesis is at its peak. Folic acid is found in high levels in green leafy vegetable, nuts, yeast and liver. Body stores last up to 4 months, therefore deficiency is not common given the fortification of foods. If one does become deficient, however, features include megaloblastic anaemia, diarrhoea, peripheral neuropathy and glossitis (classically giving a beefy tongue).

Red blood cell glutathione reductase (C) assay tests for riboflavin deficiency. Riboflavin (also known as vitamin B_2) is named after its structure – it contains a ribose sugar with a flavin ring moiety which gives it its striking yellow colour. Riboflavin is important in energy metabolism including fats, ketone bodies, proteins and carbohydrates. The assay relies on glutathione reductase (GR), an important enzyme which regenerates glutathione which acts as a buffer against oxidative damage in erythrocytes. GR activity is reliant on riboflavin; GR activity is measured *in vitro* before and after addition of riboflavin. An increased level of GR activity implies its activity is being limited by riboflavin deficiency. Clinically, riboflavin deficiency causes glossitis, mouth ulceration and dry skin. It is almost always associated with other vitamin deficiencies including iron. Treatment is with vitamin replacement.

Red cell aspartate aminotransferase (AST) activity (D) tests for pyridoxine levels (also known as vitamin B_6). This vitamin is important in neurotransmitter synthesis, histamine synthesis, haemoglobin function and amino acid metabolism – this last function is exploited in the laboratory to test for deficiency. The enzyme activity is tested before and after the addition of pyridoxine, in a similar manner to the glutathione reductase and transketolase assays. Pyridoxine is found in meats, whole grain products and vegetables. It is absorbed in the jejunum and ileum and is water soluble. Deficiency causes a seborrhoeic dermatitis-like rash, angular cheilitis and neurological symptoms including confusion and neuropathy. Treatment is with replacement. Importantly, those on isoniazid for tuberculosis infection should be supplemented with pyridoxine to prevent these symptoms.

Carbohydrate deficient transferrin (E) is used in the detection of alcohol abuse. Transferrin, normally involved in plasma iron transport, has bound carbohydrate moieties making it a glycoprotein. People who abuse alcohol have a reduction in these bound carbohydrates therefore increasing their carbohydrate deficient transferrin. The test is around 70 per cent sensitive but about 95 per cent specific for alcohol abuse. Other tests for detecting increased alcohol consumption include the presence of a macrocytic anaemia, raised gamma glutamyl transferase as well as alanine aminotransferase and AST.

Hyperkalaemia

6 B The most likely cause of this patient's hyperkalaemia is secondary to tissue injury. Potassium is the principle intracellular cation whereas sodium is the principle extracellular cation. Na–K exchange pumps require a continuous supply of adenosine triphosphate (ATP) to supply the energy required to maintain the transcellular gradient. In iscliaemic

conditions, where oxygen supply is limited, ATP production fails to meet demand via aerobic respiration alone. Therefore ATP is also generated via anaerobic respiration. This can only occur for a limited period as the anaerobic pathway is both less efficient and produces lactic acid, thereby reducing the local pH and reducing the efficiency of enzymatic activity. This patient has had a significant amount of infarcted bowel removed with a raised lactate implying anaerobic metabolism has both occurred and ultimately failed leading to cell necrosis. The cells are then unable to maintain the Na–K transporter activity leading to potassium release in the blood stream. Furthermore, surgery itself causing direct cell damage increases the intracellular potassium leak into the plasma.

Acute kidney injury (A) is not likely in this patient given the normal creatinine and urea, although this patient is at high risk of pre-renal failure. Bowel obstruction and infarction leads to so-called third space losses of fluids which can be up to litres in magnitude. The third space is within the bowel lumen where resorption of secretions has stopped owing to disrupted transport mechanisms. Acute renal failure would classically give a sharp rise in urea and creatinine and, if serious, leads to a hyperkalaemia with metabolic acidosis. This patient needs intravenous fluids with careful monitoring of input and output as well as monitoring electrolytes. Hyperkalaemia is important as it alters cardiac membrane stability making arrhythmias more likely. The classical electrocardiographic features of hyperkalaemia include tall tented T waves, small P waves, widened QRS complexes, ST depression and QT narrowing. If severe, a sinusoidal pattern emerges at which point the patient needs urgent treatment to prevent a fatal dysrhythmia.

The patient's metabolic acidosis (C) has resolved and usually the potassium abnormality associated with this resolves too. There is a close link between potassium concentration and pH – a lower pH is associated with hyperkalaemia as both K^+ and H^+ compete with each other for exchange with sodium. Thus an increased pH means increased H^+ concentration making it more available for exchange with sodium thus leaving K^+ in the extracellular space. Once the metabolic acidosis resolves, this competition no longer exists and normal potassium homeostasis resumes.

Adrenal failure (D) from metastases could lead to Addison's disease, a destruction of the zona glomerulosa and fasciculata resulting in lack of aldosterone and cortisol production. Addison's disease classically presents biochemically with hyponatraemia, hyperkalaemia and hypercalcaemia. Aldosterone acts in the distal convoluted tube and collecting duct, its intracellular receptor (aldosterone mineralocorticoid receptor) acts with specific hormone response elements on the DNA to regulate gene transcription including N^+/K^+ pumps. The aldosterone receptor is also activated by cortisol which is produced in much higher concentrations physiologically. To prevent over-stimulation of the receptor, however, a deactivating enzyme (11 beta hydroxysteroid dehydrogenase) co-localizes with the receptor to locally inactivate cortisol's effect. In hypercorisolaemia (Cushing's) this mechanism is overcome, resulting in excess aldosterone-like effects thus explaining the hypertension in these patients. Interestingly, licorice, which contains glycyrrhizic acid, inhibits this deactivating enzyme explaining its association with hypertension when eaten in excess. Adrenal metastases, although possible in this patient, are unlikely given the biochemical disparity and lack of clinical information about metastatic disease.

Overhydration with intravenous fluids (E) can cause hyperkalaemia, but the on-call doctor in this question prescribed normal saline, which alone contains 154 mmol/L sodium chloride only. Given the well known side effect of tissue injury postoperatively, some clinicians routinely omit potassium in the first postoperative bag of fluids to prevent hyperkalaemia. Hartmann's has a more physiological biochemical profile and contains 5 mmol/L potassium as well as 29 mmol/L lactate. Patients on this fluid for maintenance fluid therapy can have falsely high lactates when arterial blood samples are analyzed.

Hypernatraemia

7 E The most likely cause of hypernatraemia in this man is dehydration (E). Gastroenteritis with diarrhoea for 3 weeks causes a high rate of free water loss resulting in increased concentration of sodium in the extracellular compartment. Sodium and intravascular volume are closely linked and controlled by the renin angiotensin system and antidiuretic hormone. A reduction in renal blood flow through loss of intravascular volume results in increased renin secretion from the juxtaglomerular apparatus in the kidneys. Renin converts angiotensinogen to angiotensin I which in turn is converted to angiotensin II by angiotensin converting enzyme (which is constitutively expressed in the lungs). Angiotensin II increases the release of aldosterone from the zona glomerulosa in the adrenal cortex which acts to increase sodium retention. Retained sodium increases plasma osmolality which stimulates antidiuretic hormone (ADH) release from the posterior pituitary. ADH acts to increase free water retention, the net result being an increased intravascular volume with a normal osmolality.

Diabetes insipidus (DI) is caused by lack of ADH action. Craniogenic DI (C) implies a lack of production of ADH from the posterior pituitary whereas nephrogenic DI (B) implies a lack of sensitivity to ADH.

Craniogenic DI classically follows head injury where over 80 per cent of the descending neurones from the paraventricular and supraoptic nuclei in the hypothalamus need to be destroyed to produce clinical symptoms. It is rare and probably would have manifested earlier with polydipsia and polyuria in this patient given the head injury was at the age of 10.

Nephrogenic DI is a result of renal resistance to ADH and has numerous aetiologies. Many intrinsic renal pathologies including interstitial nephritis, polycystic kidneys, sarcoid or amyloid can cause this. However, remember nephrogenic DI means a resistance to ADH action despite normal or high levels. This does not necessarily mean there is an intrinsic kidney problem – any cause of prolonged polyuria can cause solute washout in the renal medulla reducing the action of ADH. Another important cause of nephrogenic DI is drugs. The two classical drugs associated with this are lithium and demeclocycline. The latter is sometimes used therapeutically in patients with the syndrome of inappropriate ADH (SIADH). Here the excess ADH production is counteracted by the demeclocycline which inhibits the renal response to ADH. Although demeclocycline is a type of tetracycline, prescribed tetracycline (D) (rather confusingly) is a separate drug which is not associated with nephrogenic DI. Thus the treatment this man has received is unlikely to have caused the hypernatraemia.

Conn's syndrome (A) is caused by an aldosterone secreting tumour leading to a hypertensive, hypokalaemic, metabolic alkalosis. It very rarely causes hypernatraemia. The causes of this disease include Adrenal adenoma, Bilateral nodular hyperplasia, Carcinoma of the adrenals or a Defective gene (glucocorticoid remediable aldosteronism, GRA). Adrenal ademona is by far the most common and presents with resistant hypertension and weakness (due to hypokalaemia). GRA is caused by a chimeric gene of aldosterone synthase with the 11 beta hydroxylase-1 promoter, resulting in an ACTH sensitive secretion of aldosterone. ACTH is under the negative feedback control of glucocorticoids. Exogenous administration of dexamethasone reduces ACTH levels thus reducing aldosterone expression, treating the disease!

Water deprivation test

8 C   This patient is most likely suffering from psychogenic polydipsia, an uncommon condition where excessive water drinking occurs without the physiological stimulus to drink. It was classically described in patients with schizophrenia but also occurs in children. Chronic psychogenic polydipsia can result in mineral washout of the renal interstitium resulting in a physiological inability to concentrate urine, in other words a form of nephrogenic diabetes insipidus.

The water deprivation test is a seldom used test nowadays but is useful to understand when considering these clinical problems. The test begins with the patient being completely deprived of water for 8 hours in which time the patient's weight, blood and urine osmolality and urine volume are measured. A weight loss of more than 5 per cent in adults is an indication to stop the test. After 8 hours, 2 µg of desmopressin (a synthetic analogue of vasopressin) is given. The same measurements are taken for the next 8 hours. After the desmopressin is given the patient is allowed to drink up to 1.5 times the total urine output for the first 8 hours. In this patient's case she had produced 2200 mL of urine, but drank 3000 mL of water. This therefore is acceptable and did not nullify the test making (D) an incorrect answer.

The patient's urine osmolality increased above 800 mOsmol/kg after 8 hours of water deprivation, indicating vasopressin action is functioning to appropriately retain water therefore concentrating the urine. A further 8 hours later, despite drinking 3 L of fluid, the patient's urine is still very concentrated implying the administered desmopressin and endogenous vasopressin are functioning. In patients with craniogenic DI (B), the administration of desmopressin provides the water retention signal that the kidneys are failing to concentrate the urine. The typical result for patients with craniogenic DI is a dilute urine (<300 mOsmol/kg) after the first 8 hours, but concentrated urine after the desmopressin administration (>800 mOsmol/kg). Nephrogenic DI (A) would not respond to desmopressin and would likely leave the patient with dilute urine (<300 mOsmol/kg) before and after desmopressin administration. Finally, suggesting this patient is normal given the symptomatic polyuria and polydispia is unlikely. Any patient presenting with these symptoms must be investigated with a blood glucose measurement to explore the possibility of diabetes mellitus.

Acute abdominal pain

9 A   PBG deaminase deficiency (A) causes acute intermittent porphyria, which this patient suffers from. The porphyrias are a group of seven disorders caused by enzyme activity reduction in the haem biosynthetic pathway. Haem is manufactured in both the liver and bone marrow where branched chain amino acids together with succinyl CoA and glycine are needed. The first step involves 5 aminolevulinic acid (ALA) synthesis by ALA synthase. This is the rate limiting step which is under negative feedback from haem itself.

A simplified schema of haem production is provided with the products depicted on the left, and the enzyme responsible along with the type of porphyria caused if it was deficient on the right.

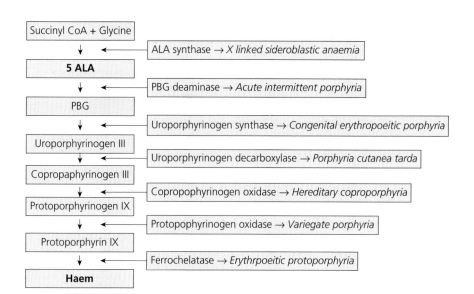

The features of porphyria can be generally classified into neurological, cutaneous and microcytic anaemia. The exact combination of symptoms depends on where in the haem pathway the deficiency occurs. Neurological symptoms, including peripheral neuropathy, autonomic neuropathy and psychiatric features, are caused by the increase of porphyrin precursors 5 ALA and prophobilinogen (PBG). Cutaneous symptoms are due to photosensitive porphyrins which are produced later on in the sequence. Finally microcytic anaemia occurs due to the deficiency of haem production.

Acute intermittent porphyria (AIP) presents without cutaneous symptoms, this is because the enzyme deficiency is further upstream from the photosensitive porphyrins which cause the cutaneous symptoms. Instead neurological symptoms of the peripheral, autonomic and psychiatric systems predominate, as in this patient. The symptoms cluster in attacks if toxins induce ALA synthase or PBG deaminase activity. These include alcohol, the oral contraceptive pill and certain antibiotics including rifampicin and pyrazinamide (two commonly used anti-tuberculosis drugs). Other common precipitants include surgery, infection and starvation. Investigations classically show urine which becomes brown or black upon standing in light as well as reduced erythrocyte PBG deaminase levels. Note there is *no* increase of faecal porphyrins in AIP. Treatment is to avoid precipitants as well as dextrose infusion and haem arginate intravenously which both inhibit ALA synthase activity.

Uroporphyrinogen synthase (B) results in congenital erythropoeitic porphyria which is one of the rarest inborn errors of metabolism. It is caused by a mutation on chromosome 10q26 and is inherited in an autosomal recessive fashion. Symptoms include vesicles, bullae and excessive lanugo hair as well as mutilating deformities of the limbs and face. Urine is classically burgundy red as well as patients having erythrodontia – red stained teeth. Treatment is to avoid sunlight and symptomatically treat the anaemia. Coproporphyrinogen oxidase (C) causes hereditary coproporphyria and is another rare type of porphyria. The symptoms are predominantly neuro-visceral. Diagnosis is confirmed with increased faecal and urinary coproporphyrinogen.

Protoporphyrinogen oxidase deficiency (D) causes variegate porphyria which is caused by an autosomal dominant mutation of chromosome 14. It is relatively rare in the world except in South Africa where its incidence is as high as one in 300 (most probably due to the founder effect from early settlers). Attacks feature neuro-cutaneous features, although not necessarily together at the same time. It is almost always precipitated by drugs making it difficult to distinguish from AIP. In variegate porphyria, however, there is increased faecal protoporphyria as well as positive plasma fluorescence scanning.

Uroporphyrinogen decarboxylase (E) causes porphyria cutanea tarda and can be inherited in an autosomal dominant manner. It is characterized by cutaneous features including bullous reactions to light, hyperpigmentation, as well as liver disease. Non-inherited causes include alcohol, iron, infections (hepatitis C and HIV) and systemic lupus erythematosus (SLE). Investigations reveal abnormal liver function tests, raised ferritin (always) and increased urinary uroporphyrinogen. This gives a characteristic pink red fluorescence when illuminated with a Wood's lamp. Treatment is to avoid precipitants as well as chloroquine which complexes with porphyrins and promotes uroporphyrin release from the liver.

Exacerbating factors for gout

10 D   Although all of these factors can contribute to hyperuricaeamia, well controlled psoriasis (D) in this patient is unlikely to contribute to this attack of gout. Gout may be acute or chronic and is caused by hyperuricaemia. Hyperuricaemia is caused either by increased urate production or decreased urate excretion.

Uric acid is a product of purine metabolism and is produced in three main ways – metabolism of endogenous purines, exogenous dietary nucleic acid and *de novo* production. *De novo* production involves metabolizing purines to eventually produce hypoxanthine and xanthine. The rate limiting enzyme in this pathway is called phosphoribosyl pyrophosphate aminotransferase (PAT) which is under negative feedback by guanine and adenyl monophosphate. The metabolism of exogenous and endogenous purines, however, is the predominant pathway for uric acid production. The serum concentration of urate is dependent on sex, temperature and pH. A patient with acute gout does not necessarily have an increased urate concentration, therefore making serum urate levels an inaccurate method of diagnosis. The diagnosis of acute gout, which most commonly affects the first metatarsophalangeal joint ('podagra') is best made by observing weakly negatively birefringent crystals in an aspirate of the affected joint. This test is performed with polarized light – urate crystals are rhomboid and illuminate weakly when polarized light is shone perpendicular to the orientation of the crystal (hence *negative* birefringence). This is in contrast with pseudogout which has positively birefringent, spindly crystals – these illuminate best when the polarized light is aligned with the crystals. X-ray of the affected joint shows soft tissue inflammation early on, but as the disease progresses, well defined 'punched out' lesions in the juxta-articular bone appear with a late loss of joint space. There is no sclerotic reaction. Treatment is with a non-steroidal anti-iflammatory (e.g. diclofenac) in the acute phase or colchicine. Aspirin (E) is avoided because it directly competes for urate acid excretion in the nephron therefore worsening hyperuricaemia. After the acute attack settles, long term xanthine oxidase inhibitors (the enzyme responsible for the final production of urate) can be inhibited by allopurinol. Alternatively, but less commonly, uricosuric drugs such as probenecid may be used (e.g. prevention of cidofovir nephropathy). Finally rasburicase, recombinant urate oxidase, is a newer pharmacological treatment in the setting of chemotherapy to prevent hyperuricaeamia.

Thiazide diuretics such as bendroflumethiazide (A) act by inhibiting NaCl transport in the distal convoluted tubule. They are contraindicated in gout as they increase uric acid concentration and are a well known precipitant of gout. Other diuretics do not have this property and therefore this patient should have his antihypertensive medication reviewed. Other side effects of thiazides include hyperglyacaemia, hypercalcaemia and increased serum lipid concentrations.

Alcohol (C) increases urate levels in two ways – first it increases adenosine triphosphate turnover thus activating the salvage pathway producing more urate. It also decreases urate excretion in the kidney as it increases organic acids which compete for urate excretion in the nephron (much like aspirin). Chemotherapy (B) involves the destruction of malignant cells, which release all of their intracellular contents into the blood stream including purines. Widespread malignancy treated with chemotherapy can dramatically increase urate concentration. Therefore some patients undergoing chemotherapy are given prophylactic allopurinal to prevent this side effect as well as being encouraged to drink plenty of fluid to essentially dilute the urate produced.

Psoriasis (D) is a dermatological condition characterized by discrete patches of epithelial hyperproliferation. There are different types including flexural, extensor, guttate, erythrodermic and pustulopalmar. Some special clinical signs associated with this condition often asked about include Koebner's phenomenon (appearance of psoriatic plaques at sites of injury) and Auspitz's sign (dots of bleeding when a plaque is scratched off representing reticular dermis clubbing with capillary dilatation). Severe psoriasis results in T-cell mediated hyperprolifera-tion and eventual breakdown of cells releasing their intracellular contents resulting in hyperuricaemia in much the same mechanism as chemotherapy. The treatment for psoriasis includes phototherapy with ultraviolet light, topical agents including tar and oral tablets including antiproliferatives.

Anion gap

11 A The anion gap is calculated using the following equation:

Anion gap = $[Na^+] + [K^+] - [HCO_3] - [Cl^-]$

It is a method of assessing the contribution of unmeasured anions in metabolic acidosis. The normal range varies between laboratories but the upper limit is usually between 10 and 18 mmol/L. It is helpful to estimate the unmeasured anions such as phosphate, ketones and lactate which are difficult to measure normally.

Metabolic acidosis in the setting of a raised anion gap implies there is an increase production or reduced excretion of fixed or organic acids. The acid produced is buffered by bicarbonate thus increasing the anion gap. Causes include raised lactate (e.g. shock, infection or tissue ischae-mia), urate (renal failure), ketones (diabetes mellitus) or drugs (metha-nol, aspirin). Furthermore there are two types of lactic acidosis – type A and type B. Type A is the most commonly associated with shock. Hypoperfusion of the tissues reduces the capacity of cells to continue aerobic respiration which leads to the formation of lactate via anaerobic respiration. Physiologically lactate concentration is around 1 mM but can rise up to 10 mM in extreme situations. It can also be falsely raised when replacing fluids which contain lactate (e.g. Hartmann's solution – a common surgical fluid used to treat hypovolaemia). This is particu-larly important when dealing with suspected bowel ischaemia where fluid resuscitation is a vital initial management step. Lactate is often used to distinguish the presence of ischaemia which could be falsely elevated if using this fluid!. Type B lactic acidosis occurs in the absence of significant oxygen delivery problems and usually occurs secondary to

the total solvent present. This gives a falsely low osmolality measurement and therefore plasma triglycerides, cholesterol and protein should be taken into account when performing this calculation. Nowadays, some laboratories take this well known effect into account, making the calculation much more accurate.

Biochemical abnormalities in chronic renal failure

13   E   Patients with chronic renal failure normally suffer from hyperphosphataemia, not hypophosphataemia (E). This is due to renal impairment of calcium metabolism which is under the control of parathyroid hormone (PTH) and vitamin D. In the evolving stages of chronic renal failure, a secondary hyperparathyroidism exists to compensate for the inability of the kidney to retain calcium and excrete phosphate. Therefore hypocalcaemia (D) is associated with chronic renal failure. This stimulates a physiological secretion of PTH by the parathyroid glands in an attempt to retain calcium. PTH is also responsible for excreting phosphate in the kidney, which is impaired due to the failure. Hyperphosphataemia also increases PTH levels as part of a negative feedback loop designed to maintain its homeostasis. Patients with chronic renal failure usually take phosphate binders (e.g. Sevelamer) which act to reduce phosphate absorption. This reduces PTH production which also reduces bone resorption thus improving renal osteodystrophy, a complex metabolic bone pathology associated with chronic renal failure. It is also important to reduce phosphate concentration to reduce ectopic calcification – if this precipitates in the tubules, this may reduce what little function there is left.

Hyperkalaemia (B) is associated with chronic renal failure and is important as it can be potentially fatal. Hyperkalaemia changes cardiac membrane excitability making it more prone to arrhythmias; other indications include. Resistant severe hyperkalaemia (>7 mmol/L) is an indication for emergency renal dialysis refractory pulmonary oedema, severe metabolic acidosis (pH <7.2 or base excess <10), uraemic encephalopathy or uraemic pericarditis. Treatment of hyperkalaemia is with calcium gluconate to stabilize the heart muscle, insulin and dextrose to reduce potassium levels as well as salbutamol or calcium resonium.

As mentioned, acidosis is also a consequence of chronic renal failure. This is due directly to the failure of acid–base handling within the renal tubules and indirectly due to hyperkalaemia causing a shift of hydrogen ions into the plasma. Acidosis impairs metabolic functions by reducing the efficacy of enzymes as well as worsening renal osteodystrophy by essentially dissolving bone. There is usually respiratory compensation with hypocapnia.

Finally, anaemia (B) is common with chronic renal failure and is normocytic normochromic in nature. It is due to the lack of erythropoietin production in the renal parenchyma. Recombinant human erythropoietin is available for this and acts as a replacement to stimulate erythropoiesis in the bone marrow. It is important to exclude iron deficiency anaemia which would produce a microcytic hypochromic picture as this is easily treatable with iron.

Thyroid function tests

14 E   Thyroid function tests are relatively easy to interpret with a basic understanding of the hypothalamic–pituitary–thyroid axis of thyroid hormone control. The pituitary produces TSH (thyroid stimulating hormone) which is released from the anterior pituitary. It is under the control of the hypothalamus which releases thyroid releasing hormone (TRH) which signals to anterior pituitary cells to release TSH. TSH travels in the bloodstream and acts on thyrocytes in the thyroid gland to stimulate production of T_4 and T_3 hormone. Specifically TSH controls the rate of iodide uptake required for thyroid hormone production, thyroid peroxidase activity, iodotyrosine reuptake into the thyrocyte from colloid and iodotyrosine cleavage to form mature hormone. T_4 is the main circulatory hormone produced in about a 10:1 ratio compared with T_3. However, free T_3 has greater efficacy; in fact circulating T_4 is converted into T_3 within cells which then binds to its hormone receptor. TSH release is under negative feedback control of T_4. In primary hypothyroidism, the thyroid does not have the ability to produce sufficient T_4 or T_3 to inhibit further TSH release. Therefore the biochemical abnormality found in primary hypothyroidism is a raised TSH with low T_4 and T_3, which is not one of the answer options (E).

A low TSH with raised free T_4 and T_3 (A) is seen in primary hyperthyroidism, the most common cause of which is Graves' disease. This is an autoimmune condition where stimulating antibodies bind to the TSH receptor to stimulate thyroid hormone production. The excessive T_4 concentration negatively feedbacks onto the hypothalamus and pituitary to reduce TSH release. The other causes of this biochemical abnormality include multinodular goitre with functional tissue, toxic nodule (also known as Plummer's disease), transient thyroiditis and De Quervain's thyroiditis. Graves' disease is unique in that it features extrathyroid features including pretibial myxoedema, exophthalmos and thyroid acropachy. Radioisotope scanning, a method using radioactive iodine to measure uptake in the thyroid gland, shows increased uptake throughout the gland.

A low or normal TSH with low free T_4 and T_3 (B) is frequently seen in patients with other non-thyroid illness. This is also known as sick euthyroid syndrome where the patient is unwell with another illness causing thyroid abnormalities. The cause is unclear but the role of inflammatory cytokines and reduced peripheral deiodination of T_4 has been implicated. Another important differential for this combination of biochemical abnormalities is secondary hypothyroidism i.e. pituitary dysfunction causing low TSH and low thyroid hormones. This differential is serious as the associated hypoadrenalism could be fatal. A pituitary tumour must be excluded by imaging (MRI brain) and endocrinological stimulation tests (i.e. short synacthen test) to exclude Addison's disease. Another explanation for these results not applicable in this patient is recently treated hyperthyroidism. There is sometimes a residual suppression of TSH following hyperthyroid treatment for up to 1 year, and if they are clinically hypothyroid replacement therapy should be prescribed.

A raised TSH with normal T_4 and T_3 (C) normally means the patient is suffering from subclinical hypothyroidism. This is an important finding as patients may have subtle symptoms and improve with treatment as well as possibly reducing deaths from cardiac events. People with TSH levels $>10\mu/L$, positive thyroid antibodies, previously treated Graves' disease or other organ specific autoimmunity (e.g. diabetes mellitus type I, myasthenia gravis) should be treated as they are at high risk of progression to clinical hypothyroidism. Other less common causes of this biochemical configuration include amiodarone therapy, recovery from sick euthyroid disease and thyroxine malabsorption in patients taking thyroxine therapy due to small bowel disease, cholestyramine or iron therapy.

A normal or raised TSH with raised T_3 and T_4 (D) is a rare disorder and usually means there is an artefact with the test. The results imply central hyperthyroidism with the hypothalamus inappropriately excreting excessive TSH stimulating the thyroid gland to overproduce T_4 and T_3. Rarely it can be caused by amiodarone therapy, thyroid receptor mutations, intermittent thyroxine overdose, or familial dysalbuminaemic hyperthyroxinaemia. This last condition is a rare abnormality of albumin which results in increased binding affinity of albumin for T_4. This interferes with the assay and shows a normal TSH and T_3 with apparently increased T_4.

Biochemical abnormalities of metabolic bone disease

15   B   Osteoporosis (B) is a common disease which affects women more than men. It is pathologically associated with a reduction in bone density but normal mineralization of bone. There are usually no biochemical abnormalities and therefore all of the parameters measured here should be normal. Given the nature of the fracture, the raised alkaline phosphatase is likely to be due to the fracture where osteoblast and osteoclast activation for remodelling and bone healing is required for bone union. Note osteoblasts produce alkaline phosphatase, not osteoclasts. The activation of the two is usually simultaneous, therefore any bone

remodelling will lead to a rise in alkaline phosphatase concentration. An important exception is in myeloma where bone lysis occurs with no rise in alkalaline phosphatase because osteoclasts are directly activated without osteoblast activity. Recently the National Institute of Clinical Excellence (NICE) have published guidelines regarding osteoporosis and its management. The risk factors of osteoporosis include:

1   Genetic factors: woman, age, Caucasion/Asian, family history

2   Nutritional factors: excessive alcohol and caffeine, low body weight

3   Life style factors: inactivity, smoking

4   Hormonal factors: nulliparous women, late menarche/early menopause, oophorectomy, post menopausal women, amenorrhoea

5   Iatrogenic factors: thyroxine replacement, steroids

The four risk factors NICE highlight are a low BMI ($<22\,\text{kg/m}^2$), chronic medical conditions including Crohn's disease, rheumatoid arthritis and ankylosing spondylitis, any condition resulting in prolonged immobility and untreated premature menopause. Investigation of osteoporosis is with a DEXA scan (dual energy X-ray absorptiometry) which uses X-rays of the spine and pelvis to calculate and compare the bone mineral density of the subject with a healthy control. This is reported as a T score; the score is a negative number and represents the number of standard deviations away the subject is from a fit and healthy 30 year old. 0 to −1 is normal, −1 to −2.5 is osteopenic whereas −2.5 or less is osteoporosis. This is different from the Z score which compares the subject's bone mineral density with an age-related control.

Osteomalacia (D) is caused by vitamin D deficiency which this patient may have a degree of. However, the question asks which is the most likely and given the fragility fracture, her age and previous risk factors, osteoporosis is a much more likely answer. Osteomalacia is the only condition where bone mineralization is reduced: in normal and osteoporotic patients demineralized bone (osteoid) accounts for about 25 per cent of bone mass whereas in osteomalacia it can approach 100 per cent. Biochemically, there is low calcium, low phosphate, high alkaline phosphatase and high PTH with low vitamin D levels. The calcium–phosphate product (that is calcium and phosphate concentration multiplied together) is diagnostically less than 2.4 where the normal value is 3. Subclinical vitamin D deficiency is becoming increasingly common, particularly in children because of reduced sunshine exposure.

Paget's disease (C) is caused by excessive and abnormal bone remodelling with a normal calcium and phosphate but markedly raised alkaline phosphatase, reflecting high osteoblastic activity. There is also increased urinary hydroxyproline which reflects osteoclast activity. Clinical features include pain, bony deformities, sensorineuronal deafness from vestibulocochlear nerve compression through the internal auditory canal or conductive deafness from osteosclerotic changes of the ossicles of the ear. Fractures are a complication of Paget's because of the disorganized remodelling of bone and patients undergoing surgery in Pagetic bone often need cross-matched blood due to the highly vascular nature of the bone. A serious complication of Paget's is osteosarcoma which occurs in 1 per cent of patients.

Malignancy usually presents with a raised calcium, phosphate, alkaline phosphatase and reduced PTH level. It is a common cause of hypercalcaemia and must be differentiated from primary hyperparathyroidism, the other common differential. The most common primary sites include breast, kidney, lung, thyroid, colon, ovary and prostate. Prostate cancer, characteristically, produces osteosclerotic changes with metastases whereas the others have an osteolytic appearance. Prostate cancer often spreads to the vertebrae first due to the venous drainage it shares with the vertebrae.

Inherited metabolic disorders

16   B   This neonate, born with cataracts, poor feeding, lethargy, conjugated hyperbilirubinaemia with hepatomegaly and reducing sugars in the urine after starting milk, is likely to have galactosaemia (B). This is a rare autosomal recessive inherited condition most commonly due to a mutation in the galactose-1-phosphate uridyltransferase gene on chromosome 9p13. It results in excessive galactose concentrations when milk, which contains glucose and galactose, is introduced into the baby's diet.

Galactose can enter the metabolic pathway through a number of steps. It must first be phosphorylated to allow its conversion into glucose-1-phosphate which eventually become glucose-6-phosphate to finally enter the metabolic cycle. Galactose-1-phosphate uridyltransferase converts galactose-1-phosphate into UDP galactose. This is the most common enzyme to be defective in galactosaemia. It is unclear exactly why the build up of galactose is so harmful, however one of the by products of its metabolism (galactitol produced by aldolase on galactose-1-phosphate) is responsible for cataract formation. The collection of gastrointestinal symptoms, hepatomegaly and cataracts on starting milk is very suggestive of this disease. Children with this disease are also more susceptible to sepsis with *Escherichia coli*. The Fehling's and Benedict's reagent tests are positive because galactose is a reducing sugar, the other important one being glucose which was excluded using glucose specific sticks. The investigation of choice is a red cell galactose-1-phosphate uridyltransferase level although this condition is sometimes screened for during the neonatal period in certain parts of the world.

Treatment is to exclude milk from the child's diet as well as eliminating other sources of galactose.

Galactokinase (C) deficiency is another cause of galactosaemia but much less common. It is due to a defective galactokinase gene on 17q24. Its function is to phosphorylate galactose to galactose-1-phosphate. Unlike classical galactosaemia as described above, severe symptoms in early life are less common. Instead, excess galactitol formation results in early cataract formation in homozygous infants. Treatment is similar to those with classical galactosaemia.

Fructose intolerance (A) is caused by fructose-1-phosphate aldolase deficiency which normally converts fructose-1-phosphate to dihydroacetone phosphate and glyceraldehyde. These products are further metabolized and can enter either glycolytic or gluconeogenesis pathways depending on the energy state of the cell. The explanation is made more complicated by the fact that there are three isoenzymes of fructose-1-phosphate aldolase (A, B and C) of which B is expressed exclusively in the liver, kidney and intestine as well as metabolizing three different reactions. Aldolase B can produce triose phosphate compounds which are central to the glycolytic pathway, but this can also be reversed making it important in gluconeogenesis. A deficiency therefore explains the hypoglycaemia experienced by these patients. Furthermore, the reduced fructose metabolism increases its blood levels which consequently changes the ATP:ADP ratio. This increases purine metabolism resulting in excess uric acid production which competes for excretion in the kidney with lactic acid. The result is lactic acidosis, hyperuricaemia and hypoglycaemia. These is also severe hepatic dysfunction, the pathophysiology of which is relatively less well understood.

Tyrosinaemia (E) is another autosomal recessive inherited disorder of metabolism which has three subtypes – types I, II and III. Type I is the hereditary form which has a specifically high incidence in Quebec, Canada and is characterized by a defect in fumarylacetoacetate hydrolase. In its most severe form it presents with failure to thrive in the first few months, bloody stool, lethargy and jaundice. A distinctive cabbage-like odour is characteristic. On examination there is hepatomegaly with signs of liver failure and subsequent survival for less than 12 months if untreated. The investigation of choice is urinary succinylacetone and treatment is to restrict dietary tyrosine and phenylalanine and to treat the liver failure, sometimes with a transplant.

Urea cycle disorders (D) normally present with a non-infective encephalopathy, along with failure to thrive and hyperventilation in the neonatal period progressing to neurological symptoms associated with protein intake. The inability to metabolize urea leads to hyperammonaemia. A blood level above 300 µM/L is associated with encephalopathy. There are also associated increases in plasma amino acids, urine amino acids and organic acids. Enzyme studies are required to differentiate it from one of the ten potential defects responsible for this group of diseases. Treatment is to use benzoate or phenylacetate or extracorporeal dialysis to remove the ammonia and a low protein diet to prevent its build up.

Neonatal jaundice

17 B This child, with a large amount of bruising (B), most probably developed unconjugated jaundice from the excess breakdown products of erythrocytes. The difficult labour requiring instrumentation has led to a large collection of bruising in the scalp which is broken down and leads to unconjugated jaundice. Neonates are susceptible to jaundice for many different reasons – reduced erythrocyte half life with increased haemoglobin levels, reduced transport in the liver (reduced ligandin is responsible for this) and increased enterohepatic circulation. Investigation of this is to rule out other causes including urinary tract infection, other haemolytic anaemias and congenital hypothyroidism which is normally tested for by the heel prick Guthrie test. Treatment is usually via phototherapy which uses light at 450 nm wavelength to solubilize (NOT conjugate) the excess bilirubin for excretion through the kidneys. This prevents passage of bilirubin through the immature blood–brain barrier which can then deposit into the basal ganglia causing kernicterus. Another method of treatment includes exchange transfusion.

Other causes of jaundice include haemolysis (C), which may be congenital or acquired. Congenital causes include G6PD deficiency which can cause severe unconjugated jaundice. The mutation in this enzyme reduces erythrocyte ability to withstand oxidative stress which can be triggered by numerous drugs (classically anti-malarials) and fava beans (hence the alternative name for this condition is favism). Other causes of haemolysis include ABO incompability where blood type O mothers sometimes express IgG anti-A-haemolysins which can cross the placental barrier resulting in haemolysis. Treatment is supportive. Rhesus haemolytic disease is serious but fortunately rare with the implementation of anti-D immunization after significant events. In this situation, a mother has anti-D antibodies which cross the placental barrier resulting in profound haemolysis, hydrops and hepatosplenomegaly. This requires previous sensitization of the mother to rhesus D antigen either by previous pregnancy or blood transfusion. Therefore all pregnant women who are rhesus D negative receive prophylactic immunoglobulins during significant events in pregnancy which may release fetal blood into the maternal circulation, e.g. abortion. The immunoglobulins effectively neutralize the fetal blood and prevent an immune response from developing. Failure to do this will risk the next rhesus positive fetus.

Urinary tract infection (A) is a common cause of unconjugated jaundice in the neonate and must be excluded because if left untreated it can lead to complicated urinary tract infection involving the kidneys and urosepsis. Sepsis in neonates does not always present with fever but instead an inability to regulate body temperature. The most common pathogen is group B streptococcus, a common commensal in the vaginal tract of the mother.

Crigler–Najar syndrome (D) is caused by a genetic defect in glucoronyl transferase which is responsible for transporting bilirubin into the hepatocyte. There are two types – type I is characterized by a complete absence of this enzyme, type II is characterized by a partial reduction of this enzyme. Type I presents with severe neonatal jaundice with kernicterus, phototherapy can reduce the levels by half and liver transplantation is the only cure. Phenobarbitone is used only in type II Crigler–Najjar syndrome. This disease is different from Gilbert's disease (E) which is relatively common but also causes a mild unconjugated hyperbilirubinaemia. The main defect is in biliribuin uridinediphosphate-glucuronyltransferase (UGT1A1) which is the enzyme responsible for conjugating bilirubin and is reduced by about 30 per cent in Gilbert's disease. It does not cause liver damage and is relatively benign. Precipitating factors include stress, fasting, fever and dehydration. Investigations aim to prove an unconjugated jaundice without haemolysis and normal plasma bile acids. There is no bilirubinuria and no increase in urobilinogen either.

Vitamin D deficiency

18　B　This man is highly likely to have osteomalacia given the history of chronic alcohol abuse and episodes consistent with chronic pancreatitis. This is significant because the pancreas is responsible for emulsification and digestion of fats which facilitate fat soluble vitamin absorption including vitamins A, D, E and K. The reduced vitamin D absorption has led to osteomalacia, the pathological syndrome caused by vitamin D deficiency after epiphyseal closure. If vitamin D deficiency occurred before epiphyseal closure, the patient would suffer from rickets.

Vitamin D metabolism involves the skin, liver and kidneys as well as the bones and gastrointestinal tract. Sources of vitamin D include sunlight exposure and diet. Sunlight converts 7-dehydrocholesterol into cholecalciferol (vitamin D_3). The latter product is what is consumed in the diet. This is then hydroxylated in the liver to form 25-hydroxy-cholecalciferol. This is then transported to the kidneys where the final hydroxylation by 1 alpha hydroxylase converts 25-hydroxy-cholecalciferol to 1,25-dihydroxycholecalciferol. This final step is stimulated by parathyroid hormone.

Therefore, this man has low 25-hydroxy-cholecalciferol levels due to reduced absorption of dietary vitamin D, but has a high level of 1,25-dihydroxy-cholecalciferol because of the reactive secondary hyperparathyroidism which converts any remaining 25-hydroxy-cholecalciferol to the activated form, hence the high levels (B). Answer (A), where there are low levels of both forms of vitamin D, could also be present in this situation but there would be a high parathyroid hormone level making this answer incorrect.

A high 25-hydroxy-cholecalciferol, low 1,25-dihydroxy-cholecalciferol, high parathyroid hormone (C) would occur in patients with chronic renal failure where there is loss of parenchymal tissue to hydroxylyze 25-hydroxy-cholecalciferol to its final activated form. There is a secondary or tertiary hyperparathyroidism depending on the stage of renal failure. Secondary hyperparathyroidism occurs early on when the kidneys retain phosphate and appropriately stimulate PTH secretion. As the renal failure continues, the gland secretes PTH autonomously despite normal or high calcium levels.

A high 25-hydroxy-cholecalciferol, high 1,25-dihydroxy-cholecalciferol, high parathyroid hormone (D) would occur in patients with vitamin D resistance where there is normal production of vitamin D but there is reduced activity due to the inability to detect vitamin D. There are two types – type 2 vitamin D dependent rickets is autosomal recessive and is caused by an end organ resistance whereas type 1 is caused by a congenital lack of 1 alpha hydroxylase giving a similar biochemical profile to that seen in chronic renal failure. Parathyroid hormone levels are high despite high vitamin D levels because PTH is under negative feedback control from calcium and phosphate levels, not vitamin D levels.

Finally a high 25-hydroxy-cholecalciferol, low 1,25-dihydroxy-cholecalciferol, low parathyroid hormone may be seen in hypoparathyroidism of which the most common cause is post-surgical intervention. There is a low PTH level and therefore low stimulation of 1 alpha hydroxylase in the kidney to covert 25-hydroxy-cholecalciferol to 1,25-dihydroxy-cholecalciferol thus explaining their levels.

Raised alkaline phosphatase

19   E   Alkaline phosphatase (ALP) is an enzyme responsible for removing phosphate groups from various molecules. It is produced in the liver, bile duct, kidney, bone and placenta. It is commonly requested as part of the liver function test panel and is used diagnostically in the approach to various conditions.

Of these answers, only myeloma does not classically cause a raised ALP. ALP is caused by osteoblast activation whereas in myeloma there is direct osteoclast activation through the release of various cytokines.

This means although there are areas of lysis on X-rays, there is little osteoblast response leading to a normal alkaline phosphatase level. This may be complicated by a fracture which will stimulate osteoblast activity leading to a raised ALP in the setting of myeloma. Paget's disease, a syndrome characterized by abnormal remodelling, normally has a very elevated level of ALP caused by increased but disorganized remodelling of the bone. On X-rays there are patches of lucency and sclerosis. There are normally no calcium or phosphate abnormalities making it different from metastatic prostatic cancer which also gives a patchy sclerotic X-ray but would raise the calcium levels.

There are various isomers of ALP which are not distinguishable on a standard liver function assay without electrophoresis. In the third trimester of pregnancy (A), placental ALP is produced leading to raised levels if one were to measure them at this time. Another isoenzyme is found in the liver and bile ducts where it is used to distinguish between an obstructive and hepatic picture in liver disease. Here, obstruction or damage to the bile ducts cause a disproportionately raised ALP compared with the AST and ALT. Another way of distinguishing whether an isolated raised ALP is originating in the liver is to look at the GGT – this often rises with bile duct injury whereas it would be normal if the ALP were of bone or placental origin.

Finally congestive cardiac failure can cause a mildly raised ALP and may be due to reduced forward flow of blood causing congestion in the liver and release of ALP into the systemic circulation. The causes of a raised ALP are many and can be categorized into the following:

1 Liver related – cholestasis, hepatitis, fatty liver, tumour

2 Drugs – phenytoin, erythromycin, carbamezepine, verapamil

3 Bones
   1 Bone disease – Paget's disease, renal osteodystrophy, fracture
   2 Non-bone disease – vitamin D deficiency, malignancy, secondary hyperparathyroidism

4 Cancer (different from metastases to bones) – breast, colon cancer and Hodgkin's lymphoma

Nutritional deficiency

20 D This man with poor diet, dermatitis, dementia and diarrhoea most likely has a niacin deficiency leading to pellagra. The other name for niacin is vitamin B_3 (D).The rash he describes is also known as Casal's necklace – a distinctive erythematous, pigmented rash in the necklace distribution named after Gaspar Casal, a Spanish physician practising in the early 1700s. Niacin is essential for most cellular processes but only usually

affects those with severe malnutrition because tryptophan can also be converted into niacin, therefore a dual deficiency is required for the full syndrome to develop. The disease is remembered by the four Ds – dementia, diarrhoea, dermatitis and death. The neurological symptoms do not exclusively manifest as dementia – other symptoms also include depression, anxiety, tremor, delusions, psychosis and even coma. The diarrhoea occurs in about half of patients furthering the malnutrition problem. Dermatitis can affect the mouth, lips, hands, arms, legs and feet. The causes are primary niacin deficiency due to poor nutrition – this is the most likely case in this question given the maize diet and the suggestion of protein malnutrition by the presence of kwashiorkor in the local population. Secondary niacin deficiency may be secondary to malabsorptive problems including prolonged diarrhoea, inflammatory bowel disease and liver cirrhosis. Iatrogenic causes are well described – implicated drugs include isoniazid and azathioprine. Treatment is with niacin replacement therapy and treatment of underlying disease if it is secondary.

Tocopherol (A) is also known as vitamin E, its deficiency causes haemolytic anaemia, spinocerebellar degeneration and peripheral neuropathy. It is rare in humans. It is one of the fat soluble vitamins (the others being A, D and K) and is important in normal reproduction, muscular development and resistance to red cell haemolysis. It is stored in the liver, adipose tissue, muscle, pituitary gland, testes and adrenals. Its levels are directly measured in the plasma. Recently in the HOPE (Heart Outcomes Prevention Evaulation) study, vitamin E was found to have no evidence of benefit in preventing the development of cardiovascular disease.

Riboflavin deficiency (B), also known as vitamin B_2, causes ariboflavinosis. Symptoms include dry mucous membranes affecting the mouth, eyes and genitalia along with a normocytic normochromic anaemia. It is usually associated with protein and energy malnutrition or alcoholism and is normally found in legumes, pulses and animal products. Riboflavin is an essential constituent in two molecules – flavin mononucleotide and flavin adenine dinucleotide (FAD). These molecules readily accept and donate electrons making them ideal coenzymes in redox metabolic reactions. Riboflavin is absorbed in the proximal small intestine, its deficiency can be tested for by assaying erythrocyte levels, or assaying the activity of erythrocyte glutathione reductase which requires FAD for its activity. Treatment of this deficiency is daily supplementation.

Retinol (C), also known as vitamin A, is another fat soluble vitamin whose function is necessary for normal epithelial tissue growth, polysaccharide synthesis and the formation of visual pigment, rhodopsin. Vitamin A deficiency can cause dry skin and hair as well as xerophthalmia (drying of the cornea with ulceration). Rarely, Bitot's spots can develop and are seen on the conjunctiva and represent an accumulation of keratin. Vitamin A deficiency can also cause night blindness due to rhodopsin abnormalities as well as a distinctive skin rash called pityriasis rubra pilaris. Treatment is with a balanced diet and supplementation. This is not without caution – vitamin A can be toxic: there are reports of Arctic explorers eating polar bear liver who developed headache, diarrhoea and dizziness. Vitamin A consumption, especially in liver, is also cautioned in pregnant women as it may be teratogenic.

Ascorbate (E) is also known as vitamin C which, if deficient, causes scurvy. The features of scurvy include anaemia, bleeding gums and induration of the calf and leg muscles. This is due to ascorbate's role in the formation of collagen including that of bone, cartilage, teeth and intercellular substance of capillaries. This explains the defective ossification and bleeding tendency. Unsurprisingly, wound healing is also poor. Vitamin C also improves the efficacy of desferrioxime, an iron chelator used in states of iron overload, which may be due to vitamin C's antioxidant action.

Therapeutic drug monitoring

21 B   Usually, drugs take between 4 and 5 half lives to reach a steady state. The half life is the time it takes for the plasma concentration of the drug to halve. Drugs such as phenytoin are monitored because underdosing will lead to no effect but overdosing will lead to toxicity. Most drugs have a wide therapeutic window – that is the difference between the minimum effective concentration and minimum toxic concentration. Drugs with narrow therapeutic windows may be suitable for drug monitoring to optimize treatment.

This figure can be calculated relatively simply. Let us consider we give a patient a single dose of a drug with a half life of 24 hours. This means 50 per cent of the medication will be eliminated in 24 hours, but 50 per cent will remain. On day 2, 24 hours after the first dose, we give another dose. On day 3 there is now 75 per cent of the original doses of drug in the patient's circulation – the original dose which has been in the system for two half lives and therefore is at 25 per cent, and the second dose which has been in the system for one half life and is therefore at 50 per cent of the original dose – giving 75 per cent. Continuing this daily, the amount of drug in steady state by day 4 is 93.75 per cent, by day 5 it is around 97 per cent. This is for a drug with a half life of 24 hours (this is approximately phenytoin's half life); but this holds true for any half life except those drugs with very short half lives.

This also explains why loading doses are used. If, say, a drug has a half life of 1 week, then it would take up to 5 weeks for the patient to be within the therapeutic range. Therefore, loading doses are used to increase the initial blood concentration and reduce the time needed to reach steady state.

Drugs which require therapeutic drug monitoring include:

- Antibiotics, e.g. gentamicin, vancomycin
- Anticonvulsants, e.g. phenytoin, lamotrigine
- Immunosuppressives, e.g. methotrexate, mycophenolate, tacrolimus
- Lithium
- Digoxin

Unfortunately, determining drug efficacy is more complicated than simply measuring its plasma concentration. The efficacy depends on both pharmacokinetic and pharmacodynamic factors. Pharmacokinetic factors relate to the absorption, distribution, metabolism and excretion of the drug. Absorptive factors include water/fat solubility of the drug or specific transport mechanisms across the mucosal lining of the gut, e.g. grapefruit juice increases ciclosporin bioavailability. Distributive factors take into account the water solubility and fat solubility of the drug as well as the amount of fat or water the patient has. A useful method of measurement of this concept is the volume of distribution which describes the volume of water required to completely account for the administered drug at the given plasma concentration. If the drug has a high fat solubility, the concentration in the plasma will be relatively low, therefore it would require a high volume at the given concentration to account for the drug given. Metabolism factors include pharmacogenetic factors, e.g. thiopurine methyltransferase mutation affects the administration of azathioprine as reduced levels are more likely to lead to toxicity. These factors also include the phase I and phase II type reactions which are involved in oxidation/reduction and solubilization of the drug, respectively. Excretive factors are mostly to do with renal function; some drugs (e.g. digoxin) can accumulate in renal failure.

The pharmacodynamic factors that must be considered include whether the drug is in the active form when administered. Some drugs are required to be metabolized before they have their therapeutic effect, e.g. azathiopurine (metabolized to mercaptopurine), enalapril (metabolized to enalaprilat) or carbimazole (metabolized to methimazole) or the drug is active but its metabolic products are also active, e.g. codeine and tramadol. Another important pharmacodynamic factor to consider is the degree of drug bound to protein. Traditionally drug levels are quoted as a total drug level which includes both bound and unbound drug but only the unbound drug is active. Drugs which are highly protein bound have an altered therapeutic effect in low protein states or if another drug has a higher protein affinity therefore displacing the former drug and increasing the proportional unbound active drug. Phenytoin is important to remember as it is highly protein bound (90–94 per cent). Others include mycophenolate and carbamazepine.

Hypoglycaemia

22 B This patient, presenting with hypoglycaemia, tiredness and hyperpigmentation with an associated autoimmune history of vitiligo, most probably has adrenal failure (Addison's disease (B)). The adrenal glands are responsible for producing cortisol, aldosterone and sex hormones. Adrenal failure is potentially lethal due to the lack of cortisol, which is an important stress hormone as well as an important gluconeogenesis stimulant at times of hypoglycaemia. An important worldwide cause is tuberculosis but in the developed world, autoimmunity is more likely. Autoimmune conditions often segregate as in this man with vitiligo, an autoimmune disease causing destruction of melanin in the skin. The patient has a tan as a by product of the lack of negative feedback in the hypothalamic–pituitary–adrenal axis. The hypothalamus releases cortisol releasing hormone (CRH) to the anterior pituitary which in turn releases ACTH (adrenocorticotropic hormone). ACTH is produced from its precursor molecule POMC (pro-opiomelanocortin) which, when cleaved, also produces MSH (melanocyte stimulating hormone). This accounts for the increased tanning seen in patients with Addison's.

In patients with hypoglycaemia, a plasma insulin and C peptide is diagnostically useful to elucidate the cause. Insulin is the main endogenous hypoglycaemic and is released from beta cells in the pancreas. C peptide is a by product of insulin production and therefore has a direct correlation with endogenous insulin production. Causes of raised insulin and C peptide concentrations are few and include islet cell hyperplasia (e.g. persistent hyperinsulinaemic hypoglycaemia of infancy, Beckwith Weidemann syndrome) or insulinoma. If insulin were exogenously administered, then the C peptide level would be low because endogenous production would be appropriately suppressed.

All of the answers given can cause hypoglycaemia with low insulin and C peptide levels. Pituitary failure (A) with TSH and ACTH failure can cause hypoglycaemia. In this patient other symptoms and signs suggesting pituitary failure would manifest, e.g. sex hormone deficiency leading to loss of libido, menopause in women; lack of growth hormone leads to muscle atrophy, abdominal obesity; lack of dopaminergic inhibition to prolactin leads to galactorrhoea, amenorrhoea and infertility; lack of TSH leads to hypothyroidism. Alcohol induced (C) hypoglycaemia occurs due to the increased production of cytosolic NADH from ethanol metabolism into acetaldehyde. NADH inhibits gluconeogenesis resulting in hypoglycaemia. Chronically, chronic alcoholism leads to malnutrition thus reducing the hepatic glycogen stores. Glycogen storage disease (D), more specifically glycogen storage disease type I (Von Gierke's disease) is caused by a mutation in the glucose-6-phosphatase enzyme. Phosphorylated glucose cannot cross cell membranes and therefore the lack of this enzyme essentially traps glucose from being transported. Patients present with stunted growth, hepatomegaly and have hypoglycaemia, lactic acidosis, high urate and high triglycerides (GLUT). Finally medium chain acyl-CoA dehydrogenase deficiency (MCADD) is caused by a genetic defect in fatty acid beta oxidation. This is important in ketone body formation in hypoglycaemia, which the brain must use to preserve function as it cannot utilize fats directly in states of neuroglycopenia. This mutation leads to hypoketotic hypogly-caemia often with hepatomegaly and cardiomyopathy.

Acute pancreatitis

23 D Hypercalcaemia is not a common consequence of acute pancreatitis, indeed hypercalcaenia is one of the causes of acute pancreatitis. Other causes of pancreatitis can be remembered by the well known mnemonic 'GET SMASHED':

- Gallstones
- Ethanol
- Trauma
- Steroids
- Mumps
- Autoimmune (polyarteritis nodosa)
- Scorpion venom (Trinidadian scorpion)
- Hypercalcaemia/Hypertriglyceridaemia/Hypothermia
- Endoscopic retrograde cholangiopancreatogram
- Drugs (including thiazides, azathioprine, valproate, oestrogens)

Corrected calcium is used instead of calcium because the latter is dependent on albumin concentration which binds 40 per cent of plasma calcium and is normally quoted by laboratory studies. The ionized non-bound calcium is the important measurement clinicians are usually interested in; therefore the corrected value is used which takes into account albumin concentration. If the laboratory has not quoted a corrected calcium, one can calculate the corrected value by subtracting 0.1 mmol/L from the calcium concentration for every 4 g/L the albumin is below 40 g/L.

The mechanism of aetiology related to hypercalcaemia is unknown. Some theorize that hypercalcaemia results in small intraductal stones in the pancreas causing blockage. Others believe hypercalcaemia directly increases pancreatic exogenous enzyme output or direct activation of trypsinogen. Pancreatitis is a potentially life-threatening disease with progression to systemic inflammatory response syndrome (SIRS) and multiorgan failure is a well recognized complication. Scoring systems which help to predict severity do exist, perhaps the most easily remembered is the modified Glasgow scoring system:

- PaO_2 <8 kPa
- Age >55 years
- Neutrophilia – white blood cells $>15 \times 10^9/L$
- Calcium <2 mmol/L
- Renal function urea >16 mmol/L
- Enzymes – LDH >600 iu/L or AST >200 ui/L
- Albumin <32 g/L
- Sugar >10 mmol/L

Scoring three or more of these criteria within 48 hours of admission should prompt early intensive care unit referral. Inspecting this list, this patient's other biochemical abnormalities can be explained from the inflammatory response to the pancreatitis. A raised white cell count (A) is due to the response of necrotic tissue in the pancreas which is being degraded by the inappropriate activation of trypsin, a powerful protease enzyme. A raised white cell count can also be secondary to the SIRS response as well as infection of the necrotic tissue. The raised sodium (B) and raised urea and creatinine (C) are likely to be secondary to dehydration which is multifactorial – nausea and vomiting and third space sequestration of fluid from the inflamed pancreas. Acute renal failure in pancreatitis is a devastating complication – one study found the risk factors for developing acute renal failure were previous renal disease, hypoxaemia and abdominal compartment syndrome. A raised glucose (E) is due to the pancreatic endocrine dysfunction where glucose monitoring and insulin release are impaired leading to hyperglycaemia. Hypocalcaemia is a complication of pancreatitis and is due to the fat saponification from the released enzymes.

Treatment of hyperkalaemia

24 C   Hyperkalaemia over 6.5 mmol/L is a medical emergency. High extracellular potassium levels increase cardiac excitability lowers the threshold of fatal dysrhythmia. Classical electrocardiographic changes include tall tented T waves, small P waves, widened QRS complexes which eventually become sinusoidal and can degenerate into ventricular fibrillation. Ten millilitres of 10 per cent calcium gluconate is the first line medication given to anyone with hyperkalaemia. It does not change the plasma potassium levels but stabilizes the myocardium to help prevent fatal dysyhythmia. It does so by increasing the threshold potential making the myocardium less excitable.

Calcium resonium (A) can be given orally or per rectum and reduces the plasma potassium levels over the longer term (around hours). This is therefore not helpful in the acute situation this patient is in, but may be considered once the potassium level is controlled. It binds potassium within the gut to increase excretion of ingested potassium therefore lowering overall potassium absorption. Its side effects unsurprisingly include gastrointestinal upset, including nausea and vomiting.

Insulin (D) along with dextrose is the main treatment to reduce potassium concentration acutely. Insulin drives potassium into cells along with glucose. Insulin must not be given alone as one could precipitate hypoglycaemia, the mechanism of action is within 20–30 minutes.

Nebulized salbutamol (E) is an example of a beta-2 receptor agonist which reduces potassium plasma concentration by activating the sodium–potassium–ATPase pump. This ubiquitous enzyme uses energy to transfer sodium and potassium to the extracellular and intracellular spaces respectively. In one recent study, it was shown that more lipophilic beta 2 agonists such as formeterol were more efficacious at reducing potassium plasma levels.

Sodium bicarbonate (B) does not directly lower plasma potassium levels, but instead neutralizes any excess acid in the blood. Bicarbonate reacts with hydrogen ions to produce carbon dioxide and water by increasing the bicarbonate levels, excess hydrogen ions are used in this reaction which raises the pH. Hydrogen and potassium compete at the cell membrane for entry into the cell; if hydrogen ion concentration decreases, a relative abundance of potassium is present making it more likely to enter the cell. This therefore lowers potassium levels, hence sodium bicarbonate indirectly can affect potassium levels.

Myocardial infarction

25 D This question is difficult as it requires both knowledge of the relative sensitivities of cardiac enzymes and their relative timelines at which they stay raised after a recent infarction. CK MB (D) is the heart isoenzyme creatine kinase which rises about 6–12 hours post-infarction and it usually peaks in concentration 24 hours later. It then reduces to normal within 48–72 hours. It is very sensitive and is diagnostic if it is >6 per cent of total creatine kinase or the CK MB mass is >99 percentile of normal. It is very useful in detecting re-infarction because of its sensitivity and rapid return to normal levels compared with troponin I and T (A and B). Troponin is the most sensitive and specific test for myocardial infarction and is traditionally taken 12 hours post-infarction. Troponin I is a better marker of myocardial infarction compared with troponin T (Trop I: sensitivity and specificity of 90 per cent at 8 hours and 95 per cent, respectively, trop T 84 per cent at 8 hours and 81 per cent, respectively). However, troponin levels take up to 10 days to normalize, making their use in re-infarction soon after a primary infarct limited. Another reason troponin is not the correct answer is that they are not strictly speaking cardiac enzymes, but rather a structural protein in the contractility mechanism. Interestingly, troponin T is also elevated

in chronic kidney disease without troponin I elevation, for reasons unknown.

AST (C) rises around 24 hours after an infarct and remains raised for 48 hours but is less sensitive and specific. It is also raised in liver disease, skeletal muscle damage (particularly in crush injury) and haemolysis. Similarly, LDH (E) rises around 48 hours after myocardial infarction and remains elevated for up to a week. It is also not very specific – it can be raised in liver disease, haemolysis, pulmonary embolism and tumour necrosis. For a summary of cardiac enzyme changes with time see the figure below.

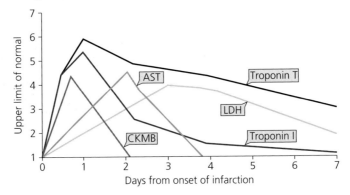

SECTION 3: HAEMATOLOGY EMQs

Questions

Answers

QUESTIONS

1. Anaemia

A	Iron deficiency anaemia	F	Vitamin B$_{12}$ deficiency
B	β-Thalassaemia	G	Renal failure
C	Anaemia of chronic disease	H	Aplastic anaemia
D	Blood loss	I	Lead poisoning
E	Alcohol		

For each scenario below, choose the most appropriate answer from the list above. Each option may be used once, more than once or not at all.

1 A 35-year-old man presents to his GP with a 1-month history of increased tiredness. The patient also admits to diarrhoea and minor abdominal pain during this period. His blood tests reveal the following:

Hb 9.5 (13–18 g/dL)
MCV 64 (76–96 fL)
Fe 12.2 (14–31 µmol/L)
TIBC 74 (45–66 µmol/L)
Ferritin 9.2 (12–200 µg/L)

Hb (haemoglobin); MCV (mean cell volume); Fe (iron); TIBC (total iron-binding capacity)

2 A 56-year-old vagrant man presents to the accident and emergency department with weakness in his legs. The patient has a history of poorly controlled Crohn's disease. His blood tests demonstrate Hb 9.4 (13–18 g/dL) and MCV 121 (76–96 fL). A blood film reveals the presence of hypersegmented neutrophils.

3 A 65-year-old man is referred to the haematology department by his GP after initially presenting with tiredness, palpitations, petechiae and recent pneumonia. His blood tests reveal Hb 9.8 (13–18 g/dL), MCV 128 (76–96 fL), reticulocyte count 18 (25–100 × 10^9/L), 1.2 (2–7.5 × 10^9/L) and platelet count 125 (150–400 × 10^9/L).

4 A 56-year-old woman presents to her GP with increased tiredness in the past few weeks. A past medical history of rheumatoid arthritis is noted. Her blood tests demonstrate the following:

Hb 8.6 (11.5–16 g/dL)
MCV 62 (76–96 fL)
Fe 10.2 (11–30 µmol/L)
TIBC 38 (45–66 µmol/L)
Ferritin 220 (12–200 µg/L)

5 A 12-year-old Mediterranean boy presents to his GP with increased tiredness over the past few weeks which is affecting his ability to concentrate at school. Examination is normal. Blood tests demonstrate the following:

Hb 9.5 (13–18 g/dL)
MCV 69 (76–96 fL)
Fe 18.2 (14–31 µmol/L)
TIBC 54 (45–66 µmol/L)
Ferritin 124 (12–200 µg/L)

2. Haemolytic anaemia

A   Hereditary sherocytosis
B   Sickle cell anaemia
C   β-Thalassaemia
D   Glucose-6-phosphate dehydrogenase deficiency
E   Pyruvate kinase deficiency
F   Autoimmune haemolytic anaemia
G   Haemolytic disease of the newborn
H   Paroxysmal nocturnal haemoglobinuria
I   Microangiopathic haemolytic anaemia

For each scenario below, choose the most appropriate answer from the list above. Each option may be used once, more than once or not at all.

1 A 48-year-old woman diagnosed with chronic lymphocytic leukaemia develops jaundice and on examination is found to have conjunctival pallor. Direct antiglobulin test is found to be positive at 37°C.

2 An 18-year-old man presents to accident and emergency after eating a meal containing Fava beans. He is evidently jaundiced and has signs suggestive of anaemia. The patient's blood film reveals the presence of Heinz bodies.

3 A 10-year-old girl presents to accident and emergency with jaundice. Blood tests reveal uraemia and thrombocytopenia. A peripheral blood film demonstrates the presence of schistocytes.

4 A 9-year-old boy from sub-Saharan Africa presents to accident and emergency with abdominal pain. On examination the child is found to have dactylitis. Blood haemoglobin is found to be 6.2 g/dL and electrophoresis reveals the diagnosis.

5 A 1-day old baby has developed severe jaundice on the neonatal ward. The mother is rhesus negative and has had one previous pregnancy. Due to having her first baby abroad, she was not administered prophylactic anti-D.

3. The peripheral blood film

A   Anisocytosis
B   Howell–Jolly bodies
C   Heinz bodies
D   Rouleaux formation
E   Spherocytes

F   Target cells
G   Cabot rings
H   Pappenheimer bodies
I   Tear-drop cells

For each scenario below, choose the most appropriate answer from the list above. Each option may be used once, more than once or not at all.

1   A 34-year-old man, who has a past medical history of splenectomy following splenic trauma, presents to his GP with malaise 2 weeks after returning from abroad. Routine blood results are found to be normal but a blood film demonstrates inclusions within erythrocytes.

2   A 66-year-old man has a gastroscopy and colonoscopy following a blood test which demonstrated a microcytic anaemia. The patient had complained of tiredness and significant weight loss over a 1-month period.

3   A 36-year-old woman presents to her GP after a 1-month history of tiredness and recurrent chest infections. Blood tests reveal a pancytopenia and a subsequent bone marrow aspirate reveals a dry tap.

4   A 3-week-old neonate is found to have prolonged jaundice with serious risk of kernicterus. Blood film demonstrates the presence of 'bite cells' as well as inclusions within erythrocytes.

5   A 45-year-old woman with known Graves' diseases presents to her GP with increased tiredness. She is found to have a megaloblastic anaemia.

4. Bleeding disorders

A   Immune thrombocytopenic
    purpura
B   Idiopathic thrombotic
    thrombocytopenic purpura
C   Disseminated intravascular
    coagulation
D   Glanzmann's thrombasthenia

E   Von Willebrand disease
F   Haemophilia A
G   Haemophilia B
H   Hereditary haemorrhagic
    telangiectasia
I   Bernard–Soulier syndrome

For each scenario below, choose the most appropriate answer from the list above. Each option may be used once, more than once or not at all.

1   A 4-year-old girl is seen by her GP due to recent onset petechiae on her feet and bleeding of her gums when she brushes her teeth. The child's platelet count is found to be 12 500 per μL. The GP prescribes prednisolone and reassures the child's mother that the bleeding will resolve.

2   A 28-year-old man attends the haematology outpatient clinic regarding a long-standing condition he has suffered from. His disorder is related to a deficiency in factor 8 and therefore requires regular transfusions to replace this clotting factor.

3   A 34-year-old man is taken to the local accident and emergency after suffering an episode of jaundice, fever and worsening headache. Blood tests reveal a low platelet count and blood film is suggestive of a microangiopathic haemolytic anaemia picture.

4   A 68-year-old man on the Care of the Elderly ward is confirmed to have Gram-negative sepsis. The patient is bleeding from his mouth and is in shock. Initial blood tests reveal a reduced platelet count, anaemia and renal failure.

5   A 2-year-old boy is taken to see the GP due to his mother noticing bruising on his arms and legs after playing in the park. The parent mentions that she has also noticed several recent nose bleeds in her son but thought he would 'grow out of it'. Investigations reveal a low APTT, low factor 8 levels and low Ristocetein cofactor activity.

5. Thrombophilia

A	Factor V Leiden	F	Prothrombin G20210A mutation
B	Antiphospholipid syndrome	G	Oral contraceptive pill
C	Malignancy	H	Buerger's disease
D	Protein S deficiency	I	Chronic liver disease
E	Antithrombin deficiency		

For each scenario below, choose the most appropriate answer from the list above. Each option may be used once, more than once or not at all.

1   A 35-year-old Caucasian man presents to accident and emergency with deep pain and swelling in his left calf. His past medical history reveals history of recurrent DVTs. The patient's notes reveal a letter from his haematologist who had diagnosed a condition caused by a substitution mutation.

2   A 38-year-old woman presents to accident and emergency with abdominal pain as well as passing blood and tissue per vagina. Ectopic pregnancy is diagnosed after ultrasound. The patient's past medical history includes a haematological condition in which a clotting factor is unable to be degraded by activated protein C.

3   A 32-year-old woman is seen by her rheumatologist to follow up her long-standing systemic lupus erythematosus (SLE). The patient has a history of recurrent miscarriages. The woman is positive for anti-cardiolipin antibodies and lupus anticoagulant.

4   A 45-year-old man, who has a 50 pack/year history of smoking, is referred to the vascular outpatient clinic by his GP after suffering intermittent claudication. A diagnostic angiogram reveals a corkscrew appearance of his lower limb arteries.

5   A 37-year-old man presents to accident and emergency with shortness of breath and severe pleuritic chest pain. A CTPA reveals the diagnosis of pulmonary embolism. The patient's haematological records state the patient has a condition that leads to the persistence of factors 5a and 8a causing increased risk of venous thrombosis.

6. Complications of transfusion

A	Immediate haemolytic transfusion reaction	F	Bacterial infection
B	Febrile non-haemolytic reaction	G	Delayed haemolytic transfusion reaction
C	Iron overload	H	Fluid overload
D	IgA deficiency	I	Graft versus host disease
E	Transfusion related lung injury		

For each scenario below, choose the most appropriate answer from the list above. Each option may be used once, more than once or not at all.

1   An 82-year-old man has just received a blood transfusion following a low haemoglobin level on the Care of the Elderly ward. He is now short of breath and is coughing up pink frothy sputum.

2   A 34-year-old HIV-positive man receives a regular blood transfusion as part of his beta-thalassaemia major treatment regimen. He soon develops diarrhoea and a maculopapular rash on his limbs.

3   A 34-year-old man requires a blood transfusion following a road traffic accident. However, soon after the transfusion, the patient is dyspnoeic and hypotensive. Investigation into the patient's past medical history reveals a history of recurrent chest and gastrointestinal infections.

4   A 56-year-old man is given a blood transfusion following severe blood loss after a hip replacement operation. Three hours after the transfusion, the patient develops shortness of breath, a dry cough and a fever of 39°C.

5   A 29-year-old woman requires an immediate blood transfusion after suffering a post-partum haemorrhage. However, 30 minutes after her transfusion she develops abdominal pain, facial flushing and vomiting. Analysis of the woman's urine reveals the presence of haemoglobin.

7. Haematological neoplasms (1)

A   Acute lymphoblastic leukaemia
B   Acute promyelocytic leukaemia
C   Chronic myeloid leukaemia
D   Chronic lymphocytic leukaemia
E   Hairy cell leukaemia

F   T-cell prolymphocytic leukaemia
G   Large granular lymphocytic leukaemia
H   Adult T-cell leukaemia
I   Acute myeloid leukaemia

For each scenario below, choose the most appropriate answer from the list above. Each option may be used once, more than once or not at all.

1   A 62-year-old woman is seen by a GP due to a recent chest infection that has been troubling her. Initial blood tests show an elevated white cell count with specifically raised granulocytes. Following referral to a haematologist, a bone marrow biopsy reveals a hypercellular bone marrow and cytogenetic screening suggests a translocation between chromosomes 9 and 22.

2   A 41-year-old man is referred to a haematologist by his general practitioner after several recent chest infections and tiredness. On examination, bruises are seen on his lower limbs as well as splenomegaly. Initial blood tests reveal a pancytopenia. Further testing demonstrates the presence of tumour cells that express tartrate-resistant acid phosphatase.

3   A 60-year-old man presents to his GP with fever, malaise and cough. On examination, the man is found to have petechiae on his legs as well as gum hypertrophy. Blood tests reveal anaemia, leukocytopenia and thrombocytopenia. A blood film demonstrates the presence of Auer rods within blast cells.

4   A 42-year-old Japanese migrant presents to his GP with generalized lymphadenopathy and nodules on his arms. On examination the patient has hepatosplenomegaly. Blood tests reveal lymphocytosis and a raised calcium level.

5   A 70-year-old man is reviewed by his GP after having felt tired and experienced weight loss over a 2-month period. The patient has lymphadenopathy on examination. Blood tests demonstrates a lymphocytosis of 4500 cells per microlitre and smudge cells can be visualized on a peripheral blood film.

8. Haematological neoplasms (2)

A   Diffuse large B-cell lymphoma
B   Burkitt lymphoma
C   Follicular lymphoma
D   Small lymphocytic leukaemia
E   Mantle cell lymphoma

F   Peripheral T-cell lymphoma
G   Mycosis fungoides
H   Angiocentric lymphoma
I   Hodgkin's lymphoma

For each scenario below, choose the most appropriate answer from the list above. Each option may be used once, more than once or not at all.

1   A 5-year-old boy is seen by a volunteer doctor at an Ethiopian refugee camp. On examination the child has a prominent swelling on the left side of his jaw. A tissue sample of the mass demonstrates a 'starry sky' appearance on light microscopy.

2   A 52-year-old man presents to his GP with painless lymphadenopathy which he describes as having fluctuated in size over the past month, as well as experiencing night sweats and weight loss. He also mentions the lumps become painful when he drinks alcohol. Further biopsy of the lumps reveals the presence of Reed–Sternberg cells.

3   A 60-year-old man presents to his GP with malaise, night sweats and weight loss. On examination the patient is found to have generalized lymphadenopathy and hepatomegaly. Cytogenetic investigation a few weeks later by a haematologist reveals a translocation between chromosomes 11 and 14, which has caused overexpression of the BCL-2 protein.

4   A 40-year-old woman is referred to a haematologist after she is found to have generalized, painless lymphadenopathy. A report on tumour cell morphology states the presence of both centrocytes and centroblasts.

5   A 62-year-old HIV-positive man presents to a haematologist with a 3-month history of weight loss and tiredness. On examination, the patient has a mass on his neck which the patient states has been rapidly growing. Staining of biopsy tissue demonstrates the present of large B cells which are positive for EBV.

9. Haematological neoplasms (3)

A	Essential thrombocythaemia	E	Polycythaemia rubravera
B	Myelofibrosis	F	Refractory anaemia with ringed
C	Chronic myelo-monocytic		sideroblasts
	leukaemia	G	Refractory anaemia
D	Refractory anaemia with excess	H	5q-Syndrome
	blasts	I	Multiple myeloma

For each scenario below, choose the most appropriate answer from the list above. Each option may be used once, more than once or not at all.

1   A 40-year-old man is referred to a haematologist after suffering an episode of petechiae on his legs followed by a burning sensation in his fingers and deep vein thrombosis a few weeks later. Blood tests reveal a platelet count of 850×10^9/L.

2   A 52-year-old woman presents to her GP due to increased tiredness. The patient also reports easy bruising and numerous bouts of pneumonia which have occurred over the past 6 months. On examination, the patient has splenomegaly. Blood tests reveal a low white cell and platelet count. Blood film reveals the presence of tear drop cells and on bone marrow aspiration there is a 'dry' tap.

3   A 60-year-old man is referred to a haematologist after complaining of back pain and tiredness as well as recent onset low mood. Urine tests reveal the presence of Bence–Jones proteins. An X-ray of the patient's spine shows the presence of lytic lesions.

4   A 72-year-old man presents with a 1-month history of fever, night sweats and weight loss. Blood tests reveal a monocyte count of 1400/mm^3 in the peripheral blood and a bone marrow biopsy demonstrates that myeloblasts constitute 16 per cent of his bone marrow.

5   A 43-year-old woman presents to her general practitioner with headaches, episodes of dizziness and a strange itching sensation after she comes out of the bath. On examination a plethoric appearance is noted. Blood tests reveal a haemoglobin of 19 g/dL and erythropoietin levels are suppressed.

10. Haematology of systemic disease

A   Temporal arteritis
B   Renal cell carcinoma
C   Colorectal cancer
D   Rheumatoid arthritis
E   Miliary tuberculosis
F   Acute pancreatitis
G   Schistosomiasis
H   Sarcoidosis
I   Epstein–Barr infection

For each scenario below, choose the most appropriate answer from the list above. Each option may be used once, more than once or not at all.

1   A 56-year-old woman visits her GP for a regular check-up for a chronic condition she suffers from. On examination, she has signs of long-term steroid therapy. There is ulnar deviation at her metacarpophalangeal joints. Blood tests reveal a microcytic hypochromic anaemia, low iron and total iron binding capacity, but a raised ferritin level.

2   A 45-year-old man presents to accident and emergency with an excruciating headache. Blood tests show an erythrocyte sedimentation rate of 110 mm/hour.

3   A 38-year-old man from Nigeria presents to his GP with progressive shortness of breath, cough and painful rashes on his lower legs. Blood tests reveal a monocytosis. Chest X-ray demonstrates bihilar lymphadenopathy.

4   A 66-year-old presents to his GP with severe weight loss over 1 month as well as tiredness. Blood tests reveal an increased erythrocyte, haemoglobin and erythropoietin count.

5   A 24-year-old man has recently returned from a trip to Kenya. He presents to his GP with abdominal pain, fever and on examination has hepatosplenomegaly. Blood tests reveal a marked eosinophilia.

ANSWERS

1. Anaemia

ANSWERS: 1) A 2) F 3) H 4) C 5) B

Iron deficiency anaemia (IDA; A) causes a hypochromic (pallor of the red blood cells on blood film due to reduced Hb synthesis), microcytic (small size) anaemia (low haemoglobin). A reduction in serum iron can be caused by a number of factors, including inadequate intake, malabsorption (coeliac disease; most likely cause in this case given diarrhoea and abdominal pain), increased demand (pregnancy) and increased losses (bleeding and parasitic infections). Further studies are required to distinguish IDA from other causes of microcytic anaemia: serum ferritin will be low, while total iron binding capacity (TIBC) and transferrin ~~will be high.~~ *high* *low*

The majority of cases of vitamin B_{12} deficiency (F) occur secondary to malabsorption: reduced intrinsic factor production due to pernicious anaemia or post-gastrectomy, as well as disease of the terminal ileum. Clinical features will be similar to those of anaemia in mild cases, progressing to neuropsychiatric symptoms and subacute degeneration of the spinal cord (SDSC) in severe cases. Vitamin B_{12} deficiency results in a macrocytic megaloblastic anaemia as a result of inhibited DNA synthesis (B_{12} is responsible for the production of thymidine). Hypersegmented neutrophils are pathognomonic of megaloblastic anaemia.

Aplastic anaemia (H) is caused by failure of the bone marrow resulting in a pancytopenia and hypocellular bone marrow. Eighty per cent of cases are idiopathic, although 10 per cent are primary (dyskeratosis congenita and Fanconi anaemia) and 10 per cent are secondary (viruses, SLE, drugs and radiation). The pathological process involves CD8+/HLA-DR+ T cell destruction of bone marrow resulting in fatty changes. Investigations will reveal reduced Hb, reticulocytes, neutrophils, platelets and bone marrow cellularity as well as a raised MCV. Macrocytosis results from the release of fetal haemoglobin in an attempt to compensate for reduced red cell production.

Anaemia of chronic disease (ACD; C) occurs in states of chronic infection and inflammation, for example in tuberculosis (TB), rheumatoid arthritis, inflammatory bowel disease and malignant disease. ACD is mediated by IL-6 produced by macrophages which induces hepcidin production by the liver. Hepcidin has the effect of retaining iron in macrophages (reduced delivery to red blood cells for erythropoiesis) and reduces export from enterocytes (reduced plasma iron levels). Laboratory features of ACD include a microcytic hypochromic anaemia, rouleaux formation (increased plasma proteins), raised ferritin (acute phase protein) as well as reduced serum iron and TIBC.

β-Thalassaemia (B) is a genetic disorder characterized by the reduced or absent production of β-chains of haemoglobin. Mutations affecting the β-globin genes on chromosome 11 lead to a spectrum of clinical features depending on the combinations of chains affected. β-Thalassaemia minor affects one β-globin chain and is usually asymptomatic, but may present with mild features of anaemia. Haematological tests reveal a microcytic anaemia but iron studies will be normal, differentiating from iron deficiency anaemia. β-Thalassaemia major occurs due to defects of both β-globin chains and results in severe anaemia requiring regular blood transfusions, as well as skull bossing and hepatosplenomegaly.

Blood loss (D) will result in a normocytic anaemia as a consequence of a reduced number of circulating red blood cells. Common causes include gastrointestinal blood loss, heavy menstrual bleeding and certain surgical procedures.

Chronic alcohol (E) consumption directly causes a non-megaloblastic macrocytic anaemia. A poor diet in such patients also leads to folate and vitamin B_{12} deficiency which exacerbates the anaemia.

Chronic renal failure (G) is caused by the reduced production of red blood cells due to diminished secretion of erythropoietin by the damaged kidneys. This results in a normocytic, normochromic anaemia.

Lead poisoning (I) causes dysfunctional haem synthesis resulting in a microcytic anaemia. Lead poisoning leads to basophilic stippling, reflecting RNA found in red blood cells due to defective erythropoiesis.

2. Haemolytic anaemia

ANSWERS: 1) F 2) D 3) I 4) B 5) G

Autoimmune haemolytic anaemia (AIHA; F) is caused by autoantibodies that bind to red blood cells (RBCs) leading to splenic destruction. AIHA can be classified as either 'warm' or 'cold' depending on the temperature at which antibodies bind to RBCs. Warm AIHA is IgG mediated, which binds to RBCs at 37°C; causes include lymphoproliferative disorders, drugs (penicillin) and autoimmune diseases (SLE). Cold AIHA is IgM mediated which binds to RBCs at temperatures less than 4°C; this phenomenon usually occurs after an infection by mycoplasma or EBV. Direct antiglobulin test (DAT) is positive in AIHA and spherocytes are seen on blood film.

Glucose-6-phosphate dehydrogenase deficiency (G6PD deficiency; D) is caused by an X-linked recessive enzyme defect. G6PD is an essential enzyme in the red blood cell pentose phosphate pathway; the pathway maintains NADPH levels which in turn supply glutathione to neutralize free radicals that may otherwise cause oxidative damage. Therefore, G6PD deficient patients are at risk of oxidative crises which may be precipitated by certain drugs (primaquine, sulphonamides and aspirin), fava beans and henna. Attacks result in rapid anaemia, jaundice and a blood film will demonstrate the presence of bite cells and Heinz bodies.

Microangiopathic haemolytic anaemia (I) is caused by the mechanical destruction of RBCs in circulation. Causes include thrombotic thrombocytopenic pupura (TTP), haemolytic uraemic syndrome (HUS; *E. coli* 0157:57), disseminated intravascular coagulation (DIC) and systemic lupus erythematosus (SLE). In all underlying causes, the potentiation of coagulation pathways creates a mesh which leads to the intravascular destruction of RBCs and produces schistocytes (helmet cells). Schistocytes are broken down in the spleen, raising bilirubin levels and initiating jaundice.

Sickle cell anaemia (B) is an autosomal recessive genetic haematological condition due to a point mutation in the β-globin chain of haemoglobin (chromosome 11); this mutation causes glumatic acid at position six to be substituted by valine. Homozygotes for the mutation (HbSS) have sickle cell anaemia while heterozygotes (HbAS) have sickle cell trait. The mutation results in reduced RBC elasticity; RBCs therefore assume a sickle shape which leads to the numerous complications associated with a crisis. Blood tests will reveal an anaemia, reticulocytosis and raised bilirubin. Haemoglobin electrophoresis will distinguish between HbSS and HbAS.

Haemolytic disease of the newborn (G) occurs when the mother's blood is rhesus negative and the fetus' blood is rhesus positive. A first pregnancy or a sensitizing event such as an abortion, miscarriage or antepartum haemorrhage leads to fetal red blood cells entering the maternal circulation resulting in the formation of anti-D IgG. In a second pregnancy, maternal anti-D IgG will cross the placenta and coat fetal red blood cells which are subsequently haemolyzed in the spleen and liver. Therefore, anti-D prophylaxis is given to at-risk mothers; anti-D will coat any fetal red blood cells in the maternal circulation causing them to be removed by the spleen prior to potentially harmful IgG production.

Hereditary spherocytosis (A) and hereditary eliptocytosis are both autosomal dominant disorders that result in RBC membrane defects and extravascular haemolysis.

β-Thalassaemia (C) results in defects of the globin chains of haemoglobin. As a consequence, there is damage to RBC membranes causing haemolysis within the bone marrow.

Pyruvate kinase deficiency (E) is an autosomal recessive genetic disorder that causes reduced ATP production within RBCs and therefore reduces survival.

Paroxysmal nocturnal haemoglobinuria (H; PNH) is a rare stem cell disorder which results in intravascular haemolysis, haemoglobinuria (especially at night) and thrombophilia. Ham's test is positive.

3. The peripheral blood film

ANSWERS: 1) B 2) A 3) I 4) C 5) G

Howell–Jolly bodies (B) are nuclear DNA remnants found in circulating erythrocytes. On haematoxylin and eosin stained blood film they appear as purple spheres within erythrocytes. In healthy individuals erythrocytes expel nuclear DNA during the maturation process within the bone marrow; the few erythrocytes containing Howell–Jolly bodies are removed by the spleen. Common causes of Howell–Jolly bodies include splenectomy secondary to trauma and autosplenectomy resulting from sickle cell disease.

Anisocytosis (A) is defined as the variation in the size of circulating erythrocytes. The most common cause is iron deficiency anaemia (IDA), but thalassaemia, megaloblastic anaemia and sideroblastic anaemia are all causative. As well as blood film analysis, anisocytosis may be detected as a raised red cell distribution width (RDW), a measure of variation in size of red blood cells. In the case of IDA, anisocytosis results due to deficient iron supply to produce haemoglobin.

Tear-drop cells (I), also known as dacrocytes, are caused by myelofibrosis. The pathogenesis of myelofibrosis is defined by the bone marrow undergoing fibrosis, usually following a myeloproliferative disorder such as polycythaemia rubra vera or essential thrombocytosis. Bone marrow production of blood cells decreases resulting in a pancytopenia. The body compensates with extra-medullary haemopoiesis causing hepatosplenomegaly. Blood film will demonstrate leuko-erythroblasts, tear-drop cells and circulating megakaryocytes. Bone marrow aspirate is described as a 'dry and bloody' tap.

Heinz bodies (C) are inclusion bodies found within erythrocytes that represent denatured haemoglobin as a result of reactive oxygen species. Heinz bodies are most commonly caused by erythrocyte enzyme deficiencies such as glucose-6-phosphate dehydrogenase (G6PD) deficiency, which may present in neonates with prolonged jaundice and NADPH deficiency (leading to accumulation of hydrogen peroxide), as well as chronic liver disease and α-thalassaemia. Damaged erythrocytes are removed in the spleen by macrophages leading to the formation of 'bite cells'.

Cabot rings (G) are looped structures found within erythrocytes which may be caused by megaloblastic anaemia, i.e. inhibition of erythrocyte production occurring as a result of reduced DNA synthesis secondary to vitamin B_{12} deficiency. Vitamin B_{12} deficiency is most commonly caused by intrinsic factor (a protein required for vitamin B_{12} absorption) deficiency as a result of pernicious anaemia. Pernicious anaemia is caused by antibody destruction of gastric parietal cells which produce intrinsic factor and may be associated with other autoimmune diseases.

Rouleaux (D) formation describes the stacks of erythrocytes that form in high plasma protein states, for example, multiple myeloma.

Spherocytes (E) are caused by hereditary spherocytosis (defect in membranous proteins, for example spectrin), which leads to haemolytic anaemia.

Target cells (F) are erythrocytes with a central area of staining, a ring of pallor and an outer ring of staining. They are formed in thalassaemia, asplenia and liver disease.

Pappenheimer bodies (H) are granules of iron found within erythrocytes. Causes include lead poisoning, sideroblastic anaemia and haemolytic anaemia.

4. Bleeding disorders

ANSWERS: 1) A 2) F 3) B 4) C 5) E

Immune thrombocytopenic purpura (ITP; A) may follow either an acute or chronic disease process. Acute ITP most commonly occurs in children, usually occurring 2 weeks after a viral illness. It is a type 2 hypersensitivity reaction, with IgG binding to virus-coated platelets. The fall in platelets is very low (less than 20×10^9/L) but is a self-limiting condition (few weeks). Chronic ITP is gradual in onset with no history of previous viral infection. It is also a type 2 hypersensitivity reaction with IgG targeting GLP-2b/3a.

Haemophilia A (F) is an X-linked genetic disorder and hence only affects men. Haemophilia A is characterized by a deficiency in factor 8. Haemophilia A is diagnosed by a reduced APTT as well as reduced factor 8. Symptoms depend on severity of disease: mild disease features bleeding after surgery/trauma; moderate disease results in bleeding after minor trauma; severe disease causes frequent spontaneous bleeds. Clinical features include haemarthrosis (causing fixed joints) and muscle haematoma (causing atrophy and short tendons).

Idiopathic thrombotic thrombocytopenic purpura (B) occurs due to platelet microthrombi. Presenting features include microangiopathic haemolytic anaemia (red blood cells coming into contact with microscopic clots are damaged by shear stress), renal failure, thrombocytopenia, fever and neurological signs (hallucinations/stroke/headache). A mutation in the ADAM-ST13 gene, coding for a protease that cleaves von Willebrand factor (vWF) allows for the formation of vWF multimers enabling platelet thrombi to form causing organ damage.

Disseminated intravascular coagulation (DIC; C) may be caused by Gram-negative sepsis, malignancy, trauma, placental abruption or amniotic fluid embolus. Tissue factor is released which triggers the activation of the clotting cascade, leading to platelet activation (thrombosis in microcirculation) and fibrin deposition (haemolysis). The consumption of platelets and clotting factors predisposes to bleeding. Plasmin is also generated in DIC which causes fibrinolysis, perpetuating the bleeding risk. The clinical manifestations of DIC are therefore linked to microthombus production (renal failure and neurological signs) and reduced platelets, clotting factors and increased fibrinolysis (bruising, gastrointestinal bleeding and shock).

von Willebrand disease (vWD; E) is an autosomal dominant condition caused by a mutation on chromosome 12. Physiologically, von Willebrand factor (vWF) has two roles: platelet adhesion and factor 8 production. Therefore, in vWD, where there is a deficiency in vWF, there is a defect in platelet plug formation as well as low levels of factor 8. Clinically, patients will present with gum bleeding, epistaxis or prolonged bleeding after surgery. Investigations will reveal a high/normal APTT, low factor 8 levels, low ristocetin cofactor activity, poor ristocetin aggregation and normal PTT,

Glanzmann's thrombasthenia (D) is caused by a mutation of GLP-2b/3a, a glycoprotein that is essential for platelet aggregation, and hence blood coagulation.

Haemophilia B (G) is an X-linked genetic disorder characterized by a deficiency in factor 9. This can lead to bleeding spontaneously or in response to mild trauma.

Hereditary haemorrhagic telangiectasia (Osler–Weber–Rendu syndrome; H) is an autosomal dominant condition characterized by telangiectasia formation on the skin and mucous membranes leading to nose and gastrointestinal bleeds.

Bernard–Soulier syndrome (I) is caused by a mutation of the glycoprotein GLP-1b, the receptor for von Willebrand factor in clot formation.

5. Thrombophilia

ANSWERS: 1) F 2) A 3) B 4) H 5) D

Prothrombin G20210A (F) is an inherited thrombophilia caused by the substitution of guanine with adenine at the 20210 position of the prothrombin gene. Physiologically, prothrombin promotes clotting after a blood vessel has been damaged. The G20210A causes the amplification of prothrombin production thereby increasing the risk of clotting, and causing a predisposition to deep vein thrombosis and pulmonary embolism. The prevalence of the mutation is approximately 5 per cent in the Caucasian population, the race with the greatest preponderance.

Factor V Leiden (A) is an autosomal dominant inherited thrombophilia. Under normal circumstances protein C inhibits factor 5. In Factor V Leiden a mutation of the *F5* gene that codes for factor 5, whereby an arginine codon is substituted for a glutamine codon, results in impaired degradation of factor 5 by protein C. As a result, patients are at risk of deep vein thrombosis and miscarriage. Diagnostic tests determine the functionality of activated protein C.

Antiphospholipid syndrome (APLS; B) is an autoimmune disorder that may present with stroke (arterial thrombosis), deep vein thrombosis (venous thrombosis) and/or recurrent miscarriages. APLS may be primary (not associated with autoimmune disease) or secondary to autoimmune disease such as SLE. Anti-cardiolipin antibodies and lupus anticoagulant bind to phospholipids on cell surface membranes of cells causing the activation of the coagulation cascade and thereby promoting clot formation. Diagnosis involves demonstrating the presence of circulating anti-cardiolipin antibodies and lupus anticoagulant.

Buerger's disease (thromboangitis obliterans; H) is a vasculitis of small/medium arteries and veins of the hands and feet; it is strongly related to smoking. Claudication may be the initial presentation but as the disease progresses there is an association with recurrent arterial and venous thrombosis leading to gangrene and amputation in severe cases. Angiograms of the upper and lower limbs are helpful in the diagnosis of Buerger's disease; a corkscrew appearance of the arteries may arise due to persistent vascular damage.

Protein S deficiency (D) is associated with the impaired degradation of factors Va and VIIIa. Protein S and protein C are physiological anticoagulants. Deficiency of protein S leads to persistence of factors 5a and 8a in the circulation and hence patients have a susceptibility to venous thrombosis. Three types of protein S deficiency exist: type I (quantitative defect) and types II and III (qualitative defect). Since protein S is a vitamin K dependent anticoagulant, warfarin treatment and liver disease may also lead to venous thrombosis in rare cases (the majority of cases show increased bleeding).

Malignancy (C) may predispose to thrombosis due to venous thrombosis. Some tumour cells also express tissue factor, most notably pancreatic cancer cells.

Antithrombin deficiency (E) is an inherited cause of venous thrombosis. Under physiological conditions antithrombin inhibits clotting factors thrombin and factor 10a.

The oral contraceptive pill (G) may cause venous thrombosis secondary to increased circulating oestrogens, amplifying the synthesis of clotting factors by the liver.

Chronic liver disease (I) results in reduced clotting factor production by the liver as well as abnormalities of platelet function.

6. Complications of transfusion

ANSWERS: 1) H 2) I 3) D 4) E 5) A

Fluid overload (H) is an immediate complication of blood transfusion. Clinical features suggestive of fluid overload will include dyspnoea, distended neck veins and pink frothy sputum. Usually fluid overload occurs in situations where the blood transfusion rate is too fast; a transfusion would generally have to run at more than 2 mL/kg/hour to induce fluid overload. Patients with pre-existing cardiac or renal failure are prone to fluid overload as a result of blood transfusion.

Graft versus host disease (GVHD; I) occurs due to the transfer of donor lymphocytes to the recipient in a blood transfusion in patients who are immunosuppressed. Normally, the immune system is strong enough to detect and destroy donor lymphocytes. However, in immunosuppression (stem cell transplant patients/chemotherapy/malignancy/HIV) the donor lymphocytes cannot be destroyed; these foreign lymphocytes persist and target host tissue, especially the gastrointestinal tract and skin. Symptoms of GVHD include diarrhoea, maculopapular rash and skin necrosis. To minimize GVHD, donor blood is irradiated to remove lymphocytes.

IgA deficiency (D) leads to recurrent mild infections of the mucous membranes lining the airways and digestive tract. In affected patients serum IgA levels are undetectable but IgG and IgM levels are normal. IgA is found in mucous secretions from the respiratory and gastro-intestinal tracts and plays a key role in mucosal immunity. IgA deficient patients are also predisposed to severe anaphylactic reactions to blood transfusions due to the presence of IgA in donor blood.

Transfusion-related lung injury (TRALI; E) is characterized by acute non-cardiogenic pulmonary oedema that occurs within 6 hours follow-ing blood transfusion. The pathogenesis of TRALI involves the presence of anti-white blood cell antibodies in the donor blood that attack host leukocytes; sensitizing events in donors include previous blood transfu-sion or transplantation. Clinical features of TRALI are dry cough, dysp-noea and fever.

Immediate haemolytic transfusion reaction (IHTR; A) is characterized by ABO incompatibility and occurs 1–2 hours post-transfusion. Clinical features include abdominal pain, loin pain, facial flushing, vomiting and haemoglobinuria. Host IgG and IgM target donor red blood cells which are subsequently removed by the reticuloendothelial system. The most severe reaction occurs if a group O patient is transfused with group A blood.

Febrile non-haemolytic reaction (B) occurs after pregnancy when anti-leukocytic antibodies can form; this causes a reaction to leukocytes in subsequent transfusions. Low fever and rigors are characteristic.

Iron overload (C) may occur in patients who have regular blood transfusions for conditions such as thalassaemia or sickle cell disease. Features include a bronzed discolouration to the skin, short stature and heart failure.

Bacterial infection (F) caused by blood transfusion is categorized by high fevers, rigors and hypotension. Organisms that can be transmitted if the blood is not screened include hepatitis B, hepatitis C and HIV.

Delayed haemolytic transfusion reaction (G), also known as non-ABO transfusion reaction, occurs more than 24 hours after the transfusion. Clinical effects are milder than immediate haemolytic transfusion reaction.

7. Haematological neoplasms (1)

ANSWERS: 1) C 2) E 3) I 4) H 5) D

Chronic myeloid leukaemia (CML; C) is most prevalent in the elderly population and is commonly suspected secondary to routine blood tests. Blood results will show an elevated level of granulocytes (neutrophils, basophils and eosinophils). Blood film will demonstrate myeloid cells at different stages of maturation. Bone marrow biopsy in CML patients suggests hypercellularity. Ninety-five per cent of cases are caused by the Philadelphia chromosome, a chromosomal translocation between chromosomes 9 and 22; this results in the BCR-Abl fusion oncogene that has tyrosine kinase activity. Recent novel therapies for CML include imatinib, a BCR-Abl inhibitor.

Hairy cell leukaemia (HCL; E) is a haematological malignancy of B lymphocytes and a subtype of chronic lymphocytic leukaemia. It most commonly occurs in middle-aged men. The cancer derives its name from the fine hair-like projections that are seen on tumour cells on microscopy. Cell surface markers include CD25 (IL-2 receptor) and CD11c (adhesion molecule). Diagnosis can be confirmed by the presence of tartrate-resistant acid phosphatase (TRAP) on cytochemical analysis. Clinical features relate to invasion of the spleen (splenomegaly), liver (hepatomegaly) and bone marrow (pancytopenia).

Acute myeloid leukaemia (AML; I) is characterized by more than 20 per cent myeloblasts in the bone marrow. AML also causes proliferation of megakaryocytes and erythrocytes. Mutations that can cause AML include internal tandem duplications of the FLT3 gene (coding for a tyrosine kinase) and t(8;21) (a translocation causing a compressor complex to inhibit haematopoietic differentiation. Primary causes include Down's syndrome; secondary causes include myeloproliferative disease. Blood tests will reveal a variable white cell count, anaemia, thrombocytopenia and reduced neutrophil count. Auer rods on blood film are pathognomonic, which will also be leuko-erythroblastic. Immunophenotyping of CD13, CD33 or CD34 can also aid diagnosis.

Adult T-cell leukaemia (adult T-cell lymphoma; ATL; H) is a rare haematological malignancy with poor prognosis. It is caused by human T-cell leukaemia virus type 1 (HTLV-1), endemic in Japan and the Caribbean. Tumour cells express the cell surface protein CD4 and will contain the HTLV-1 virus within; the nuclei of ATL cells have a characteristic cloverleaf appearance. Clinical features include lymphadenopathy, hepatosplenomegaly, skin lesions and hypercalcaemia.

Chronic lymphocytic leukaemia (CLL; D) is a B-cell neoplasm characterized by a lymphocyte count of over 4000 cells per microlitre. CLL most commonly occurs in elderly men. The cancer presents primarily in the lymph nodes with small lymphocytes containing irregular nuclei mixed with larger prolymphocytes. Prolymphocytes may aggregate to form pathognomonic proliferation centres. Blood film may reveal the presence of smudge cells. Clinical features are non-specific and include tiredness and weight loss. Hypogammaglobulinaemia is an associated immune phenomenon. CLL may convert into more aggressive forms including prolymphocytic transformation and diffuse-large B-cell lymphoma (Richter's syndrome).

Acute lymphoblastic leukaemia (ALL; A) is the most common paediatric cancer, characterized by the presence of greater than 20 per cent lymphoblasts in the bone marrow due to suppressed maturation and uncontrolled proliferation.

Acute promyelocytic leukaemia (APML; B) is the M3 subtype of acute myeloid leukaemia. It is caused by a translocation mutation forming PML-RAR leading to proliferation of promyelocytes.

T-cell prolymphocytic leukaemia (T-PLL; F) is an aggressive T-cell leukaemia. The most common causative mutation is an inversion in chromosome 14: inv 14(q11;q32).

Large granular lymphocytic leukaemia (G) is characterized by the presence of large lymphocytes in the blood stream and bone marrow that contain azurophilic granules.

8. Haematological neoplasms (2)

ANSWERS: 1) B 2) I 3) E 4) C 5) A

Burkitt lymphoma (BL; B) is a haematological cancer of B lymphocytes caused by latent Epstein–Barr viral (EBV) infection and is most prevalent in Africa, affecting children and teenagers. Subtypes of BL include endemic, sporadic and immunodeficiency-associated disease. Endemic BL presents with a mandibular mass whereas non-endemic types present with an abdominal mass. All forms are highly associated with translocations of the c-*myc* gene on chromosome 8 (the most common with the Ig heavy chain on chromosome 14). A 'starry sky' appearance is characteristic when viewing BL cells under microscopy.

Hodgkin's lymphoma (I) results from the proliferation of B cells from the germinal centre. The pathogenesis is linked to EBV infection which activates NF-κB, preventing apoptosis of infected cells. Release of IL-5 from B-cells activates eosinophils, prolonging the life of B cells further. Histologically, Hodgkin's lymphoma is characterized by the presence of Reed–Sternberg cells (binucleate/multinucleate cells with abundant cytoplasm, inclusion-like nucleoli and surrounded by eosinophils). Lymphadenopathy associated with Hodgkin's lymphoma is usually painless, asymmetrical, fluctuates in size and is painful with alcohol intake. Other clinical features include fever, night sweats, weight loss and Pel–Ebstein fever (intermittent fever every 2 weeks). Unlike non-Hodgkin's lymphoma, extra-nodal involvement is rare.

Mantle cell lymphoma (MCL; E) is an aggressive B-cell lymphoma primarily affecting elderly men. The most common cause is a translocation between chromosomes 11 and 14, involving the BCL-1 locus and Ig heavy chain locus, therefore leading to over-expression of cyclin D1. Over-expression of cyclin D1 leads to dysregulation of the cell cycle. Clinically, generalized lymphadenopathy, as well as bone marrow and liver infiltration, are common. Hodgkin's lymphoma can be split into classical and lymphocyte predominant nodular (LPN) subtypes.

Follicular lymphoma (C) is caused most commonly by a translocation between chromosomes 14 and 18, leading to over-expression of the BCL-2 protein. Over-expression of BCL-2 causes inhibition of apoptosis, promoting the survival of tumour cells. Tumour cells in follicular lymphoma are characterized by centrocytes (small B cells with irregular nuclei and reduced cytoplasm) and centroblasts (larger B cells with multiple nuclei). Clinical features include painless, generalized lymphadenopathy. Follicular lymphoma usually presents in middle-aged patients and has a non-aggressive course but is difficult to cure.

Diffuse large B-cell lymphoma (DLBL; A) is a haematological malignancy most commonly affecting the elderly, characterized by large lymphocytes which have a diffuse pattern of growth. Common chromosomal abnormalities which contribute to the development of DLBL include the t(14;18) translocation which is characteristic of follicular lymphoma; this suggests that follicular lymphoma may undergo a degree of transformation to cause DLBL in such circumstances. Tumour cells that have follicular lymphoma morphology may be present at other sites. Two subtypes of DLBL have been described, both of which are associated with immunodeficiency: immunodeficiency-associated large B-cell lymphoma (linked to latent EBV infection) and body cavity-based large cell lymphoma (linked to HHV8 infection).

Small lymphocytic lymphoma (SLL; D) is indistinguishable from chronic lymphocytic leukaemia (CLL) in terms of genetics and morphology. SLL more commonly presents with greater peripheral blood lymphocytosis than CLL.

Peripheral T-cell lymphomas (F) are a group of heterogeneous mature T-cell lymphomas that are not easily classified. They usually present in adulthood and have an aggressive course.

Mycosis fungoides (G) is a cutaneous T-cell lymphoma most commonly occurring in elderly men. It can present with rash-like lesions that may appear similar to eczema or psoriasis.

Angiocentric lymphoma (H) presents in adulthood as cutaneous masses most commonly in the nasal area. Tumour cells will express NK-cell markers and commonly may be infected with EBV.

9. Haematological neoplasms (3)

ANSWERS: 1) A 2) B 3) I 4) C 5) E

Essential thrombocythaemia (A) results in a high platelet count, which quickly become dysfunctional; it is characterized by periods of bleeding or thrombosis. Clinical features of bleeding events include gastrointestinal bleeding, bruising, petechiae and/or menorrhagia. Thrombotic events manifest as erythromelalgia (erythema, swelling, pain and/or burning sensation in the extremities), digital ischaemia, cerebrovascular accident, deep vein thrombosis and Budd–Chiari syndrome. Blood tests will demonstrate a platelet count of over 600×10^9/L and the bone marrow will be hypercellular with giant platelets, as well as megakaryocyte clustering and hyperplasia. Treatment options include hydroxyurea or anagrelide.

In myelofibrosis (B) the bone marrow undergoes fibrosis, the cause of which is unknown. The body compensates with extra-medullary haemopoiesis causing enlargement of the spleen and liver. The underlying pathogenesis is related to abnormal megakaryocytes releasing PDGF and TGF-β which stimulate fibroblast proliferation. Blood tests will show an initial rise in white cell and platelet counts during the compensatory phase; as fibrosis progresses the bone marrow reduces white cell and platelet production. Blood film will be leukoerythroblastic, with tear-drop cells and circulating megakaryocytes (fibrosis causes ejection of megakaryocytes from the bone marrow). Bone marrow aspirate will demonstrate a 'dry' or bloody tap.

Multiple myeloma (I) is defined as the proliferation of plasma cells in the bone marrow (>10 per cent plasma cells). Myeloma cells release monoclonal antibodies (most commonly IgG or IgA) and/or light chains (paraproteins); IgA production significantly increases the viscosity of the blood. Diagnosis is based on paraprotein bands of greater than 30 g/L on electrophoresis. Blood tests will demonstrate an increased

ESR and calcium levels as well as rouleaux formation on blood film. Bence–Jones proteins (immunoglobulin light chains) may be present in the urine. Plasma cells visualized from bone marrow biopsy are atypical, with multiple nuclei, prominent nucleoli and cytoplasmic granules (containing immunoglobulin). X-rays may reveal punched-out lytic lesions.

Chronic myelo-monocytic leukaemia (CMML; C) is a myelodysplastic/ myeloproliferative disease which most commonly affects the elderly population, defined by a monocytosis of >1000/mm^3 and increased number of monocytes in the bone marrow. Myeloblasts make up <5 per cent of the peripheral blood and <20 per cent of the bone marrow. Eosinophilia may be present in CMML associated with a t(5;12) translocation. The Philadelphia chromosome BCR/ABL fusion gene is not responsible for causing CMML. Commonly, patients will present with fever, fatigue, night sweats; on examination hepatomegaly and/or more commonly splenomegaly may be present.

Polycythaemia rubra vera (PRV; E) is characterized by proliferation of erythroid, granulocytic and megakaryocyte lines. Many PRV cases are due to a V167F mutation on exon 2 of the JAK2 gene, leading to uncontrolled stem cell proliferation. Clinical features include hyperviscosity (headaches, dizziness and stroke), hyper-mast-cell degranulation (pruritis after hot baths, plethoric skin and peptic ulceration) and increased cell turnover (gout). Blood tests will reveal a haemoglobin concentration above 18 g/dL, leukocytosis and thrombocytosis. Erythropoietin levels are low due to a negative-feedback response from increased erythrocyte production.

Refractory anaemia with excess blasts (D) is a myelodysplastic disease that may be classified into type 1 (5–9 per cent myeloblasts in the bone marrow) or type 2 (10–19 per cent myeloblasts in the bone marrow).

Refractory anaemia with ringed sideroblasts (F) is a myelodysplastic disease characterized by fewer than 5 per cent myeloblasts in the bone marrow, but greater than 15 per cent erythrocyte precursors stuffed with iron in their mitochondria.

Refractory anaemia (G) is defined by fewer than 5 per cent myeloblasts present in the bone marrow.

5q-Syndrome (H) is caused by deletion of the long arm of chromosome 5. Features include hypo-lobulated megakaryocytes and an increased/ normal platelet count.

10. Haematology of systemic disease

ANSWERS: 1) D 2) A 3) H 4) B 5) G

Rheumatoid arthritis (RA; D) is an inflammatory disease that mainly affects the small joints of the hands but systemic involvement can be a feature, manifesting in the lungs (fibrosis), heart (pericarditis) and eyes (scleritis). RA is a cause of anaemia of chronic disease (ACD), which is mediated by IL-6 produced by macrophages. IL-6 induces hepcidin production by the liver which has the effect of retaining iron in macrophages (reduced delivery to red blood cells for erythropoiesis) and decreases export from enterocytes (reduced plasma iron levels). Laboratory features of ACD include a microcytic hypochromic anaemia, rouleaux formation and raised ferritin (acute phase protein).

Temporal arteritis (A) is a vasculitis most commonly affecting the medium and large arteries of the head. It is also known as giant cell arteritis due to the inflammatory cells that are visualized on biopsy. Prominent temporal arteries with regional tenderness, coupled with an erythrocyte sedimentation rate (ESR) of more than 60 mm/hour is highly suggestive of temporal arteritis. ESR may be raised due to increase plasma proteins (fibrinogen, acute phase proteins or immunoglobulin) or due to reduced packing of red blood cells (anaemia). Other causes of a raised ESR include myeloma, polymyalgia rheumatica and autoimmune disease.

Sarcoidosis (H) is a granulomatous disease characterized by the presence of non-caseating granulomas in multiple organs, most commonly affecting the lungs. Diagnosis of sarcoidosis is usually a matter of excluding other diseases but chest X-ray (bihilar lymphadenopathy), CT scanning and lung biopsy can all help. Blood tests commonly reveal a monocytosis; monocytes are contributory to the pathogenesis of granulomatous disease. Other causes of monocytosis include brucellosis, typhoid, varicella zoster infection and chronic myelo-monocytic leukaemia (CMML).

Renal cell carcinoma (RCC; B) is the most common type of renal cancer. Secondary polycythaemia may be associated with RCC as a result of increased erythropoietin (EPO) production. Secondary polycythaemia can be distinguished from primary polycythaemia as in the former there is an increase in blood EPO levels, whereas in the latter EPO levels decrease. Other causes of secondary polycythaemia include chronic hypoxia (high altitude, smoking, lung disease, cyanotic heart disease), renal disease (cysts, renal artery stenosis, hydronephrosis) and solid tumours (renal cell carcinoma and hepatocellular carcinoma).

Schistosomiasis (G) is a parasitic disease caused by *Schistosoma* spp. It is particularly common in Asia, Africa and South America. The risk of bladder cancer is increased in urinary forms of schistosomiasis. The immune response to parasitic infection involves eosinophils and hence a marked eosinophilia is characteristic. Other causes of eosinophilia besides parasitic infection include allergic disease (asthma, rheumatoid arthritis, polyarteritis), neoplasms (Hodgkin's lymphoma, non-Hodgkin's lymphoma) as well as certain drugs (NSAIDs).

Colorectal cancer (C) may result in iron deficiency anaemia (IDA) secondary to bleeding. IDA will demonstrate a microcytic anaemia, reduced ferritin and iron count and raised total iron binding capacity.

Miliary tuberculosis (E) may cause infiltration of the bone marrow leading to a leuko-erythroblastic picture on blood film. Other causes of a leuko-erythroblastic film include myelofibrosis, leukaemia, lymphoma and non-haemopoietic cancers (for example, breast cancer).

Acute pancreatitis (F) can result in a neutrophilia as a result of tissue inflammation. Other causes of neutrophilia include ulcerative colitis and corticosteroids.

Epstein–Barr virus (EBV; I) results in a reactive lymphocytosis. Other causes include cytomegalovirus, toxoplasmosis, hepatitis, rubella and herpes virus infection. Autoimmune disorders and neoplasia can also be causative.

SECTION 4: HAEMATOLOGY SBAs

Questions

19. Platelet count (2)
20. Obstetric haematology
21. Vitamin K dependent clotting factors
22. Deep vein thrombosis
23. Thrombocytopenia
24. Erythrocyte sedimentation rate
25. Polycythaemia
26. Haemolysis
27. Secondary polycythaemia
28. von Willebrand's disease (1)
29. Myeloproliferative disease
30. Lymphoma
31. Hodgkin's lymphoma
32. Glucose-6-phosphate dehydrogenase deficiency
33. Anaemia (6)
34. Splenomegaly
35. Hodgkin's lymphoma staging
36. Acute leukaemia
37. Treatment of chronic myeloid leukaemia
38. von Willebrand's disease (2)
39. Myelodysplastic syndrome
40. Factor V Leiden

Answers

QUESTIONS

1. Blood transfusion (1)

A 22-year-old motorcyclist is involved in a road traffic accident, and is transfused two units of blood. Four hours later he develops acute shortness of breath and hypoxia, and despite attempts at ventilation deteriorates rapidly and goes into respiratory arrest. An autopsy shows evidence of massive pulmonary oedema with granulocyte aggregation within the pulmonary microvasculature. The most likely diagnosis is:

A   Anaphylaxis
B   ABO incompatible blood transfusion
C   Fluid overload
D   Transfusion related acute lung injury
E   Air embolism

2. Blood transfusion (2)

A 43-year-old woman is transfused three units of blood as an emergency following prolonged haematemesis. A few minutes later she becomes restless, and complains of chest pain. On examination she is pyrexial and tachycardic with a blood pressure of 95/60. There is bleeding at the site where her cannula is inserted, and urinalysis reveals haemoglobinuria. The most likely diagnosis is:

A   Anaphylaxis
B   ABO incompatible blood transfusion
C   Myocardial infarction
D   Graft versus host disease
E   Bacterial contamination

3. Blood transfusion (3)

An 83-year-old woman with myelodysplasia is found to have a haemoglobin of 6.2 on admission. She is transfused two units of blood, and is discharged 2 days later. Six days after her admission her carer calls the GP with concerns that she is feverish and her skin looks slightly yellow. She is readmitted to hospital where blood tests reveal the following: bilirubin 35, ALT 15 (N 5–35), ALP 82 (N 20–140), Hb 7.3 g/dL, platelets 264×10^9/L. The most likely diagnosis is:

A   Febrile haemolytic transfusion reaction
B   Hepatitis B
C   Graft versus host disease
D   Post-transfusion purpura
E   Delayed haemolytic transfusion reaction

4. Haemolytic anaemia (1)

An 8-year-old boy is brought to his GP by his father, who reports that he has been feeling progressively more tired over the past few months. On examination the GP notices a slight yellowing of his sclera, and the presence of splenomegaly. His father recollects that he himself was told he had a problem with his blood cells as a child, but has never been affected by it. A peripheral blood film shows a raised reticulocyte count and spherocytes. He is likely to have a positive:

A   Coombs test
B   Osmotic fragility test
C   G6PD test
D   Sickle cell screen
E   Schilling test

5. Haemolytic anaemia (2)

A 33-year-old Turkish man presents with extreme tiredness and shortness of breath after being started on a course of anti-malarial tablets. A full blood count reveals an Hb of 6.8. His Coombs test is negative. The cell type most likely to be found on his blood film is:

A   Heinz bodies
B   Pencil cells
C   Target cells
D   Spherocytes
E   Sickle cells

6. Infectious mononucleosis

A 25-year-old student is treated for infectious mononucleosis following a positive Paul Bunnell test. A blood film reveals target cells, Howell–Jolly bodies and atypical lymphocytes. Together, these suggest that he has features of:

A   Bone marrow suppression
B   Hyposplenism
C   Disseminated intravascular coagulation
D   Haemolytic anaemia
E   Liver failure

7. Haemoglobinopathies in children (1)

A 4-year-old Afro-Caribbean boy has chest and abdominal pain. His blood tests reveal an Hb of 6.1 g/dL, with an MCV of 65. A blood film shows the presence of sickle cells. The most likely diagnosis is:

A   Sickle cell trait
B   Sickle cell anaemia
C   Sickle cell/β-thalassaemia
D   Sickle cell/haemoglobin C
E   β-Thalassaemia

8. Haemoglobinopathies in children (2)

A 7-year-old child has known sickle cell disease. He presents with a 5-day history of fever, shortness of breath and extreme fatigue. His mother reports that
his younger brother, who also has sickle cell disease, has been feeling unwell too
recently. A blood test for the patient reveals a severe anaemia and low reticulocyte count. He has most likely developed:

A   Splenic sequestration
B   Pneumococcal infection
C   Vaso-occlusive crisis
D   Folic acid deficiency
E   Parvovirus B19 infection

9. Anaemia (1)

A 26-year-old pregnant woman is found to have an Hb of 9.5 g/dL on a routine blood test, with an MCV of 70. Serum electrophoresis reveals an Hb A2 of
3.9 per cent and Hb A of 96.1 per cent. Her ferritin levels are normal. The most
likely diagnosis is:

A   Iron deficiency anaemia
B   Cooley's anaemia
C   β-Thalassaemia intermedia
D   β-Thalassaemia minor
E   α-Thalassaemia

10. Anaemia (2)

A 24-year-old unemployed man presents to his GP with a 4-week history of
flu-like symptoms and a persistent dry cough. On examination he has a maculopapular rash. A blood film reveals a haemolytic anaemia, and he is positive for
cold agglutinins. The most likely organism implicated is:

A   *Streptococcus pneumoniae*
B   *Mycoplasma pneumoniae*
C   *Legionella pneumophilia*
D   *Chlamydophila psittaci*
E   *Borrelia burgdorferi*

11. Anaemia (3)

A 7-year-old boy is taken ill from school on a cold December day, with a presumed viral infection. On returning home that day, he beings to feel even more unwell with a very high fever, headache and abdominal pain. His father begins to worry that his skin has taken on a yellow tinge, and the boy says his urine is now a dark reddy-brown colour. He is taken to the GP and after several tests the presence of 'Donath–Landsteiner antibodies' is reported. This child is suffering from:

A   Paroxysmal cold haemoglobinuria
B   Paroxysmal nocturnal haemoglobinuria
C   Sickle cell disease
D   Acute intermittent porphyria
E   Epstein–Barr virus

12. Anaemia (4)

A 21-year-old student has recently been diagnosed with coeliac disease. She presents to her GP complaining of increased tiredness and shortness of breath on climbing stairs. Which of the following are most likely to be raised in this patient?

A   Serum iron
B   Haematocrit
C   Transferrin
D   Ferritin
E   Mean cell haemoglobin

13. Anaemia (5)

A 34-year-old woman with known Addison's disease is brought to the GP by her husband, as he is concerned that she keeps falling over at night. On examination the GP notes that she has conjunctival pallor. A thorough neurological examination reveals absent knee jerks, absent ankle jerks and extensor plantars bilaterally. Which of the following is the most sensitive test for the condition she has developed?

A   Anti-intrinsic factor antibodies
B   Anti-endomysial cell antibodies
C   Anti-smooth muscle antibodies
D   Anti-parietal cell antibodies
E   Anti-voltage gated calcium channel antibodies

14. Macrocytic anaemia

A 58-year-old woman is referred to a haematology clinic following repeated chest infections and epistaxis. On examination the doctor notes that she has conjunctival pallor and some petechial rashes on her forearms, but no organo-megaly. Her blood tests reveal a pancytopenia, and an MCV of 112. Her drug history includes omeprazole, carbamazepine, gliclazide, metformin, paracetamol, and simvastatin. A bone marrow biopsy reveals a hypocellular marrow. The most likely diagnosis is:

A   Aplastic anaemia
B   Myelodysplasia
C   Hypothyroidism
D   Chronic myeloid leukaemia
E   Myeloma

15. Hepatomegaly

A 50-year-old diabetic man sees his GP complaining of generalized tiredness and a painful right knee. He is found on examination to have five finger breadths of hepatomegaly. An X-ray of his right knee is reported as showing chondrocalci-nosis. His blood tests are likely to reveal:

A   Raised MCV
B   Raised total iron binding capacity
C   Reduced serum ferritin
D   Reduced iron level
E   Raised transferrin saturation

16. Plasma cell disorders (1)

A 64-year-old woman is seen in the haematology clinic with generalized bone pain and recurrent infections. Following a set of blood tests, a skeletal survey reveals multiple lytic lesions and a bone marrow biopsy reports the presence of >10 per cent plasma cells. Her blood tests are most likely to have shown:

A   Raised calcium, normal alkaline phosphatase, raised ESR
B   Normal calcium, raised alkaline phosphatase, normal ESR
C   Raised calcium, raised alkaline phosphatase, raised ESR
D   Raised calcium, normal alkaline phosphatase, raised CRP
E   Normal calcium, normal alkaline phosphatase, raised CRP

17. Plasma cell disorders (2)

A 67-year-old woman presented with polyuria and polydipsia on a background of ongoing bone pain. Her blood tests revealed a high calcium, and a serum electrophoresis was sent. Her serum paraprotein was 25 g/L and a bone marrow biopsy revealed 6 per cent clonal plasma cells. The most likely diagnosis is:

A   Plasma cell dyscrasia
B   Monoclonal gammopathy of undetermined significance
C   Smouldering myeloma
D   Multiple myeloma
E   Hypercalcaemia with no evidence of underlying malignancy

18. Platelet count (1)

A 39-year-old motorcyclist is admitted following a road traffic accident complicated by severe burns. Several days later he is due to go home, when ooz-
ing is noted from his cannula site and he has several nose bleeds. Repeat blood
tests reveal an Hb of 12.2 g/dL, WCC of 11.2 × 10⁹/L, and platelets of 28 × 10⁹/L.
A coagulation screen shows a prolonged APTT and PT. He also has a reduced
fibrinogen and raised D-dimers. The most likely diagnosis is:

A   Liver failure
B   Disseminated intravascular coagulation
C   Thrombotic thrombocytopenic purpura
D   Aplastic anaemia
E   Heparin induced thrombocytopenia

19. Platelet count (2)

A 46-year-old woman is brought to accident and emergency by her daughter,
who reports that she had been feeling unwell for a few days with a fever and is
now hallucinating. On examination she has a temperature of 38.9°C, is noted to
be pale and has widespread purpura over both arms. Blood tests reveal an Hb of
9.1 g/dL, platelet count of 60 × 10⁹/L, creatinine of 226 and urea 16.7. A blood film
is reported as showing the presence of shistocytes. The most likely diagnosis is:

A   Weil's disease
B   Glandular fever
C   Idiopathic thrombocytopenic purpura
D   Thrombotic thombocytopenic purpura
E   Haemolytic uraemic syndrome

20. Obstetric haematology

A 28-year-old woman in her 29th week of pregnancy comes to accident and
emergency with epigastric pain, nausea and vomiting. She also complains that
her hands and feet have been swelling up. On examination her blood pressure
is 165/96, HR 125 bpm, and she is apyrexial. She is noted to have yellowing of
her sclera and right upper quadrant tenderness. Blood tests reveal an Hb of 10.1,
platelets 96, WCC 11.3, LDH 820 (N 70–250), AST 115 (N 5–35), and ALT 102
(N 5–35). Her coagulation screen is normal and a blood film is reported as
showing the presence of schistocytes. The most likely diagnosis is:

A   Hepatitis
B   Thrombotic thrombocytopenic purpura
C   Pre-eclampsia
D   Acute fatty liver of pregnancy
E   HELLP syndrome

21. Vitamin K dependent clotting factors

A 56-year-old woman with known cirrhosis presents with falls. On examination she is clinically jaundiced and rectal examination reveals malaena. Blood tests reveal an INR of 2.2. She is diagnosed with decompensated chronic liver disease. Which of the following is not a vitamin K dependent clotting factor?

A   Thrombin
B   Factor VII
C   Factor VIII
D   Protein C
E   Factor X

22. Deep vein thrombosis

A 46-year-old man presents with pain and swelling in the right calf 2 weeks after being fitted with a plaster cast to his leg after a fall. The calf is tender, erythematous and swollen. He is also a heavy smoker and slightly overweight. His admitting physician suspects a deep vein thrombosis (DVT) and books an ultrasound of the calf. A deep vein thrombosis is confirmed and 5 mg warfarin is started the next day. Two days later, the same patient develops pain and swelling in the other calf, an ultrasound confirms a further deep vein thrombosis in the contralateral leg. What factor is least likely to contribute to the development of the second DVT?

A   Smoking
B   Warfarin
C   Previous DVT
D   Being slightly overweight
E   Plaster cast

23. Thrombocytopenia

A 54-year-old man presents with haematemesis. He has known varices and is currently vomiting large amounts of bright red blood. The admitting doctor takes some blood for fast analysis and confirms a haemoglobin of 4 g/dL. The patient's haematemesis continues and he is transfused a total of 20 units of blood and eight units of fresh frozen plasma in the next 24 hours. The patient underwent gastroscopy which revealed bleeding oesophageal varices which were successfully treated by endoscopic banding. His post-transfusion bloods are the following:

Hb 9.2 g/dL
White cells 8.0×10^9/L
Platelets 57×10^9/L
Prothrombin time normal
Activated partial thromboplastin time normal
Fibrinogen >1.0 g/L

What is the most likely cause of his thrombocytopenia?

A   Disseminated intravascular coagulopathy
B   Alcohol excess
C   Massive blood transfusion
D   Megaloblastic anaemia
E   Hypersplenism

24. Erythrocyte sedimentation rate

Which of the following is not often associated with a very high (>100 mm/hour) erythrocyte sedimentation rate (ESR)?

A   Myeloma
B   Anaemia
C   Leukaemia
D   Aortic aneurysm
E   Malignant prostatic cancer

25. Polycythaemia

A 62-year-old man presents with shortness of breath. This has been gradually getting worse for the last few years and is associated with chronic productive cough. He is a heavy smoker. His chest X-ray reveals a hyperexpanded chest with no other abnormalities. His bloods tests are normal except for a raised haemoglobin and raised haematocrit. What is the most likely cause for this?

A   Polycythaemia rubra vera
B   Idiopathic erythrocytosis
C   Secondary polycythaemia
D   Gaisbock's disease
E   Combined polycythaemia

26. Haemolysis

A 25-year-old black man develops jaundice and dark red urine 2 days after starting primaquine, an anti-malarial. His blood tests reveal a macrocytic anaemia with raised bilirubin and urine dipstick is positive for blood. A peripheral blood film reveals 'bite cells' and Heinz bodies. The most likely diagnosis is:

A   Hereditary spherocytosis
B   Glucose-6-phosphate dehydrogenase deficiency
C   Paroxysmal nocturnal haemoglobinuria
D   Microangiopathic haemolytic anaemia
E   Autoimmune haemolytic anaemia

27. Secondary polycythaemia

What are the likely laboratory findings for a patient with renal cell carcinoma with secondary polycythaemia who is not dehydrated?

A   Normal red cell count, normal red cell mass, increased erythropoietin concentration
B   Increased red cell count, increased red cell mass, increased erythropoietin concentration
C   Decreased red cell count, decreased red cell mass, normal erythropoietin concentration
D   Increased red cell count, decreased red cell mass, increased erythropoietin concentration
E   Decreased red cell count, increased red cell mass, decreased erythropoietin concentration

28. von Willebrand's disease (1)

von Willebrand's disease is characterized by abnormal platelet aggregation when they are exposed to:

A   Streptomycin
B   Aspirin
C   Fibrinogen
D   Collagen
E   Ristocetin

29. Myeloproliferative disease

An 18-month-old child with Down syndrome presents with recurrent infections and petechial bleeding. A blood film was analyzed showing a particular distinctive feature of haematological malignancy. What is the most likely diagnostically helpful finding seen in this patient?

A   Smudge cell
B   Reed Sternberg cell
C   Auer rod
D   Pelger Huet anomaly
E   Hairy cell

30. Lymphoma

An 8-year-old African boy presents with a large jaw mass which has been growing rapidly over the last few weeks. A histological sample was taken and a classical 'starry sky' appearance was observed. The most likely diagnosis is:

A   Follicular lymphoma
B   Marginal zone lymphoma
C   Burkitt's lymphoma
D   Diffuse large B cell lymphoma
E   Mantle cell lymphoma

31. Hodgkin's lymphoma

A 35-year-old Afro-American man presents with painless lymphadenopathy which he noticed after shaving. He denies any recent infections, fevers, weight loss or night sweats. A biopsy is performed which shows lymphocytic and histiocytic cells. A haematologist calls to confirm the diagnosis of non-classical Hodgkin's lymphoma. Which subtype is this?

A   Nodular sclerosis
B   Mixed cellularity
C   Nodular lymphocytic
D   Lymphocytic rich
E   Lymphocytic depleted

32. Glucose-6-phosphate dehydrogenase deficiency

A 17-year-old boy with glucose-6-phosphate dehydrogenase (G6PD) deficiency presents with tiredness and is noticed to be jaundiced. These features have developed since he was diagnosed with a chest infection 1 week ago. What is the most likely haematological finding?

A   Positive direct antiglobulin test
B   Low mean cell volume
C   Reduced reticulocyte count
D   Haemoglobinuria
E   Increased haptoglobin concentration

33. Anaemia (6)

A 35-year-old Asian woman presents with tiredness. The full blood count shows:

Haemoglobin: 10.1 g/dL (11.5–16.5)
Platelet count: 160×10^9 (150–400×10^9)
White cell count: 6.6×10^9 (4–11×10^9)
Mean cell volume: 62 fL (80–96 fL)
Hb A$_2$: 6.3 per cent (2–3 per cent)

Which of the following is the most likely diagnosis?

A   Sickle cell disease
B   Acute myeloid leukaemia
C   β-Thalassaemia major
D   β-Thalassaemia trait
E   Hereditary spherocytosis

34. Splenomegaly

A 62-year-old man presents with bruising and tiredness. Examination reveals moderate splenomegly and his a reveal a normocytic anaemia with blood tests platelet count of 900×10^9/L, neutrophilia, basophilia, numerous myelocytes and 4 per cent myeloblasts. The neutrophils have low leukocyte alkaline phosphatase levels. Which of the following is likely to be present in this patient?

A   t(9;22)
B   t (8;14)
C   BCR-Abl fusion gene only
D   V617F point mutation in JAK2
E   5q-Syndrome

35. Hodgkin's lymphoma staging

Which of the following patients has the worse prognosis?

A   25-year-old man with inguinal lymphadenopathy
B   25-year-old woman with mediastinal and inguinal lymphadenopathy
C   25-year-old woman with mediastinal and inguinal lymphadenopathy and night sweats
D   25-year-old woman with mediastinal and inguinal lymphadenopathy with 5 per cent weight loss in last 6 months
E   25-year-old man with cervical and mediastinal lymphadenopathy

36. Acute leukaemia

A patient presents with acute promyelocytic leukaemia. What is the most likely mechanism of underlying leukaemogenesis?

A   Telomere shortening
B   Aberrant fusion of two genes
C   Impaired protein degredation
D   Over-expression of cellular oncogene
E   Post-translational modification

37. Treatment of chronic myeloid leukaemia

A 64-year-old man presents with lethargy, weight loss and abdominal fullness. He is found to have chronic myeloid leukaemia. He is started on imatinib as part of the initial treatment to control his disease. What is the mechanism of action of imatinib?

A   Proteosome inhibitor
B   Tyrosine kinase inhibitor
C   IL-6 inhibitor
D   p53 inhibitor
E   Human epidermal growth factor receptor 2 protein inhibitor

38. von Willebrand's disease (2)

A 16-year-old girl with mild von Willebrand's disease is scheduled for a dental extraction. She has had one previously where she required two units of blood transfused. What is the most appropriate treatment for this patient prior to surgery?

A   Cryoprecipitate
B   Desmopressin
C   Fresh frozen plasma
D   Vitamin K
E   Recombinant factor VIII concentrate

39. Myelodysplastic syndrome

An 80-year-old man presents with tiredness and lethargy. After initial work-up, a diagnosis of myelodysplastic syndrome is suspected. Which of the following is true about this condition?

A   A blood film will typically show neutrophil toxic granulation
B   If there are 1 per cent blasts of the total white cell count, this represents leukaemic transformation
C   Cytotoxic chemotherapy is first line treatment
D   Mortality is more likely to be from infection than leukaemic transformation
E   Absence of the short arm of chromosome 5 is a subtype

40. Factor V Leiden

A middle-aged woman comes to the dermatology clinic with a suspicious mole on her back. You decide excision is required and during the history she says 'I have Factor V Leiden'. Which of the following best describes the pathophysiology of Factor V Leiden mutation?

A   Prothrombin mutation
B   Activated protein C resistance
C   Antithrombin III deficiency
D   Protein C deficiency
E   Protein S deficiency

ANSWERS

Blood transfusion (1)

1 D   Transfusion related acute lung injury (TRALI) (D) is rare but is one of the leading causes of transfusion related mortality. It can present with acute shortness of break and hypoxia, as in this case, typically within 6 hours of receiving the transfusion. The classic presentation to look out for is that of non-cardiogenic pulmonary oedema, i.e. pulmonary oedema that is not due to fluid overload.

The underlying mechanism is not fully understood, but it is thought to involve HLA antibodies in the blood donor reacting with corresponding HLA antigens on the patient's white blood cells. This leads to the formation of aggregates of white blood cells which become stuck in small pulmonary capillaries. The release of proteolytic enzymes from neutrophils and toxic oxygen metabolites causes lung damage, and subsequent non-cardiogenic pulmonary oedema which can be fatal. Treatment is essentially supportive, and includes stopping the transfusion, giving IV fluids and ventilation if needed. TRALI can occur with platelets and FFP, as well as with packed red cells as in this case. You might find it helpful to remember the mechanism by rearranging 'TRALI' to form the word 'TRAIL', and think of the blood donor leaving a 'trail' of antibodies in the recipient.

An anaphylactic reaction (A) can also present immediately following a blood transfusion, but look out for clues such as a rash, urticaria and a wheeze to point you towards this diagnosis. ABO incompatible transfusions (B) present with symptoms and signs of acute intravascular haemolysis, such as restlessness, chest or loin pain, fever, vomiting, flushing, collapse and haemoglobinuria. Shortness of breath and acute hypoxia are less common with this, and the pathological description given here at autopsy is characteristic of TRALI. The use of the term 'pulmonary oedema' in the question may have misled you to think of fluid overload (C). Whilst fluid overload is much more common, this patient has only received two units of blood and fluid overload would be less likely to cause such a rapid deterioration. These patients might have pedal oedema and bilateral crepitations on examination, and can be treated with diuretics. An air embolism (E) can rarely occur if air is introduced into the blood bag, and can present with circulatory collapse. Again, the findings on autopsy from this case would not correlate with this diagnosis.

Blood transfusion (2)

2   B   An ABO incompatible blood transfusion (B) can occur immediately
after a transfusion has been given. For example, if group A, B or AB
blood is given to a group O patient, the patient's anti-A and anti-B
antibodies attack the blood cells in the donor blood. The most severe
form of reaction is thought to occur if group A red cells are transfused
to a group O patient. Even just a few millilitres of blood can trigger a
severe reaction within a few minutes. These reactions can also occur
with platelets or fresh frozen plasma because they also contain anti-red
cell antibodies.

Symptoms can include chills, fever, pain in the back, chest or along
the IV line, hypotension, dark urine (intravascular haemolysis), and
uncontrolled bleeding due to DIC. In this case, the management involves
stopping the transfusion immediately and taking blood samples for
FBC, biochemistry, coagulation, repeat x-match, blood cultures and
direct antiglobulin test, and contacting the haematology doctor as soon
as possible. The blood bank should also be urgently informed because
another patient may have also been given incompatible blood. These
patients require fluid resuscitation and possibly inotropic support. They
should be transferred to ICU if possible.

These reactions can be prevented through measures such as proper identification of the patient from sample collection through to administering
the blood product and careful labelling of the samples. If the patient is
unconscious, then careful monitoring of observations before, during and
after the transfusion can help to detect signs of a reaction as early as
possible.

An anaphylactic reaction (A) can also present immediately following
a blood transfusion, but look out for clues such as a rash, urticaria
and a wheeze to point you towards this diagnosis. A myocardial
infarction (C) is less likely in this setting, and would not cause intravascular haemolysis. Graft versus host disease (D) is a rare form of a
delayed transfusion reaction which can occur in immunosuppressed
patients, where lymphocytes from donor blood can attack the host.
This can result in liver failure, diarrhoea, skin rashes and bone marrow failure. Bacterial contamination (E) would also cause a fever and
may lead to hypotension and tachycardia, so can be difficult to differentiate from ABO incompatibility. However, these reactions would
not typically cause pain or haemoglobinuria. Usually a very high
fever, rigors, and profound hypotension can be clues to this diagnosis
in the question.

Blood transfusion (3)

3 E Delayed haemolytic transfusion reactions (E) can occur more than 24 hours after a transfusion is given. They occur when patients are sensitized from previous transfusions or pregnancies, and therefore have antibodies against red cell antigens which are not picked up by routine blood bank screening if they are below the detectable limits. The most frequent causes are the antibodies of the Kidd (Jk) and Rh systems.

Clinical features might include falling haemoglobin concentration, a smaller rise in haemoglobin than expected following a transfusion as in this case, fever, jaundice and rarely haemoglobinuria or renal failure. A blood film may show a raised reticulocyte count. Management of these reactions includes monitoring renal function, sending a repeat group and antibody screen and cross-match and further transfusion if needed. The blood bank should be notified too, and further specific treatment might not be needed unless renal failure develops.

Febrile haemolytic transfusion reactions (A) typically occur less than 24 hours after the transfusion. These reactions are thought to be due to antibodies in the patient reacting with white cell antigens in the donor blood, or due to cytokines which build up in the blood products during storage. These reactions usually only warrant slowing the transfusion, and giving an anti-pyretic if needed. Hepatitis B (B) can occur after a blood transfusion, but blood products are usually screened for this virus as well as for the hepatitis C antibody and RNA, HIV antibody, HTLV antibody, and syphilis antibody. A high ALT would be expected if the patient had been infected with a hepatitis virus. Graft versus host disease (C) is a rare form of delayed reaction which can occur in immuno-suppressed patients, where lymphocytes from donor blood can attack the host. This can result in liver failure, diarrhoea, skin rashes and bone marrow failure. Post-transfusion purpura (D) is a rare but potentially lethal reaction which occurs 5–9 days after a transfusion. Patients can develop a severe thrombocytopenia with bleeding. Treatment is usually with IV immunoglobulin therapy.

Haemolytic anaemia (1)

4 B Hereditary spherocytosis is a type of autosomal dominant inherited haemolytic anaemia. It occurs due to an increase in the fragility of the red blood cell membrane due to dysfunctional skeletal proteins in the membrane, such as spectrin, ankyrin and band 4.2. Most patients develop a haemolytic state that is partially compensated. Clinical features can include tiredness from anaemia, as in this case, and the presence of jaundice and splenomegaly on examination. They can also develop pigment gallstones from the haemolysis. As with this child, there is often a positive family history.

A blood film can show the presence of spherocytes and reticulocytes, and a Coombs test is negative. They may have a positive osmotic fragility test (B), but remember that this is just used to confirm that there are spherocytes present, not that the cause is hereditary spherocytosis. With this test, because the membrane is more permeable to salt and water, the spherocytes rupture in a mildly hypotonic solution. Do not forget that spherocytes may also be found in autoimmune haemolytic anaemia.

To go back to basics, remember that common laboratory features of all haemolytic anaemias might include:

- anaemia
- reticulocytosis
- raised bilirubin (unconjugated)
- raised LDH
- reduced haptoglobins (a plasma protein that binds free haemoglobin)

It is then worth classifying haemolytic anaemias as inherited or acquired to help you remember the different types. Hereditary anaemias can be thought of as due to defects in the red cell, such as the membrane (such as in spherocytosis and elliptocytosis), the haemoglobin itself (structural defects in sickle cell disease (D) or quantitative defects in thalassaemias), or of the enzymes inside the cell (such as in glucose-6-phosphate deficiency (C)).

Acquired haemolytic anaemias can be immune or non-immune. Immune haemolytic anaemias can include autoimmune haemolytic anaemia, which might result in the formation of spherocytes and is direct antiglobulin test (DAT) or Coombs test positive (A). In the Coombs test, red blood cells are washed and incubated with Coombs reagent (anti-human globulin). In a positive test, this produces agglutination of the red blood cells (RBCs) which indicates that antibodies or complement proteins have become bound to the red blood cell membrane. So spherocytes can occur both in hereditary spherocytosis and in AIHA, with the latter being Coombs test positive.

Other immune haemolytic anaemias can occur in the presence of underlying autoimmune disease or lymphomas. Non-immune acquired haemolytic anaemias can occur due to infections such as malaria, or microangiopathic haemolytic anaemia.

The Schiling test (E) is used for vitamin B_{12} deficiency to determine if the cause is pernicious anaemia.

Haemolytic anaemia (2)

5 A This man is suffering from glucose-6-phosphate dehydrogenase (G6PD) deficiency, an X-linked recessive disorder that is common in people from the Mediterranean, South East Asia, Middle East and West

Africa. This enzyme is responsible for maintaining levels of glutathione from the pentose phosphate pathway, which protects against oxidant free radicals. Oxidative stress, for example in the form of chemicals, food or infection, can put people with this condition at risk of severe haemolytic anaemia. Drugs to be avoided in these patients include anti-malarials, such as primaquine, and others such as sulphonamides, vitamin K and dapsone. The exam favourite of broad beans can lead to a reaction called favism in these patients.

Heinz bodies (A) are characteristically found on the blood film during a crisis: these are small inclusions within the red cell due to denatured haemoglobin. Remember that the blood count can actually be normal in between crises. The level of G6PD itself can also be assayed, but can be falsely negative during active haemolysis so may be delayed until a few weeks after an acute episode.

Pencil cells (B) are a type of elliptocyte that occur in iron deficiency anaemia, thalassaemia and pyruvate kinase deficiency. Target cells (C) have a central dense area with a ring of pallor, and can occur in the three Hs: hepatic pathology, hyposplenism and haemoglobinopathies. Spherocytes (D) are found in hereditary spherocytosis, where an increase in the fragility of the red blood cell membrane occurs due to dysfunctional skeletal proteins in the membrane, such as spectrin, ankyrin and band 4.2. They can also be found in haemolytic anaemia. Sickle cells (E) are found in sickle cell anaemia, but not in sickle cell trait.

Infectious mononucleosis

6 B   Up to half of all patients might develop splenomegaly in infectious mononucleosis. This does not often cause symptoms but can lead to splenic rupture, either spontaneously or following minor trauma, and may necessitate treatment with splenectomy. Postoperatively a combination of features on a blood film might suggest hyposplenism:

- Howell–Jolly bodies: these are small fragments of non-functional nuclei that are normally removed by the spleen, so might be seen on a blood film in hyposplenism. They may also be seen in megaloblastic and iron-deficiency anaemias
- Target cells: these have a central dense area with a ring of pallor, and can occur in the three Hs: hepatic pathology, hyposplenism and haemoglobinopathies
- Occasional nucleated red blood cells
- Lymphocytosis
- Macrocytosis
- Acanthocytes: spiculated red cells that are found in hyposplenism, α-β-lipoproteinaemia, chronic liver disease and α-thalassaemia trait

Atypical lymphocytes are large lymphocytes which vary in size and shape, and might be seen in infectious mononucleosis (even if the patient has not developed hyposplenism).

Other causes of hyposplenism can be classified as follows:

1   Traumatic, i.e. following an accident or during surgery

2   Planned splenectomy – prophylactically in massive splenomegaly or hypersplenism (e.g. hereditary spherocytosis or elliptocytosis)

3   Physiological hyposplenism, e.g. in sickle cell anaemia, coeliac disease, or ulcerative colitis

To remember in which haematological diseases a splenectomy may provide a substantial benefit, the following mnemonic may be useful: The PIIES = Thalassaemia, Pyruvate kinase deficiency, Immune haemolytic anaemia, Idiopathic thrombocytopenic purpura, Elliptocytosis, and Spherocytosis (hereditary).

Importantly, splenectomy patients are at increased risk of sepsis from capsulated organisms. They therefore require lifelong:

1   Penicillin V prophylaxis

2   Pneumococcal conjugate vaccine

3   Human influenza b (Hib) vaccine

4   Meningococcal vaccine

Haemoglobinopathies in children (1)

7   B   This boy is suffering from sickle cell anaemia (B), an autosomal recessive haemoglobinopathy. The term sickle cell disease actually comprises several different states: sickle cell anaemia, but also compound heterozygous states including sickle cell/haemoglobin C (D) and sickle cell/β-thalassaemia (C).

Do not forget that the haemoglobin molecule consists of four chains, and there are three different forms: haemaglobin A ($\alpha2\beta2$), haemoglobin A2 ($\alpha2\delta2$) and haemoglobin F ($\alpha2\Upsilon2$). The proportions of the different forms vary with age – haemoglobin F predominates before birth, but concentrations of haemaglobin A and A2 increase after birth, with haemoglobin A predominating. In sickle-cell anaemia a point mutation in the β-globin chain of haemoglobin (found on chromosome 11) results in the hydrophilic amino acid glutamic acid being replaced by the hydrophobic amino acid valine at the sixth position. This promotes aggregation of the haemoglobin chains in conditions of low oxygen, distorting the red blood cells so they adopt a sickle shape. These cells become adherent to the endothelieum of post capillary venules, causing retrograde capillary obstruction which can lead to painful crises.

Sickle cell trait is not the same as sickle cell disease – they have one abnormal allele of the β-haemoglobin gene, but are asymptomatic and have no sickle cells on the blood film unlike in this case.

Sickle cell/β-thalassaemia is a variant of sickle cell anaemia, where an individual inherits one haemoglobin gene from a parent who is a carrier of β-thalassemia and and the other from a parent who is a carrier of sickle cell anaemia. The exact β-thalassaemia mutation inherited will determine the severity of the disease. A similar situation occurs in sickle cell/haemoglobin C, where the patient has one gene coding for haemoglobin C – these patients may have a mild splenomegaly and haemolytic anaemia. Haemoglobin C is similar to haemoglobin S in that it comprises two normal alpha chains and two variant beta chains in which lysine has replaced glutamic acid at position 6. Both sickle cell/β-thalassaemia and sickle cell/haemoglobin C are much less likely in this scenario than sickle cell disease.

Haemoglobinopathies in children (2)

8   E   Aplastic crises caused by parvovirus B19 infection (E) can occur in patients with sickle cell disease. They can present with acute worsening of the patient's baseline anaemia, which might manifest as shortness of breath and fatigue as in this case. The fever points to an infectious cause.

The virus affects erythropoiesis by invading erythrocyte precursors and destroying them. Infants and children with sickle cell disease initially have no immunity to parvovirus B19, and their first exposure can lead to pure red cell aplasia. In a normal individual the virus blocks red cell production for 2 or 3 days with little consequence, but it can be life threatening in sickle cell patients in whom the red cell life span is already shortened. This can lead to profound anaemia over the course of just a few days, and a dramatic drop in the reticulocyte count. Serum IgM antibodies to parvovirus B19 can confirm the diagnosis, and blood transfusion may be required.

Splenic sequestration (A) is a potentially fatal emergency caused by the acute pooling of a large percentage of circulating red cells in the spleen when it is enlarged. It would not present in the way described in this case, but with an abdomen that can become bloated and hard with signs of circulatory failure. This is less common in older children and adults because recurrent infarction has often left the spleen small and fibrotic, but is a possibility in younger children.

Sickle cells can also become adherent to the endothelieum of post capillary venules, causing retrograde capillary obstruction which can lead to painful vaso-occlusive crises (C). Pain would be a more significant feature of the presentation than in this case, and a severe anaemia and reticulocytopenia would not normally occur as a consequence. Patients with sickle cell disease are at high risk of pneumococcal infection (B) after a splenectomy, and this would not typically cause a low reticulocyte count. Folic acid deficiency (D) is more common in sickle cell patients due to hyperplastic erythropoesis, and is a particular problem in children who require folic acid for growth spurts. This is less likely to present as acutely as in this case, and the fact that the patient's sibling is also affected makes an infectious trigger more plausible.

Anaemia (1)

9 D β-Thalassaemias are a group of genetic haemoglobinopathies that essentially result in reduced or absent formation of the beta chains of haemoglobin leading to anaemia of varying degrees of severity. They are prevalent in the Middle East, Central, South and South East Asia, Southern China and around the Mediterranean. There are three main forms: thalassaemia major, thalassaemia intermedia and thalassaemia minor.

In β-thalassaemia minor (D) only one of the β-globulin alleles is mutated, so these individuals usually only have a well-tolerated microcytic anaemia (Hb >9 g/dL) which is clinically asymptomatic. They might be picked up on a routine blood test, with a low MCH and significantly low MCV (<80 fL). They also have an increase in the fraction of Hb A2, as in this case. In most people the fraction of Hb A2 ($\alpha2\delta2$) will be 1.5–3.5 per cent, but in β-thalassaemia minor the proportion of Hb A2 is >3.5–4 per cent to compensate for the reduced amount of normal haemoglobin, and they might have a slight increase in Hb F. It can worsen in pregnancy, as in this case.

β-Thalassaemia intermedia (C) is a condition that lies in between the minor and major forms. These patients often have a moderate anaemia and sometimes have splenomegaly, but do not require blood transfusions.

Cooley's anaemia (B), or β-thalassaemia major, is the homozygous form. These patients would present much earlier than in this case, usually in the first year of life with failure to thrive and a severe microcytic anaemia. Hepatosplenomegaly and bossing of the skull may occur due to extramedullary haemopoesis (i.e. red blood cells being produced outside the bone marrow). Treatment includes lifelong blood transfusions with iron chelators to prevent overload, splenectomy if hypersplenism persists and bone marrow transplant can offer the chance of a cure.

α-Thalassaemia (E) affects the genes coding for the α-haemoglobin chains on chromosome 16. There are varying forms which would not cause the increase in Hb A2 as in this case. If one of the four α-haemoglobin genes is deleted, the patient is clinically normal. If two are deleted, the patient has a low MCV but is asymptomatic. If three are deleted the disease is called Hb H, and they might have features of haemolysis (such as hepatosplenomegaly and jaundice), as well as anaemia of moderate severity. If all four genes are deleted, this is known as 'Bart's hydrops', and death occurs *in utero*. Iron deficiency anaemia (A) can cause a low Hb and MCV as in this case, but the ferritin would usually be reduced.

Anaemia (2)

10 B Autoimmune haemolytic anaemia is a form of mainly extravascular haemolysis, which is mediated by autoantibodies. It is classified into warm and cold autoimmune haemolytic anaemia, according to the optimal temperature at which the antibodies bind to red blood cells. This activates the classical pathway in the complement system, resulting in haemolysis. Cold AIHA is mediated by IgM antibodies, and as the name suggests these antibodies bind optimally at lower temperatures (28–31°C), resulting in anaemia that is aggravated in cold conditions. In severe cases, patients may suffer from Raynaud's or acrocyanosis (purplish discolouration of peripheries). Most cases are idiopathic, but there are some specific causes worth remembering, as 'Cold LID':

- Lymphoproliferative disease, e.g. CLL, lymphomas
- Infections – mycoplasma, as in this case (B), EBV
- Do not know, i.e. idiopathic!

This patient has typical features of mycoplasma pneumonia including a protracted history of flu-like symptoms (such as myalgia, arthralgia, headache) and a non-productive cough. Treatment includes avoiding cold conditions, use of chlorambucil, and treating the underlying cause. The other infectious agents listed here do not typically cause a cold haemolytic anaemia.

Warm AIHA on the other hand is mostly IgG mediated, and these antibodies have maximal reactivity at body temperature of 37°C. These antibodies attach to the membrane of red blood cells, and the 'Fc' portion is recognized by splenic macrophages. These remove part of the red blood cell membrane, which leads to the formation of spherocytes. Secondary causes may again include lymphoproliferative disease, but also drugs such as penicillin and autoimmune diseases such as SLE. Treatment options include steroids, immunogolobulins and possibly splenectomy.

Anaemia (3)

11 A Paroxysmal cold haemoglobinuria (A) is a rare form of autoimmune haemolytic anaemia. It usually affects children in the acute setting after an infection, and the key in this case is the presence of sudden haemoglobinuria and jaundice after exposure to a cold temperatures. IgG autoantibodies usually form after an infection, and bind to red blood cell surface antigens, inducing variable degrees of intravascular haemolysis in the cold. The antibodies are known as 'Donath–Landsteiner antibodies'.

Analysis of the urine will confirm the presence of haemaglobinuria, and blood tests often reveal a normocytic or macrocytic anaemia. It is possible to test indirectly for the IgG antiglobulins at a low temperature, as in this case. Blood transfusion may be required if the anaemia is severe, but in children who have an acute onset with an antecedent infection, it is usually a transient and self limiting condition.

Paroxysmal nocturnal haemoglobinuria (B) is another rare acquired disease, but one that is potentially life threatening. The resulting defect in the red cell membrane leads to intravascular haemolysis. The disease has three aspects: the most common way for it to present is with a haemolytic anaemia, which may cause haemoglobinuria, especially overnight. The second aspect is thrombophilia, which can present with visceral thrombosis (e.g. CNS, pulmonary, mesenteric). The third aspect is deficient haematopoiesis which can cause a pancytopenia with aplastic anaemia. You can remember this as PNH = Pancytopenia – New thrombus – Haemolytic anaemia. The latest diagnostic test is flow cytometry, which can detect absent membrane proteins on red blood cells. This has largely replaced the 'Ham's test' (which was used to show that a patient's erythrocytes are lysed if the blood is acidified). Treatment is with thromboprophylaxis, and the monocolonal antibody eculizumab may have a role.

Sickle cell disease (C) can lead to vaso-occlusive crises precipitated by the cold, but this would present with severe pain due to microvascular occlusion and Donath Landsteiner antibodies would not be present. Acute intermittent porphyria (D) is an autosomal dominant condition caused by deficiency of an enzyme involved in haem synthesis (porphobilinogen deaminase). This can lead to accumulation of toxic haem precursors, which cause neurovisceral symptoms. The urine can characteristically turn a deep red colour on standing. Epstein–Barr virus (E) alone would not cause the symptoms described in this case, though it can trigger paroxysmal cold haemoglobinuria.

Anaemia (4)

12 C This patient is suffering from iron deficiency anaemia, a common complication in coeliac disease. The tiredness and shortness of breath are common symptoms. Causes can include blood loss (e.g. upper or lower GI bleeding, menstruation), malabsorption (as in this case), dietary deficiency (rare in adults but can be seen in children) or infestation with parasitic worms (the most common cause worldwide). Blood tests characteristically reveal a low mean cell volume, mean cell haemoglobin (E) and mean cell haemoglobin concentration. A blood film may reveal hypochromic red blood cells with anisocytosis (variation in cell size) and poikilocytosis (variation in cell shape). The red blood cell distribution width (RDW) (a measure of the variation of the width of red blood cells) may be increased initially.

Serum iron levels (A) can be measured directly, but are unreliable and may be increased if the patient has started on iron supplements, as the levels increase straight away. Levels of ferritin (D), the intracellular protein that stores iron, may also be low and this is the most sensitive test. However, it is also an acute phase protein, and so may be falsely elevated in the presence of inflammation or malignancy which coexists with the iron deficiency anaemia (therefore a normal ferritin level cannot exclude IDA). The haematocrit (B) is the percentage of red blood cells in the blood, and it may be reduced in IDA.

Transferrin (C) is a glycoprotein that binds to iron in the blood, and levels may be increased in IDA as the liver produces greater amounts (you can think of this as the liver trying to compensate for the little iron it has available, so it makes more of the binding carrier for iron). Total iron-binding capacity (TIBC) is a laboratory test used to give a measure of the capacity of the blood to bind iron with transferrin, and it too would be raised in IDA. The TIBC is reduced in anaemia of chronic disease, possibly because the body produces less transferrin to prevent the pathogens that require iron for metabolism obtaining it.

IDA can be treated with oral iron supplements, with an expected rise in the haemoglobin of 1 g/dL per week. Do not forget that iron supplements characteristically lead to production of black stools.

Anaemia (5)

13 D This woman has developed pernicious anaemia leading to vitamin B_{12} deficiency. It can be associated with other autoimmune conditions, such as Addison's disease or thyroid disease. Specifically, she has developed a condition called subacute combined degeneration of the cord (SACD) which has led to symmetrical loss of dorsal columns (resulting in loss of touch and proprioception leading to ataxia, and LMN signs) and corticospinal tract loss (leading to UMN signs), with sparing of pain and temperature sensation (which is carried by spinothalamic tracts). The ataxia and loss of joint position sense have resulted in her falling at night, which may be exacerbated by optic atrophy – another manifestation of vitamin B_{12} deficiency.

Remember that vitamin B_{12} is found in meat, fish and dairy products. More common causes of vitamin B_{12} deficiency can be related to diet (e.g. vegans) or to malabsorption. It is absorbed in the terminal ileum after binding to intrinsic factor produced by the parietal cells in the stomach. Causes of malabsorption can therefore be related to the stomach (e.g. post gastrectomy, pernicious anaemia), or due to the terminal ileum (e.g. Crohn's, resection of the terminal ileum, bacterial overgrowth).

Pernicious anaemia is caused by an autoimmune atrophic gastritis when autoantibodies are produced against parietal cells and intrinsic factor itself. The lack of B_{12} impairs DNA synthesis in red blood cells, leading to the production of large, megaloblastic erythrocytes.

Blood tests and a blood film may reveal several features that are worth remembering:

- Low haemoglobin
- High MCV
- Low platelets and WCC if severe
- Low serum B_{12}
- Hypersegmented neutrophils
- Megaloblasts in the bone marrow
- Cabot rings in RBCs (remnants of the nuclear membrane seen in pernicious anaemia, lead poisoining and other forms of megaloblastic anaemia)

Intrinsic factor antibodies (A) can be found in approximately 50 per cent of patients, and are specific for pernicious anaemia but not as sensitive as anti-parietal cell antibodies (D) which are found in >90 per cent of patients. However, anti-parietal cell antibodies can also be found in approximately 10 per cent of normal people, and 40 per cent of people who have atrophic gastritis without pernicious anaemia. The Schilling test is no longer commonly used for diagnosis.

Anti-endomysial cell antibodies (B) are found in coeliac disease (with a specificity of approximately 95 per cent), anti-smooth muscle cell antibodies (C) are found in autoimmune hepatitis and primary biliary cirrhosis, and anti-voltage gated calcium channel antibodies (E) are found in Lambert–Eaton syndrome (a variant of myasthenia gravis).

Macrocytic anaemia

14 A Causes of macrocytosis can be divided into:

1   Megaloblastic, e.g. folate and B_{12} deficiency

2   Non-megalobastic, causes of which can be remembered as **RALPH** = reticulocytosis (e.g. in haemolysis), alcohol, liver disease, pregnancy and hypothyroidism)

3   Other haematological disorders, e.g. myelodysplasia, aplastic anaemia, myeloma, myeloproliferative disorders

This woman is suffering from aplastic anaemia (A), where the bone marrow stops producing cells leading to a pancytopenia. Bone marrow examination is needed to confirm the diagnosis, and shows a hypocellular bone marrow. Causes of aplastic anaemia can be primary or secondary. Primary causes can be congenital (e.g. Fanconi's anaemia) or idiopathic acquired aplastic anaemia. Secondary causes include drugs (all the Cs – cytotoxics, carbamazepine, chloramphenicol, anticonvulsants such as phenytoin), ionizing radiation and viruses (e.g. hepatitis, EBV). This woman's aplastic anaemia is secondary to long-term carbamazepine therapy for hypothyroidism. Hypothyroidism (C) alone may lead to macrocytosis, but is not the underlying cause for her pancytopenia. Patients with aplastic anaemia can present with features of the pancytopenia, such as recurrent infections (from a low white cell count), bleeding and petechial rashes (from a low platelet count) and features of anaemia.

Treatment of aplastic anaemia is with supportive therapy, such as red cell transfusions and platelets, allogenic bone marrow transplant which can be curative, or immunosuppression with, for example, ciclosporin and antithymocyte globulin (ATG).

Myelodysplasia (B) is a group of disorders caused by ineffective haematopoeisis, so results in pancytopenia with increased marrow cellularity. Chronic myeloid leukaemia (D) would typically result in a very high white blood cell count, and a hypercellular bone marrow as there is active production of cells. Myeloma (E) can also cause a macrocytic or normocytic anaemia, but a bone marrow biopsy would show increased plasma cells.

Hepatomegaly

15 E This man has hereditary haemachromatosis, an inherited disorder of iron metabolism. It is particularly common in those of Celtic descent, and the gene responsible for the majority of cases is the HFE gene on chromosome 6.

Increased iron absorption leads to deposition to multiple organs including:

- the liver (hepatomegaly, deranged LFTs)
- joints (arthralgia, chondrocalcinosis)
- pancreas (diabetes)
- heart (dilated cardiomyopathy)
- pituitary gland (hypogonadism and impotence)
- adrenals (adrenal insufficiency)
- skin (slate grey skin pigmentation)

Blood tests can show deranged LFTs as in this case, as well as a raised serum ferritin, raised serum iron, reduced or normal total iron binding capacity and raised transferrin saturation (E) (>80 per cent).

Remember that the TIBC measures the blood's capacity to bind iron with transferrin. The transferrin saturation is the ratio of serum iron to TIBC ×100, and represents the percentage of iron binding sites on transferrin that are occupied by iron. It is typically 20–40 per cent, but is raised in haemachromatosis. This is because TIBC is usually low or normal whilst serum iron levels are high, so the percentage of transferrin occupied by iron is increased.

The following table summarizes the common laboratory findings for various conditions:

Condition	Iron	TIBC/transferrin	% Transferrin saturation	Ferritin
Iron deficiency anaemia	Low	High	Low	Low
Haemachromotosis	High	Low or normal	High	High
Anaemia of chronic disease	Low	Low	Low	High
Chronic haemolysis	High	Low	High	High

Liver biopsy with Perl's staining or Prussian blue staining can demonstrate iron overload in haemachromatosis. This can be used to quantify iron loading and determine the severity of the disease. MRI is also a less invasive way to accurately gauge iron concentrations in the liver.

Treatment options include lifetime regular venesection to reduce iron levels, maintenance of a low iron diet, and treatment with iron chelators if venesection is not possible. Patients with haemachromatosis who have developed liver cirrhosis are at increased risk of developing hepatocellular carcinoma.

Plasma cell disorders (1)

16 A   This woman has multiple myeloma, a cancer of plasma cells. The symptoms can be remembered using the mnemonic BRAIN: Bone pain (due to osteoclast activation leading to hypercalcaemia and the presence of lytic lesions on a skeletal survey, characteristically with a 'pepperpot skull' appearance), Renal failure (which can be secondary to one or a combination of: hypercalcaemia, tubular damage from light chain secretion, or secondary amyloidosis), Anaemia (typically normocytic), Infections (particularly pneumonias and pyelonephritis), and Neurological symptoms (such as a headache and visual changes from hyperviscosity, or confusion and weakness from the hypercalcaemia).

The diagnostic criteria for symptomatic myeloma are as follows:

- Clonal plasma cells >10 per cent on bone marrow biopsy
- A paraprotein in the serum or urine – most commonly IgG
- Evidence of end-organ damage related to the plasma cell disorder (commonly referred to by the acronym 'CRAB'):
  - Calcium – high
  - Renal insufficiency
  - Anaemia
  - Bone lesions (e.g. lytic lesions, or osteoporosis with compression factors)

Blood tests may reveal a high calcium but the alkaline phosphatase is often normal (A) (in contrast to other malignancies, with osteolytic metastases and raised alkaline phosphatase).

The bone disease in myeloma is thought to be mediated by over-expression of the 'RANK ligand' by bone marrow stroma, which activates osteoclasts. Peripheral blood films can reveal the presence of rouleaux formation (stacks of red blood cells which occur because high plasma protein concentrations make the cells stick to each other, which also causes the high ESR).

Beta 2 microglobulin levels (a component of MHC class 1 molecules) can also be measured, and are an important prognostic indicator. Along with albumin levels, the level of beta 2 microglobulin forms part of the International Staging System for myeloma.

Treatment of multiple myeloma includes high dose chemotherapy, with the possibility of stem cell transplantation in younger patients.

Plasma cell disorders (2)

17   D   This question tests your understanding of the diagnostic criteria for plasma cell disorders. Do not forget that:

1   Symptomatic myeloma (D):
  • Clonal plasma cells on bone marrow biopsy
  • Paraprotein in either serum or urine
  • Evidence of end-organ damage attributed to the plasma cell disorder, commonly remembered using the acronym 'CRAB' (Calcium – high, Renal insufficiency, Anaemia and Bone lesions)

2   Asymptomatic (smouldering) myeloma (C):
  • Serum paraprotein >30 g/L AND/OR
  • Clonal plasma cells >10 per cent on bone marrow biopsy AND
  • NO myeloma-related organ or tissue impairment

3   Monoclonal gammopathy of undetermined significance (MGUS) (B):
  • Serum paraprotein <30 g/L AND
  • Clonal plasma cells <10 per cent on bone marrow biopsy AND
  • NO myeloma-related organ or tissue impairment

This woman has multiple myeloma because she has evidence of end organ damage in the form of hypercalcaemia. You can automatically exclude asymptomatic myeloma and MGUS on this basis!

MGUS itself is usually asymptomatic and does not normally require treatment. Patients will undergo regular blood tests to check their paraprotein levels because of the small risk of transformation to multiple myeloma (approximately 1–2 per cent per year).

Plasma cell dyscrasia (A) is a more general term for cancers of the plasma cells, of which MGUS is the most common. This term also encompasses multiple myeloma, solitary plasmacytoma of bone, extramedullary plasmacytoma, and Waldenström's macroglobulinaemia amongst others. A plasmacytoma is a discrete neoplastic mass of plasma cells within the bone marrow or elsewhere (extra-medullary). There is no evidence of myeloma in this condition, but a serum paraprotein is sometimes present (usually IgM).

Waldenström's macroglobulinaemia is a chronic, indolent disorder, also known as 'lymphoplasmacytic lymphoma'. It is essentially a clonal disorder of B cells, characterized by a high level of IgM. This leads to features of hyperviscosity and vascular complications. Because of the high IgM levels it used to be thought of as related to multiple myeloma, but is now classified as a lymphoproliferative disease (similar to a low grade non-Hodgkins lymphoma).

Platelet count (1)

18   B   This man has developed disseminated intravascular coagulation (DIC) (B) following his severe burns. DIC is widespread pathological activation of the clotting cascade in response to various insults. The cascade is activated in various ways: one mechanism is the release of a transmembrane glycoprotein called 'tissue factor' in response to cytokines or vascular damage. This results in fibrin formation, which can eventually cause occlusion of small and medium sized vessels and lead to organ failure. At the same time, depletion of platelets and coagulation proteins can result in bleeding (as in this case).

It can be caused by a wide range of factors, which can be remembered using the mnemonic 'I'M STONeD!': Immunological (e.g. severe allergic reactions, haemolytic transfusion reactions), Miscellaneous (e.g. aortic aneurysm, liver disease), Sepsis, Trauma (including serious tissue injury, burns, extensive surgery), Obstetric (e.g. amniotic fluid embolism, placental abruption), Neoplastic (myeloproliferative disorders as well as solid tumours such as pancreatic cancer), and Drugs and toxins.

Patients with DIC can present with rapid onset of shock, widespread bleeding, bruising and renal failure, or more insidiously (for example in the cases of malignancy). Blood tests will typically reveal a thrombocytopenia, raised PT and APTT, decreased fibrinogen and increased D dimers. D dimers are fibrinogen degradation products, which form from intense fibrinolytic activity. The blood film may show the presence of schistocytes (broken red blood cells).

The following table may help you to differentiate between the blood test results for various conditions. Liver failure (A) is less likely to cause a thrombocytopenia, reduced fibrinogen and raised D dimers, and the history of burns points more towards DIC. TTP (C) would not typically result in raised D dimers either, and the PT and APTT are not normally prolonged. This condition usually has other clinical features too, including a fever and fluctuating CNS signs. Aplastic anaemia (D) does not typically cause abnormalities in clotting, and heparin induced thrombocytopenia (HIT) (E) is most likely to present paradoxically with thrombosis rather than bleeding.

Condition	INR/PT	APTT	Thrombin time	Platelet count	Bleeding time
DIC	↑↑	↑↑	↑↑	↓	↑
Vit K deficiency/warfarin	↑↑	↑	N	N	N
Liver disease	↑	↑	N/↑	N/↓	N
Heparin use	↑	↑↑	↑↑	N	N
Platelet defect	N	N	N	N	↑
von Willebrand's disease	N	↑	N	N	↑
Haemophillia	N	↑	N	N	N

Platelet count (2)

19 D This woman has thrombotic thrombocytopenic purpura (TTP) (D), a rare but potentially fatal haematological emergency. It consists of six key features:

1 MAHA

2 A fever

3 Renal failure

4 Fluctuating CNS signs, e.g. seizures, hallucinations, hemiparesis, decreased consciousness

5 Haematuria/proteinuria

6 Low platelet count

You can remember these as 'MARCH with low platelets'.

TTP typically affects adults and is thought to occur due to a deficiency of a protease that is responsible for cleaving multimers of von Willebrand factor. The resulting formation of large vWF multimers stimulates platelet aggregation and fibrin deposition in small vessels. This in turn causes microthrombi to form in blood vessels, impeding the blood supply to major organs such as the kidneys, heart and brain. Haemolysis occurs and shistocytes form because of the sheer stress on red blood cells as they pass through the microscopic clots.

Urgent plasma exchange can be lifesaving in patients with TTP, so it is important to consider this diagnosis early in patients who have unexplained thrombocytopenia and anaemia. The mortality rate is reported as >95 per cent if untreated.

Idiopathic thrombocytopenic purpura (C) is an autoimmune disorder caused by IgG antibodies against platelets in most cases. Treatment depends on the platelet count and the presence of bleeding, but includes steroids, anti-D, immunosuppressants and splenectomy. Haemolytic uraemic syndrome (D) typically affects young children infected with a specific strain of *E. coli* called O157, which produces a verotoxin that attacks endothelial cells and results in MAHA. The anaemia, thrombocytopenia, renal failure and presence of shistocytes could be caused by HUS in this question, but it is less likely given the patient's age, the presence of neurological symptoms and the absence of preceding symptoms of gastroenteritis.

The presence of a fever may have led you to consider an infectious cause such as Weil's disease (A) or glandular fever (B). Weil's disease is caused by the spirochaete *Leptospira interrogans*, and is spread by infected rat urine. Although it can cause an abrupt onset of renal failure and a fever, it would not typically result in thrombocytopenia or features of MAHA. Glandular fever is also unlikely in this scenario: whilst it can cause palatal petechiae, it does not typically present with hallucinations or purpura, and a thrombocytopenia and anaemia are again less likely.

Obstetric haematology

20 E 'HELLP' syndrome (E) is a potentially fatal occurrence in pregnancy, characterized by a triad of features:

1   H – haemolysis

2   EL – elevated liver enzymes

3   LP – low platelet count

In a similar way to DIC, generalized activation of the clotting cascade is triggered which can only be terminated with delivery. Platelet consumption and MAHA occurs, and liver ischaemia can lead to periportal necrosis and, in severe cases, formation of a subcapsular haematoma which can rupture.

It usually presents in the third trimester, but can happen even up to a week after delivery. Often patients with HELLP have had pregnancy-induced hypertension or pre-eclampsia prior to its development. Common symptoms are often vague, and can include nausea and vomiting, epigastric pain, peripheral swelling, paraesthesia, headaches and visual problems. On examination patients may be noted to have peripheral oedema, upper abdominal tenderness, jaundice and hepatomegaly. Complications can include liver and renal failure, pulmonary oedema,

DIC and placental abruption. Clotting studies may be normal as in this case, unless DIC has occurred. The only effective treatment is delivery, but other supportive treatment includes control of the hypertension, seizure prophylaxis and corticosteroid use.

Hepatitis (A) can result in jaundice, right upper quadrant tenderness and abnormal LFTs, but is less likely to cause a marked thrombocytopenia and the presence of schistocytes (indicating haemolysis) in an apyrexial patient as in this case. A leukocytosis is also more likely. TTP (B) is characterized by the classic sextet of symptoms as described previously, but deranged LFTs are not typical of this condition. Haemolysis and abnormal LFTs are also rare in pre-eclampsia (C), and mild thrombocytopenia is present in only 10–15 per cent of cases. Acute fatty liver of pregnancy (D) is a life-threatening rare complication of pregnancy that can also present non-specifically with deranged LFTs, but is often accompanied by abnormal coagulation, leukocytosis and hypoglycaemia.

Vitamin K dependent clotting factors

21　C　The vitamin K dependent clotting factors include II, VII, IX and X. Vitamin K is also required for the production for protein C, protein S and protein Z, although these are strictly not clotting factors, rather anticoagulant factors. Vitamin K is a fat soluble vitamin found in green leafy vegetables such as spinach, cabbage and cauliflower. It is absorbed in the small bowel and is important in the production of functional clotting factors in the liver. This patient's acute chronic liver failure has meant she is no longer producing functional clotting factors, represented as a raised INR.

Vitamin K is recycled in the liver and its oxidation is coupled with the post-translational modification of glutamate residues to form gamma-carboxyglutamate. Vitamin K is firstly reduced by vitamin K epoxide reductase to form vitamin K hydroquinone. This reduced form is oxidized by vitamin K dependent carboxylase to form vitamin K epoxide. This reaction is coupled with gamma-glutamyl carboxylase; the enzyme responsible for post-translational modification of the vitamin K dependent factors. Vitamin K epoxide is then reconverted to vitamin K by vitamin K epoxide reductase; thus completing the cycle. If the patient were to be given vitamin K metabolism antagonists, e.g. warfarin, the clotting factors produced would still be immunologically identical (these are also known as Proteins Induced by Vitamin K Absence/Antagonism – PIVKA) but would lack efficacy as they are unable to interact with calcium or platelet factor 3.

Factor VIII is not a vitamin K dependent clotting factor, it is synthesized by endothelium and sinusoidal cells of the liver and is found in the plasma as well as non-covalently bound to von Willebrand factor (vWF). It is classically described to be a part of the intrinsic pathway of

APTT

the clotting cascade which is tested by the use of the ~~prothrombin time~~.
Factor VIII is a procofactor activated by thrombin during the amplification phase of the coagulation cascade. Once active, it binds to factor IXa on the platelet which together activate factor X with Va. Factors Va, Xa, phospholipids and calcium together form the prothrombinase complex which leads to a thrombin burst where thrombin production is rapidly amplified.

Thrombin (A) is the penultimate product of the coagulation cascade, its functions include cleaving fibrinogen to form fibrin, activating platelets, activating procofactors V and VIII and activating zymogens VII, XI and XIII. It also acts to control fibrinolysis by binding to endothelial-bound thrombospondin thus activating protein C (D) and protein S. This complex inhibits cofactors V and VIII and acts as a negative feedback control on the coagulation cascade.

Factor VII (B) is a vital part of the extrinsic clotting cascade which is activated by tissue factor, a factor expressed by damaged endothelial cells. Within this *initiation phase*, factor VIIa activates downstream factors IX and X. Factors Xa and Va bind to the damaged area providing the base site of coagulation activity where the *amplification phase* begins. Here, the Xa/Va complex activates prothrombin to thrombin which then acts to activate XI, VIII and V. The end result is the prothrombinase complex; a structure consisting of factor Va heavy and light chains, Xa, phospholipids and calcium which explodes with thrombin generating activity in order to produce fibrin rapidly and stabilize the platelet clot. This final phase is thus called the *propagation phase*.

Deep vein thrombosis

22 D   All of the factors except being slightly overweight probably directly contributed to this patient developing a second deep vein thrombosis. The risk factors for developing venous thrombosis may be categorized to mechanisms affecting the blood vessel wall, the blood flow and the blood itself, i.e. Virchow's triad.

Smoking (A) increases thrombotic risk by inducing endothelial damage and increasing thromboxane A2 production, which stimulates platelet aggregation, and perhaps increasing platelet dependent thrombin generation. The link between smoking and venous thrombosis is well established although the risk reduction over time once someone quits is not fully understood.

Previous DVT (C) is probably one of the strongest risk factors for DVT with a five-fold increase over baseline risk. This, along with a recent fitting of a plaster cast (E) and associated immobility, represents the highest risk for this patient in developing a second DVT. Other important risk factors include major surgery, particularly involving the abdomen or lower limb, cancer, prothrombotic states, some chemotherapeutic agents, myocardial infarction and congestive heart failure, pregnancy and combined oral contraceptive pill.

Warfarin (B), a commonly used anticoagulant, probably contributed to a second DVT in this situation. Warfarin antagonizes vitamin K epoxide reductase; a liver enzyme responsible for recycling vitamin K to its reduced state. Warfarin thus antagonizes the production of vitamin K dependent factors including factors II, VII, IX, X, protein C and protein S. The latter two are anticoagulant factors which provide a negative feedback on the coagulation cascade by inhibiting procofactor V and VIII activation. Protein C and S have a shorter half life than the other coagulant factors thus when their production is inhibited by warfarin, a state of transient hypercoagulability is formed in the first few days after starting warfarin. Normally, clinicians will cover this problem by the use of concomitant heparin until the therapeutic range is obtained. In this patient, the admitting physician unfortunately did not give any heparin, and thus transiently increased the thrombotic risk of this already high risk patient.

Although obesity is associated with risk of development of DVT, this man is described as slightly overweight (D). Thus, in comparison to the other risk factors presented, it probably represents the lowest attributable risk to the second DVT.

Thrombocytopenia

23 C Although all of the given options are causes of thrombocytopenia, the most likely cause in this patient is massive blood transfusion without replacement of platelets (C). Massive blood loss may be defined as losing one's entire circulating blood volume in 24 hours. Other definitions include losing 50 per cent of one's blood volume in 3 hours or a rate of loss of greater than or equal to 150 mL/min. This patient has been transfused 20 units of blood in the space of 24 hours, thus fulfilling the criteria for massive haemorrhage. Massive transfusion has its own particular complications, including thrombocytopenia. This is because this patient was only given packed red cells and fresh frozen plasma. These two blood products contain very few platelets and in general, a platelet count of around 50×10^9/L is to be expected when approximately two blood volumes have been replaced, as is the case in this patient. In this situation, the expert consensus is to keep the platelet level above 50×10^9/L, but there is marked interindividual variation therefore some consider using 75×10^9/L as the trigger value for platelet transfusion.

Disseminated intravascular coagulopathy (DIC) (A) is a feared complication of massive blood transfusion and carries with it a high mortality. It can be thought of as the loss of haemostatic control resulting in consumption of coagulant factors, platelets and fibrinogen. Widespread clotting ensues with microvascular structures becoming ischaemic, resulting in potential end organ failure. Once coagulation factors and platelets are depleted bleeding becomes apparent making this disorder a concomitant bleeding and clotting problem. Those at particular risk include patients with prolonged hypoxia or hypovolaemia with cerebral or extensive muscle damage, or those who become hypothermic from infusion of cold resuscitation fluids. It is biochemically detected by a rising prothrombin time, activated thromboplastin time in excess of that expected by dilution together with significant thrombocytopenia and low fibrinogen (<1.0 g/L). This is not the case with this patient, although he should be monitored closely to look out for this complication.

Alcohol excess (B) can cause thrombocytopenia; it is a direct bone marrow suppressant thereby inhibiting megakaryocyte development and platelet production. Cirrhosis, of any aetiology including alcohol, can cause portal hypertension thus causing splenomegaly and a potential hypersplenism (E). The normal human spleen contains about one-third of the circulating platelets, if it engorges in size due to portal hypertension it may sequester more platelets; this is the difference between hypersplenism (increased function) and splenomegaly (increased physical size). This is less likely in this case given the massive haemorrhage and the lack of clinical evidence of splenomegaly in the question, despite there being evidence of portal hypertension as there are oesophageal varices present.

Megaloblastic anaemia (D) is caused by B_{12} or folate deficiency which is classically macrocytic in nature, although the mean cell volume will be difficult to interpret now given the patient has had a blood transfusion. It is most commonly caused by pernicious anaemia, an autoimmune condition where antibodies are directed against stomach parietal cells or intrinsic factor. The blood film classically shows megaloblasts – nucleated red blood cells along with polychromasia (where red cells have multiple colours due to premature release from bone marrow), basophilic stippling (peripheral dots which represent rRNA and is always pathological) and Howell–Jolly inclusion bodies (clusters of DNA within erythrocytes). This could potentially be true in this patient, but it is not the most likely answer given the circumstances of massive blood loss.

Erythrocyte sedimentation rate

24　B　ESR is a commonly used laboratory test to detect the presence of inflammation in general. It is performed by adding a sample of anticoagulant to a blood sample and adding this mixture to a calibrated vertical tube (Westergren tube). As the red cells fall with gravity and accumulate, they lie in the bottom of the tube, and are called sediment. The rate at which they accumulate is therefore the erythrocyte sedimentation rate.

Factors which influence the ESR include age, sex and pathological processes which increase plasma proteins or the number of red cells. Women generally have a higher ESR than men and it also increases with age. Depending on the exact reference range for your particular lab, women and men over 50 can have an ESR of up to 30 and 20 mm/hour, respectively, and still be normal. Conditions which increase plasma proteins such as fibrinogen, acute phase proteins and immuno-globulins can increase the ESR as these proteins reduce the ionic resistance between erythrocytes leading to an increased fall rate. They also promote rouleaux formation of erythrocytes which is the characteristic stacking of erythrocytes seen under the microscope. The most important protein to promote rouleaux formation is fibrinogen. The number of red cells in a given volume also influences ESR; in severe anaemia ESR is falsely raised as the reduced ionic repulsion between erythrocytes allow faster sedimentation. However, this rarely leads to an ESR of >100 mm/hour, making anaemia (B) the correct answer.

The other conditions listed can all raise ESR above 100 mm/hour. Myeloma (A) and leukaemia (C) do this by the production of increased plasma proteins including immunoglobulins which promote rouleaux formation as well as reduce ionic erythrocyte repulsion. Aortic aneurysms (D) can cause a very raised ESR, particularly when they are of the inflammatory type. Patients with chronic abdominal pain, weight loss, raised ESR with a known abdominal aneurysm should prompt the thought of an inflammatory aneurysm subtype. In these patients the inflammatory process sometimes encases the nearby ureters causing obstruction and eventually hydronephrosis. Malignant prostate cancer (E) raises ESR by virtue of raising fibrinogen levels in the blood. Quantative *in vitro* studies have found a direct relationship between fibrinogen concentration and ESR. Fibrinogen is an important part of the clotting cascade; its activation to fibrin is important in binding to platelets and stabilizing the platelet plug to maintain haemostasis. As mentioned, fibrinogen increases rouleaux formation as well as reducing ionic repulsion between erythrocytes, thus increasing ESR.

Sometimes patients present with a persistently raised ESR but a normal C reactive protein – another marker of inflammation which rises and falls more acutely. There are a few important conditions to note with this configuration of test results: systemic lupus erythematosus, multiple myeloma, lymphoma, anaemia and pregnancy.

Polycythaemia

25   E   Combined polycythaemia (E), also known as smoker's polycythaemia, has multiple aetiological factors. Cigarettes contain high concentrations of carbon monoxide gas which bind avidly to haemoglobin, thus displacing oxygen. This leads to increased erythropoietin (EPO) secretion from the hypoxic renal interstitium. EPO promotes erythrocyte

proliferation and differentiation and prevents their apoptosis in the bone marrow, thus increasing red cell mass. Smoking is also a significant risk factor for chronic obstructive pulmonary disease, which is what this man suffers from. The obstructed airways reduce oxygen delivery to the alveoli and pulmonary vessels they supply thus causing a reduction of oxygen supply furthering the hypoxia. Finally, smokers also have an associated reduced plasma volume, thus increasing the relative concentration of haemoglobin. This is therefore 'combined' because of the presence of both increased red cell mass and reduced plasma volume.

Polycythaemia rubra vera (PRV) (A) is a chronic myeloproliferative disorder characterized by a V617F point mutation in exon 14 of the JAK2 gene (E). It is present in 95–97 per cent of patients with PRV, but the finding of this mutation is not specific to this condition (it also occurs in a substantial proportion of patients with essential thrombocythaemia and myelofibrosis). Crucially, these patients will have an increased red cell mass. It is important to realize that a raised haemoglobin, raised haematocrit or raised red blood cell count alone is not the same as a raised red cell mass. Haemoglobin may be raised with relative deficiency of plasma (i.e. relative or apparent polycythaemia, historically known as Gaisbock's disease (D)). This is also the same with haematocrit, which is a measurement of the proportion of a centrifuged test tube red cells occupy compared with the entire sample. If there is a relative deficiency of plasma, e.g. secondary to dehydration, there is a relative increase in the haematocrit. The red cell mass is an absolute measure and is assessed by isotope dilution studies. This is sometimes used to differentiate between true and apparent polycythaemia. Idiopathic erythrocytosis (B) is the label given to those with polycythaemia secondary to JAK2 mutation, but not with the V617F exon 14 mutation, e.g. exon 12 mutations.

Secondary polycythaemia (C) is where there are circulating plasma factors stimulating erythropoeisis, usually EPO but sometimes anabolic steroids (e.g. testosterone). It can also be secondary to an EPO secreting tumour – the five most common of which include hepatocellular carcinoma, renal cell carcinoma, haemangioblastoma, phaechromocytoma and uterine myomata. Oxygen sensitive EPO response may be appropriate, for example in chronic hypoxia when living at altitude or inappropriate, e.g. post transplant erythrocytosis where other hormones act to increases erythropoiesis and the EPO concentration is not elevated.

Haemolysis

26 B   G6PD deficiency (B) (also known as favism) is an X-linked condition where the lack of this enzyme increases the oxidative damage sustained by red blood cells. It is part of the pentose phosphate pathway which maintains levels of reduced glutathione – an important erythrocyte antioxidant. People with this condition have erythrocytes with less reduced

glutathione and are thus more sensitive to oxidative stress resulting in haemolysis. There are many variants of G6PD of differing severity. It is unlike some X-linked conditions where women can also be affected if they are homozygous. Precipitating factors include anti-malarials, primaquine, nitrofurantoin, dapsone, sulphonylureas and sulphonamides. Its alternate name, favism, relates to the fact that fava beans (broad beans) can trigger a haemolytic attack. The haemolysis released intracellular haemoglobin causing jaundice in this patient and haemoglobinuria, which caused a positive dipstick result. It is important to note that the differential for a positive dipstick for blood includes haemoglobinuria and myoglobinuria. Macrocytosis occurs from the raised reticulocyte production from increased bone marrow activity. Heinz bodies are seen due to the denatured haemoglobin which gets removed by macrophages in the spleen leaving 'bite' cells. A G6PD assay is useful in this patient but less so in the acute setting as the new reticulocytes can contain normal G6PD levels, thus giving a false negative result.

Hereditary spherocytosis (A) is an autosomal dominant disorder characterized by erythrocyte cytoskeletal abnormalities. The most common is due to a spectrin protein defect which is responsible for binding to protein 4.1, thus joining the intracellular cytoskeleton to the external membrane based proteins. The abnormal cell structure results in reduced erythrocyte flexibility giving it its characteristic shape but also making it more vulnerable to splenic sequestration and extravascular haemolysis. The erythrocyte vulnerability is exploited by the osmotic fragility test which strains the erythrocyte in varying solution concentrations to determine how fragile the cells are.

Paroxysmal nocturnal haemoglobinuria (C) is an acquired clonal stem cell disorder characterized by an abnormal erythrocyte sensitivity to the lytic complement pathway. There is a deficiency of glucosyl phosphatidyl inositol (GPI) linked proteins namely CD55 (decay-accelerating factor) and CD59 (membrane inhibitor or reactive lysis). The nocturnal nature of haemolysis is thought to be due to the relative acidosis created during sleep, thus causing haemolysis and red urine in the morning. There is also an association with thrombosis particularly Budd–Chiari syndrome (hepatic vein thrombosis).

Microangiopathic haemolytic anaemia (D) refers to haemolysis of red cells caused by narrowing microvasculature seen in patients with mechanical heart valves, disseminated intravascular coagulopathy, thrombotic thrombocytopenic purpura or haemolytic uraemic syndrome. Autoimmune haemolytic anaemia (E) occurs when autoantibodies directed at erythrocytes trigger haemolysis. The origin of the antibody might be due to a systemic disease (e.g. systemic lupus erythematosus, chronic lymphocytic leukaemia), infection (mycoplasma related cold agglutinins) or drugs (penicillins). Primaquine does not often cause an autoimmune haemolysis.

Secondary polycythaemia

27 B This question tests your understanding of erythropoeisis physiology and your understanding of laboratory measurements in a standard full blood count analysis. Red cell count is measured as the number of erythrocytes in a quantum of plasma, whereas red cell mass is determined by isotope studies quoted as mL/kg. It is a measure of absolute red cell mass and is therefore not affected if someone is dehydrated, for example, where the relative plasma volume is reduced giving a falsely high red cell concentration. There are many situations where the red cell concentration and red cell mass do not parallel each other, e.g. vomiting, diarrhoea or overuse of diuretics. If a patient has increased red cell concentration this may therefore be absolute or relative – the latter being secondary to reduced plasma volume thus making the polycythaemia secondary to haemoconcentration. Absolute polycythaemia may be primary or secondary. In this case there is secondary polycythaemia where the renal cell carcinoma is inappropriately producing too much EPO, thus overstimulating bone marrow erythropoeisis. Secondary polycythaemia is not always inappropriate – people with cyanotic heart disease, lung disease, haemoglobinopathies with high oxygen affinity or those living at altitude can get appropriate secondary polycythaemia as a physiological response to chronic hypoxaemia.

If polycythaemia were to be primary, then the EPO levels would be low with the other parameters being high. This would be the case in patients with polycythaemia rubra vera where virtually all of these patients have a *V617F* gene mutation of exon 14 of the Janus Kinase 2 enzyme. These patients are at risk of thrombosis due to the marked increased in red cell mass, and development of hyperuricaemia from high cell turnover. Patients also develop high basophil and eosinophil numbers – the increased histamine release from the former may results in intense pruritus and peptic ulceration.

von Willebrand's disease (1)

28 E von Willebrand's disease (vWD) is characterized by a quantitive or qualititative defect in von Willebrand factor (vWF). Ristocetin, an antibiotic no longer used clinically, causes vWF to bind the platelet receptor glycoprotein Ib (GlpIb) through an unknown mechanism. If ristocetin is added to platelets with defective vWF or defective GlpIb (called Bernard–Soulier syndrome) then platelet aggregation does not occur. It will occur, however, with other pro-aggregative factors including collagen (D) and fibrinogen (C). If vWF or GlpIb is absent, aggregation does not occur with collagen as there is no molecular link between collagen and the platelet. However, this is the case with all patients with vWF.

Furthermore, cryoprecipitate which contains vWF will correct defects in vWD but not in Bernard–Soulier syndrome.

Platelet disorders may be inherited or acquired. Inherited disorders include Glanzmann's thrombasthenia (an inherited lack of GlpIIb/IIIa) where fibrinogen cannot cross-link platelets during the initial platelet aggregative stage of thrombosis. Understanding these receptors and their importance in platelet aggregation has led to the development of powerful antiplatelet medications including adciximab, eptifibatide and tirofiban. Other inherited platelet diseases include storage pool diseases, e.g. grey platelet syndrome, Quebec platelet disorder, Hermansky–Pudlak syndrome and Chediak–Higashi syndrome. These refer to defects of the alpha and dense granules in the platelet which are released to promote platelet aggregation. Acquired platelet defects include aspirin (B) and uraemia. Aspirin irreversibly inhibits cyclooxygenase thus reducing levels of thromboxane A2, a powerful aggregative factor.

Myeloproliferative disease

29   C   The Auer rod (C) is pathognomonic of acute myeloblastic leukaemia (AML). Children with Down syndrome are at higher risk of this disease due to chromosome 21 duplication where a 'dosage' effect is theorized to increase the expression of proto-oncogenes. This may also explain the increased risk of AML in Warkany syndrome type 2 (trisomy 8). Another dosage effect example, also in Down syndrome, is the increased risk of Alzheimer's disease with beta amyloid, which accumulates in Alzheimer's disease and is coded for on chromosome 21. Epidemiologically, children with Down syndrome are more likely to get AML than ALL in the first 3 years of their life, but thereafter are more likely to get ALL, similar to those without Down syndrome. Auer rod's are pathognomonic for AML and are found in the cytoplasm. They represent stacked granules in myeloblasts and are azurophilic. They are particularly common in the M3 subtype of AML (according to the French American British classification).

Smudge cells (A) are seen in chronic lymphocytic leukaemia, the most common leukaemia and generally a disease of elderly people. Smudge cells represent the fragility of B-cell CLL upon mechanical manipulation and considered characteristic of CLL. CLL is characterized by the failure of B-cell apoptosis and the cells have undergone cell cycle arrest in the G0/G1 phase. White cell counts of over 100 are typical in patients who may be completely asymptomatic.

Reed–Sternberg cells (B) are pathognomonic for Hodgkin's lymphoma. These cells are actually uncommonly found when looking at histological samples from patients with Hodgkin's lymphoma. Recent advances looking at the origin of the Reed–Sternberg cell reveal it is most likely derived from germinal centre B cells, but they have characteristically lost their phenotypic features. Furthermore, routine stains for leukocyte common antigen, T cell and B cell markers are usually negative.

The Pelger–Huet anomaly (D) is caused by a benign dominantly inherited defect of terminal neutrophil differentiation. It is due to a mutation in the lamin-B receptor gene. The nucleus is bilobed and dumbbell-shaped with a narrow bridge connecting the two. This anomaly can also be acquired secondary to colchicine and sulphonamides which is reversible (so called pseudo-Pelger cells).

Hairy cells (E) are found in hairy cell leukaemia. This is an uncommon chronic B-cell lymphoproliferative disorder and is so named due to the prominent irregular cytoplasmic projections. It is now considered an indolent non-Hodgin lymphoma. It can present with splenomegaly, constitutional symptoms, bone marrow failure or incidentally with abnormal blood counts. The nuclei are variable in configuration and the cytoplasmic outline is often indistinct but best seen with phase-contrast microscopy.

Lymphoma

30 C Burkitt's lymphoma (C) is one of the most aggressive malignancies known to man. It is a type of non-Hodgkin's lymphoma (NHL) which arises from lymph node germinal centres. It is associated with Epstein–Barr virus and there are three subtypes – endemic, sporadic and immunodeficiency related. It is associated with translocation and dysregulation of the *c-myc* gene on chromosome 8 including t(8;14), t(2;8) and t(8;22). Histologically, there is profound proliferation. The starry sky appearance reflects islands of macrophages ingesting necrotic tumour cells as they have outgrown their own blood supply. Clinically, the endemic form affects younger men and classically presents with a jaw mass which spreads to extranodal sites including mesentery, ovary, testis, bone marrow and meninges.

Follicular lymphoma (A) is the most common indolent NHL. It is defined as a lymphoma of the follicle centre B cells (centrocytes). It usually presents with painless adenopathy with a prolonged history of waxing and waning lymphoadenopathy. Histologically, a nodular growth pattern with a mixture of centrocytes and centroblasts is characteristic. The proportion of centroblasts found determines the tumour grade which has therapeutic implications. These cells are CD10 and BCL-6 positive in the majority. It is usually indolent but can transform into a high grade lymphoma.

Marginal zone lymphoma (B) arises mainly at extranodal sites due to chronic antigenic stimulation and malignant transformation. It is a B-cell NHL arising from marginal cells in the lymph node. There are clinically three subtypes: extranodal marginal zone B-cell lymphoma of mucosa associated lymphoid tissue (MALT); nodal marginal zone B-cell lymphoma; and splenic marginal zone B-cell lymphoma. MALT lymphoma can occur in the stomach, lung, thyroid, breast, synovium and lacrimal or salivary glands. Associated conditions with MALT lymphoma include autoimmune conditions (e.g. Sjögren's disease, Hashimoto's thyroiditis, relapsing polychondritis) and *Helicobacter pylori* infection in the stomach. In fact, early treatment of *H. pylori* infection can induce regression.

Diffuse large B-cell lymphoma (D) is a subtype of B-cell NHL which usually affects elderly men presenting with lymphadenopathy and constitutional 'B' symptoms (weight loss, fever, drenching night sweats) in one-third. It is the most common histological subtype of NHL. The diagnosis is usually made with an excisional biopsy demonstrating pan-B cell markers, e.g. CD20, and CD79a. Histologically, there is effacement of normal architecture by sheets of atypical lymphoid cells. The cell of origin is the centroblast. There is some overlap with Burkitt's lymphoma as diffuse large B-cell lymphoma can have high proliferative indexes and t(8;14) mutations also seen in Burkitt's.

Mantle cell lymphoma (E) is another B-cell NHL, whose precursor cell is the mantle cell in the pre-germinal area. It typically affects middle-aged men with lymphadenopathy and gastrointestinal tract involvement including spleen and Waldeyer's ring. It usually presents with advanced disease and involves any region of the GI tract occasionally presenting as multiple intestinal polyps. Nuclear staining for cyclin D1 is present in 95 per cent of cases and is strongly associated with the t(11;14) (q13;q32) mutation – a translocation between cyclin D1 locus and immunoglobulin heavy chain locus. This is not specific, however, for Mantle cell lymphoma and has been seen in multiple myeloma.

Hodgkin's lymphoma

31 C Nodular lymphocytic (C) Hodgkin's lymphoma is often called the non-classical subtype of Hodgkin's lymphoma. It is so called due to the atypical nature of the Reed–Sternberg cell which characterizes all Hodgkin's lymphomas. This cell is known as the lymphocytic and histiocytic cell or L&H variant. Sometimes these cells are referred to as 'popcorn' cells because their nucleus resembles an exploded popcorn kernel. This subtype of HL accounts for 5 per cent of cases and has a bimodal age distribution – children and adults between the ages of 30 and 40. Unlike common HL, this type is more common in African American men compared with Caucasians in the US. Clinically, patients often present with peripheral lymphadenopathy without B symptoms (namely fever, night sweats and weight loss). It is generally thought of as a more indolent form of HL.

Nodular sclerosis classical HL (A) is characterized by at least a partially nodular grown pattern, with fibrous bands separating nodules. Mixed cellularity (B) classical HL is a heterogeneous group with a diffuse or vaguely nodular growth patter without band-forming sclerosis.

Lymphocytic rich (D) most commonly has a nodular growth pattern. In this subtype, cells resembling L&H variants may be present making the distinction from non-classical lymphoma more difficult. The background infiltrate consists predominantly of lymphocytes, with rare eosinophils or neutrophils. Lymphocyte depleted (E) subtype has a diffuse growth pattern and appears hypocellular with a lack of inflammatory cells. This subtype has a poor prognosis.

Questions about lymphoma are often difficult as detailed knowledge of subtypes is difficult to digest. The clinical clues in questions pointing to lymphoma include B symptoms, alcohol induced painful lymphadeno-pathy (although clinically rare), and the even rarer cyclical fever lasting 1–2 weeks termed the Pel–Ebstein fever.

Glucose-6-phosphate dehydrogenase deficiency

32 D   This patient has glucose-6-phosphate dehydrogenase (G6PD) deficiency; a common X-linked condition where the reduction of G6PD function leads to haemolysis when erythrocytes are exposed to oxidative stress. Less commonly there is a chronic haemolysis when enzymatic activity is less than 10 per cent of normal. Unlike some other X-linked conditions, women can be affected due to the random nature of X chromosome inactivation (lyonization) which leads to some cells being vulnerable to oxidative stress. G6PD is important in the pentose phosphate shunt which critically regenerates NADPH, a cofactor important in glutathione metabolism. Reduced glutathione is the primary buffer against oxidative stress. Haemoglobinuria (D) occurs due to intravascular haemolysis in the face of oxidative stress in a susceptible patient. Red cells undergo intravascular and extravascular haemolysis leading to haemoglobinae-mia and haemoglobinuria. Common precipitants include intercurrent infection but also drugs, the most notorious of which are dapsone, pri-maquine and nitrofurantoin. Classically, haemolysis can be triggered by fava beans (hence its alternate name 'Favism') as well as naphthalene (found in moth balls and henna).

A positive direct antiglobin test (A) indicates an immunological cause for haemolysis. This is not true of G6PD deficiency as there is oxida-tive damage causing denatured erythrocyte proteins and haemolysis mostly via the reticuloendothelial system. This test, also known as the direct Coombs test, involves washing red cells and adding antiserum or monoclonal antibodies against various immunoglobulins (particu-larly IgG and C3d). A positive test results in red cell agglutination. It will therefore detect if antibodies or complement have bound to the red blood cell antigen. The indirect Coombs test is where antibodies or complement taken from the patient's plasma will react to donor red blood cells. The indirect test is used for compatibility testing in blood transfusion.

A low mean cell volume often reflects decreased haemoglobin content and is often associated with a reduced mean cell haemoglobin. This is represented in the blood film as a hypochromic microcytosis. The most common cause is reduced iron availability (iron deficiency, anaemia of chronic disease or rarely copper deficiency). Other causes include reduced haem synthesis (lead poisoning, sideroblastic anaemia) or reduced globin production (thalassaemia or other haemoglobinopathies). Practically, an older patient with microcytic anaemia should be investigated for bowel cancer as this is a serious and common cause of chronic occult blood loss. With haemolysis, the mean cell volume normally increases – this is mainly due to the presence of reticulocytes which are larger than red cells. Thus one would expect a raised reticulocyte count and not a reduced count (C).

Finally, haptoglobin concentration is reduced during haemolysis, not increased (E). Haptoglobin circulates in the plasma and avidly binds to free haemoglobin to be later removed by the reticuloendothelial system. It is therefore reduced in intravascular haemolysis only. Extravascular haemolysis occurs mainly in the spleen where free haemoglobin is not released into the circulation and therefore haptoglobin levels are generally unchanged.

Anaemia (6)

33 D This woman presents with microcytic anaemia, the most common cause of which is iron deficiency. However, the mean cell volume is disproportionally reduced compared with the degree of anaemia indicating there might be a haemoglobinopathy present. The presence of increased Hb A_2 confirms the diagnosis of β-thalassaemia trait. Unfortunately the nomenclature surrounding β-thalassaemia is relatively confusing but an attempt to clarify it will be made here. Firstly, thalassaemia is the reduction or absence of a type of globin gene. Normal haemoglobin is a tetramer of two alpha and two beta globin proteins. The ratio of alpha to non-alpha globin production is tightly controlled. There are two alpha genes located on chromosome 16, whereas only one beta gene on chromosome 11. β-Thalassaemia implies a reduction or absence of the beta chain. Beta (0) thalassaemia refers to an absence of beta globin production. This encompasses over 40 genetic mutations. Patients with this are often described as having β-thalassaemia major (C), however, confusingly some patients can produce beta globin genes but to such a poor extent they behave very similar clinically, as if they had no production. Within the first year of life they have profound life-long transfusion dependent anaemia. This is therefore not compatible in this patient's case.

β-Thalassaemia trait (D), also known as β-thalassaemia minor, includes patients who have beta (+) thalassaemia. This means patients produce beta globin but to a lesser degree, and can produce some normal Hb A.

It is usually asymptomatic and picked up during blood tests for other reasons, such as in this case. Hb A$_2$ is increased due to the imbalance of alpha globin production compared with beta globin production. A rare situation where HbA$_2$ is not increased is in the setting of β-thalassaemia trait with concomitant delta thalassaemia trait. β-Thalassaemia intermedia are patients who are compound heterozygotes of two thalassaemia variants, e.g. β-thalassaemia trait plus Hb E variant.

Sickle cell disease (A) is caused by a valine to glutamic acid substitution in the 6th position of the beta globin gene. This reduces haemoglobin solubility once deoxygenated giving the characteristic sickle cell appearance and therefore causing microvascular occlusion resulting in ischemia and sickle crises. There is usually a chronic haemolysis with a normochromic normocytic anaemia. It may become microcytic if there is concomitant iron deficiency or coexistent α- or β-thalassaemia.

Hereditary spherocytosis (E) is a disorder of erythrocyte cytoskeleton giving a characteristic spherocyte appearance in the blood film. The mean cell volume is normal or low, but is confounded by the presence of reticulocytes which increases the average mean cell volume. This is reflected in an increased red cell distribution width (RDW) which is a standardized measure of the degree of anisocytosis. The most useful red cell index is the mean cell haemoglobin concentration (MCHC) which is normally elevated reflecting membrane loss and cell dehydration. A raised RDW with increased MCHC is very suggestive of this condition.

Acute myeloid leukaemia (B) is unlikely to present with these features and would normally have raised white cell counts with blasts as well as features of bone marrow failure.

Splenomegaly

34   A   This patient exhibits features of chronic myeloid leukaemia as evidenced by raised myeloid lineage cells including neutrophils, myelocytes and basophils. The neutrophils are morphologically normal but cytochemically different – a laboratory test sometimes used to differentiate between reactive or leukaemoid neutrophilia and CML is the leukocyte alkaline phosphatase. It is normal or high in the former, but characteristically low in CML. Absolute basophilia is a universal finding in CML, with absolute eosinophilia found in 90 per cent of cases. A raised platelet count is also common in CML; a low platelet count, however, should make one reconsider the diagnosis, e.g. myelodysplastic syndromes.

Up to 95 per cent of patients with chronic myeloid leukaemia have the Philadelphia chromosome – a fusion chromosome between the long arms of chromosomes 9 and 22 (A). The formation of the BCR-Abl fusion gene acts as a constitutively active tyrosine kinase, but the induction of leukaemogenesis is complicated and mediated through both tyrosine dependent and independent pathways. It is known, however, that the tyrosine kinase activity of the BCR-Abl gene is absolutely required for transformation. BCR-Abl fusion genes alone (C) can occur without the t(9;22) translocation but this is much less common. This Robertsonian translocation is worth remembering as it is frequently asked about in examinations.

The t(8;14) translocation occurs in Burkitt's lymphoma: a highly aggressive lymphoma where *cmyc*, an oncogene, is under the influence of an immunoglobulin promoter, which is highly expressed. The V617F point mutation in JAK2 (D) is found in up to 99 per cent of cases of polycythaemia rubra vera. JAK2 is involved in downstream processing of the erythropoietin receptor signalling. This mutation causes constitutive activation of downstream STATS molecules leading to uncontrolled gene transcription. 5q- is a subtype of myelodysplasic syndrome (MDS) in the World Health Organization classification. The nomenclature means there is a deletion in the long arm of chromosome 5. It is the most common chromosomal abnormality seen in MDS (up to 15 per cent).

Hodgkin's lymphoma staging

35 C   This question relies on the candidate's knowledge and understanding of the Ann Arbor staging system. This clinical staging system is relatively intuitive – stages are between I and IV either in the absence or presence of 'B symptoms'. A simplified version of the classification is as follows:

- Stage I: involvement of a **single** lymph node region
- Stage II: involvement of two or more lymph node regions on the **same side of the diaphragm**
- Stage III: involvement of lymph nodes on **both sides of the diaphragm**
- Stage IV: **extranodal spread** (not spleen however, this is taken as a lymph node)

The definition of B symptoms includes significant unexplained fever, night sweats or unexplained weight loss of over 10 per cent during 6 months prior to diagnosis. The presence of B symptoms is denoted by a B subscript after the stage number, the absence is denoted by an A subscript. Patient A would therefore be classified as Ia, patient B as IIa, patient C as IIIb, patient D as IIIa, technically as she does not quite fulfil the 10 per cent loss in 6 months and finally patient E as stage IIa. Note that in Hodgkin's lymphoma, the disease always spreads contiguously whereas in non-Hodgkin's lymphoma this is not always the case. Further investigations for clinical staging include an upright chest

X-ray, integrated positron emission tomography/computer tomography of the chest/abdomen/pelvis and sometimes a unilateral bone marrow aspirate and biopsy for those with stage III or IV with B symptoms.

Acute leukaemia

36 B   Acute promyelocytic leukaemia is interesting for a number of reasons. There is a reciprocal translocation between the long arms of chromosomes 15 and 17 giving the PML-RARA fusion gene (B). This links the retinoic acid receptor alpha (RARA) gene on chromosome 17 with the promyelocytic leukaemia (PML) gene on chromosome 15. RARA is a member of a family of retinoin-binding transcription factors that regulate gene expression. It heterodimerizes with retinoid X receptor (RXR) and binds to retinoic acid response elements to influence gene transcription. In the absence of retinoic acid, the RARA/RXR dimer interacts with another protein (nuclear corepressor) to repress gene transcription. Therefore, addition of retinoic acid stimulates gene transcription. In the setting of promyelocytic leukaemia, retinoic acid induces myeloid differentiation which is abnormally halted thus providing remission by encouraging cell differentiation rather than cell death. The second reason this type of leukaemia is interesting is its association with disseminated intravascular coagulopathy. The pathogenesis is not completely understood but recognizing it early is important as treatment with retinoic acid plus supportive therapy can lead to rapid improvement in the coagulopathy.

Telomeres (A) are nucleoprotein end caps on chromosomes which provide protection of the chromosomal ends which are not copied fully during mitosis. It has been theorized that aging cells are more vulnerable to DNA damage due to shortened telomeres as they have undergone more mitosis and therefore have shorter telomeres.

The mechanisms for chromosomal mutations in leukaemia include:

- chromosomal translocation where there is creation of a fusion gene or damage to a differentiation gene
- chromosomal duplication where there is a potential dosage effect, e.g. Down syndrome and its association with acute myeloid leukaemia
- chromosomal loss or deletion can lead to the loss of tumour suppressor genes

Normally two types of gene mutation occur for acute leukaemia to occur – the first is type I mutation which promotes proliferation and survival whereas type II mutations block differentiation (which would normally be followed by apoptosis).

Treatment of chronic myeloid leukaemia

37 B   Imatinib is a tyrosine kinase inhibitor (B) and is used in the treatment of chronic myeloid leukaemia. It is a rational therapy which acts to inhibit the BCR-Abl tyrosine kinase thus blocking proliferation and inducing apoptosis in BCR-Abl positive cell lines. The BCR-Abl fusion is most commonly secondary to a balanced Robertsonian translocation between chromosomes 9 and 22. Imatinib is also used for gastrointestinal stromal tumour (GIST). Other tyrosine kinase inbitors include dasatinib and nilotinib. They do not cure CML but provide long-term control in the majority of patients, thus they are the initial treatment of choice for almost all newly diagnosed patients with CML.

Proteosome inhibitors (A) such as bortezomib inhibit 26S proteosome. This molecule is essential in the ubiquitin–proteosome pathway important for the degradation of intracellular proteins. Proteosome 26S inhibition leads to apoptosis via disruption of the NF kappa B pathway. Bortezomib is used in multiple myeloma and certain types of lymphoma.

IL-6 inhibitors (C) such as tocilizumab are biologic agents used in the treatment of rheumatoid arthritis. Blocking IL-6 prevents various immunological responses such as production of certain cytokines and acute phase proteins. It is not used in any malignancies.

Inhibitors of p53 (D) do not exist as p53 is a key inducer of apoptosis in cells with damaged DNA. Diseases where there is p53 mutation (e.g. Li–Fraumeni syndrome) result in a wide range of malignancies which develop at an unusually early age. It is also known as Sarcoma, Breast, Leukaemia and Adrenal gland (SBLA) cancer syndrome. Finally a human epidermal growth factor receptor 2 (HER2) protein antagonist, i.e. trastuzumab, is used in HER2 positive patients with breast cancer and sometimes in metastatic gastric cancer.

von Willebrand's disease (2)

38 B   This woman has mild von Willebrand's disease (vWD) which can be treated with desmopressin (B). There are three types of vWD – type I is a quantitative deficiency of von Willebrand Factor (vWF), type II is a qualitative defect in vWF whereas type III results in profound deficiency in vWF. There are four subtypes of type II vWF (2A, 2B, 2M and 2N). vWF is important in two ways; first it acts as a bridge between platelets and between platelets and subendothelial structures at the site of injury; and second it carries factor VIII which is a key molecule in the clotting cascade. Desmopressin acts to increase vWF and factor VIII concentration by encouraging its release from endothelial cell storage sites. Desmopressin is efficacious in type I and most type II disease but

not in type III. This woman is known to have 'mild' disease thus making desmopressin a viable option. Interestingly, desmopressin in patients with type 2B will lead to a transient worsening of their thrombocytopenia. Patients with type 2B vWD have increased binding of the abnormal vWF to platelets causing sequestration and clearance of platelets. This is worsened for desmopressin, if only for a few hours. Despite this, there have been reports of patients benefiting from desmopressin.

Cryoprecipitate (A) is produced from freezing fresh plasma and thawing it at 4°C. The precipitate left is centrifuged and contains high concentrations of factor VIII, fibrinogen, fibronectin, factor XIII and vWF. It is not recommended in this patient as she has mild disease and the risk of viral transmission from blood products, although low, is not therefore justified.

Fresh frozen plasma (C) is prepared from whole blood or plasma collected by special techniques which is frozen with 8 hours of acquisition. It contains all of the coagulation factors and proteins present in the original blood. It is generally an overused resource but is useful for when complicated clotting issues need to be corrected quickly, e.g warfarin overdose, liver disease, disseminated intravascular coagulopathy.

Vitamin K (D) is used to reverse warfarin overtreatment or in decompensated liver disease. Vitamin K is used for the synthesis of clotting factors II, VII, IX and X. It does not increase vWF which is required in this patient. Recombinant factor VIII (E) is used in life-threatening surgery or emergency surgery in patients with haemophilia type A, not in mild vWD. If factor replacement were contemplated in patients with severe vWD (usually type III), then recombinant vWF would be used instead.

Myelodysplastic syndrome

39 D The myelodysplastic syndromes are a heterogeneous group of conditions characterized by an abnormal clone of stem cells with impaired proliferation and differentiation. The result is a peripheral cytopenia, qualitative abnormalities in erythroid, myeloid and megakaryocyte maturation, as well as increased risk of leukaemic transformation. The abnormalities, both quantitative and qualitative, in neutrophils mean susceptibility to bacterial infection is high and thus a corresponding increased likelihood of mortality (D). Skin infections are particularly common and resistant to treatment.

The peripheral blood film would not show toxic granulation (A) unless there is concomitant infection. 'Toxic granulation' is a term referring to the appearance of dark blue, coarse granules representing azurophilic granules with abnormal staining. Dohle bodies are light blue in colour and are found in the periphery of neutrophils in patients with infections but also myelodysplasia. They represent areas of rough endoplasmic reticulum with bound ribosomes. Another characteristic neutrophil change seen in MDS is the Pelger–Huet abnormality where there is a reduction in lobule number.

A blast content of 1 per cent would not be considered as a leukaemic transformation. Refractory anaemia with an excess of blasts (RAEB) describes a type of MDS where there is an increased blast load implying progression to leukaemic transformation. Type I indicates a blast percentage between 5 and 10, whereas type II has a blast load of 10–19 per cent. Twenty per cent blasts or more is therefore considered leukaemic transformation.

Absence of the *long* arm of chromosome 5 is a specific subtype of MDS. There is an interstitial deletion and it most commonly affects elderly women. It may respond quite dramatically to lenolidamide, a thalidomide derivative. Deletion of the short arm of chromosome 5 is associated with Cri du chat syndrome – a genetic disorder unrelated to MDS, named due to the characteristic cat cry made by affected children ('*cri du chat*' from French meaning 'call of the cat').

Cytotoxic therapy (C) is not usually used first line unless they are symptomatic or high risk using the International Prognostic Scoring system. Most treatment is supportive with the use of blood products, antibiotics to treat infection and growth factors such as eryhropoeitin or granulocyte-colony stimulating factor.

Factor V Leiden

40 B Factor V Leiden is an autosomal dominantly inherited point mutation where arginine is replaced by glutamine in the 506th position. Factor V normally circulates in plasma as an inactivated factor and is activated by thrombin which then acts as a co-factor, with factor Xa, to convert prothrombin to thrombin. Factor Va is inactivated by cleavage of its heavy chain; firstly at position Arg506, which causes conformational change to reveal a further two cleavage sites (Arg306 and Arg 679). This inactivation is performed by the activated protein C complex, and thus the Leiden mutation confers resistance (B). The prothrombotic consequence of Factor V Leiden is actually two-fold – first Factor V is degraded more slowly thus there is more generation of thrombin in the prothrombinase complex and second, once factor V is cleaved at the first Arg506 site, it is thought to play a role, with protein S, to support activated protein C in Factor VIIIa degradation too.

Prothrombin mutation (A) where there is a guanine to adenine transition at the 20210 in the 3′ untranslated region of the prothrombin gene is related to factor V Leiden. It is, however, another cause of inherited hypercoagulability. It is thought the mutation may alter the efficiency of mRNA processing or increase the prothrombin mRNA half life. Antithrombin III deficiency (B) is caused by a mutation in the long arm of chromosome 1 where a lack of antithrombin III leads to a hypercoaguable state. This is because antithrombin III is an important anticoagulant acting to inhibit thrombin and factors Xa and IXa. Its activity is increased 4000-fold by heparin. Protein C (D) and Protein S (E) deficiency are other types of inherited hypercoagulable states not related to Factor V Leiden. Protein C is the key component in the activated protein C complex which degrades factors Va and VIIIa. The activated protein C complex effect is markedly increased by the presence of protein S, hence its importance in anticoagulation.

SECTION 5: IMMUNOLOGY EMQs

QUESTIONS

1. Immunodeficiency (1)

A   Kostmann syndrome
B   Severe combined immunodefi-
     ciency
C   Hyper IgM syndrome
D   Leukocyte adhesion deficiency

E   Protein-losing enteropathy
F   Cyclic neutropenia
G   Bruton's agammaglobulinaemia
H   Di George's syndrome
I   AIDS

For each scenario below, choose the most appropriate answer from the list above. Each option may be used once, more than once or not at all.

1   A 4-month-old girl is referred to a paediatrician with failure to thrive, after suffering from recurrent infections since birth, especially recurrent candida infections of her skin and mouth. Blood tests reveal a diminished T-cell count; further lymphocyte testing demonstrates non-functional B cells.

2   A 5-month-old boy is referred to a paediatrician after suffering with recurrent infections since his birth. His mother has noticed increased irritability. Blood tests reveal a neutrophil count of 350/μL. NBT test is normal.

3   A 4-year-old girl is referred to a paediatrician after experiencing recurrent chest infections. Blood tests demonstrate a reduced B-cell count as well as low IgA, IgM and IgG levels.

4   A 48-year-old woman presents to her GP with a history of diarrhoea for 3 weeks, which occasionally contains blood. She has felt increasingly tired and feverish. The patient has had similar episodes in the past which were treated with mesalazine. She also reports recurrent chest infections since her first episode of diarrhoea.

5   A 3-year-old girl is seen by a GP due to recurrent mild chest infections. The doctor notices the girl has a cleft lip. Blood tests reveal a reduced T-cell count as well as hypocalcaemia.

2. Immunodeficiency (2)

A   Selective IgA deficiency disease
B   Common variable immuno-
     deficiency
C   Nephrotic syndrome
D   Bare lymphocyte syndrome
     deficiency

E   Sickle cell anaemia
F   Chronic granulomatous
G   Reticular dysgenesis
H   Wiskott–Aldrich syndrome
I   Interferon-gamma receptor

For each scenario below, choose the most appropriate answer from the list above. Each option may be used once, more than once or not at all.

1 A 4-year-old boy is referred to a paediatrician after suffering recurrent chest infections over the preceding few months. The boy has a history of eczema as well as recurrent nose bleeds. Blood tests reveal a reduced IgM level but raised IgA and IgE levels.

2 A 20-year-old man presents to his GP with signs of a mild pneumonia. The patient states he has had several similar episodes in the past. Further investigations by an immunologist reveal the patient has a genetic condition caused by a mutation of MHC III.

3 A 3-year-old girl is referred to a paediatrician after concerns about recurrent skin infections she has suffered from since birth. A nitro-blue-tetrazolium test is negative (remains colourless).

4 A 4-year-old boy is referred to a paediatrician after a period of mild but chronic diarrhoea. On examination the child is found to have icteric sclera and hepatomegaly. Following blood tests, the doctor has a high suspicion that the child could have a defect in MHC I.

5 A 22-year-old woman visits her GP after several chest infections in the past few years. As well as the chest infections, the patient reports that she has had several bouts of diarrhoea over the same time period.

3. Transplantation

A	HLA-matching	F	OKT3
B	Corticosteroids	G	IL-2 receptor antibody
C	Cyclosporine A	H	Tacrolimus
D	Azathioprine	I	Anti-lymphocyte antibody
E	Sirolimus		

For each scenario below, choose the most appropriate answer from the list above. Each option may be used once, more than once or not at all.

1 A 48-year-old man has undergone a kidney transplant operation as a result of renal failure caused by long-standing diabetes mellitus. However, despite immunosuppression, signs of organ rejection become evident just 1 hour after the procedure.

2 A 45-year-old man undergoes a heart transplant due to end-stage heart failure. Seventy-two hours after the operation, the patient shows signs of organ rejection which is resistant to corticosteroid therapy. A mouse monoclonal antibody is administered to save the transplant.

3   A 32-year-old woman undergoes a bone marrow transplant for chronic lympho-
     blastic leukaemia. She is prescribed a medication that inhibits calcineurin. On
     examination, the patient has gum hyperplasia.

4   A 62-year-old man who has undergone a kidney transplant was started on an
     immunosuppressive agent prior to the operation. The patient is warned that he
     will only be on the medication for a short period due to long-term side effects
     such as osteoporosis.

5   A 62-year-old man who is undergoing a liver transplant as a result of cirrhosis
     is prescribed a medication that inhibits DNA synthesis in an attempt to prevent
     proliferation of T cells.

4. Autoimmune antibodies (1)

A	Anti-smooth muscle	F	Anti-double stranded DNA
B	p-ANCA	G	Anti-parietal cell
C	Anti-Jo1	H	Anti-thyroid stimulating
D	Anti-cyclic citrullinated protein		hormone
E	Anti-centromere	I	Anti-topoisomerase

For each scenario below, choose the most appropriate answer from the list above.
Each option may be used once, more than once or not at all.

1   A 56-year-old woman presents to the rheumatologist with pain in her hands.
     On examination there are obvious deformities of her proximal interphalyngeal
     joints and metacarpophalyngeal joints. Swan-neck deformities are seen but the
     patient has retained functionality of her fingers.

2   A 45-year-old woman is referred to a hepatologist after suffering an episode of
     jaundice, fatigue and fever. Liver function tests reveal an increased AST. Biopsy
     of the liver reveals cirrhosis and an autoimmune pathology is suspected.

3   A 42-year-old woman presents to the rheumatologist with weakness in her
     proximal muscles and describes how she is finding it difficult to climb stairs.
     On examination, a rash is observed surrounding both eyes. A high resolution CT
     scan reveals a pulmonary fibrosis picture.

4   A 43-year-old man is referred to the rheumatologist after experiencing paleness
     in his fingers, especially when exposed to cold weather. The patient also com-
     plains of recent onset difficulty in swallowing solid food.

5   A 42-year-old woman presents to the rheumatologist with joint pain and stiff-
     ness. On examination, the patient appears to have a tight mouth and fine end
     inspiratory crackles on auscultation of the lungs. The woman also has a wide-
     spread itchy rash on her body.

5. Autoimmune antibodies (2)

A	Anti-mitochondrial	F	Anti-Ro
B	c-ANCA	G	Anti-nuclear
C	Anti-cardiolipin	H	Anti-intrinsic factor
D	Anti-ribonucleoprotein	I	Anti-endomysial
E	Anti-glutamic acid decarboxylase		

For each scenario below, choose the most appropriate answer from the list above. Each option may be used once, more than once or not at all.

1   A 25-year-old woman presents to her GP with a dry mouth and eyes for a period of 2 weeks. The patient also complains of joint pains over this time-course.

2   A 52-year-old man is referred to a gastroenterologist with itchy skin and malaise. On examination, the man has bruising on his arms and legs.

3   A 10-year-old girl is brought to see a GP. Her mother describes how she has recently been urinating with greater frequency than previously as well as feeling thirsty and has lost several kilograms in weight in the recent weeks.

4   A 42-year-old man presents to accident and emergency with haemoptysis. The patient also describes how he has been experiencing nose bleeds with increasing frequency in recent weeks. The patient is noted to have a saddle-shaped nose.

5   A 22-year-old woman presents to her GP with recent onset diarrhoea and abdominal cramping after she has eaten meals containing wheat.

6. Hypersensitivity (1)

A	TSH receptor	F	*Chlamydia trachomatis*
B	Nuts	G	Mouldy hay
C	DNA	H	Grass pollen
D	Nickel	I	Pancreatic β-cell proteins
E	Type IV collagen		

For each scenario below, choose the most appropriate answer from the list above. Each option may be used once, more than once or not at all.

1   An 11-year-old girl presents to the GP with increased thirst and urinary frequency. Urine dipstick demonstrates the presence of glucose.

2   A 13-year-old girl eats a slice of cake at a birthday party and quickly develops swollen lips, itchy skin and difficulty breathing. A shot of intramuscular adrenaline is immediately administered.

3   A 56-year-old farmer presents to his GP with a 2-month history of worsening shortness of breath. He mentions that he has experienced periodic fevers, malaise and mild shortness of breath, which has recently become so bad that he has had to stop work.

4   A 45-year-old man presents to accident and emergency with a sudden onset of haemoptysis. His wife mentions that the patient had noticed some blood in his urine a few days previously but had thought nothing of it.

5   A 12-year-old boy experiences a runny nose, itchiness of his eyes and nasal congestion. His GP suggests he has a seasonal condition, and should begin taking anti-histamines to help relieve him of his symptoms.

7. Hypersensitivity (2)

A	Stony fruit	F	Peanuts
B	HBsAg	G	Antiserum
C	Myelin basic protein	H	Synovial membrane antigens
D	Rhesus antigens	I	Poison ivy
E	Glycoprotein IIb–IIIa		

For each scenario below, choose the most appropriate answer from the list above. Each option may be used once, more than once or not at all.

1   A 26-year-old woman at a work dinner has ordered a curry. Soon after eating the meal, she feels short of breath and wheezy. Her husband who is present swiftly administers an intramuscular shot of adrenaline.

2   A 35-year-old woman presents to the GP with blurry vision and weakness in her legs. Cerebrospinal fluid demonstrates oligoclonal bands of IgG on electrophoresis.

3   A 34-year-old man who has been taking amoxicillin for pneumonia has developed tiredness and palpitations since taking the medication. Blood tests reveal a normocytic anaemia and direct antiglobulin test is positive.

4   A 34-year-old man, who is a known intravenous drug user, presents to accident and emergency with a 1-week history of fever, fatigue and abdominal pain. The patient also has associated joint pain. An angiogram reveals the presence of multiple aneurysms.

5   A 45-year-old man with diagnosed systemic lupus erythematosus (SLE) presents to the GP with a recent onset of nose bleeds and bleeding of his gums when he brushes his teeth. Blood tests reveal a very low platelet count.

8. Immune-based therapies

A   Cyclophosphamide
B   Mycophenolate mofetil
C   Basiliximab
D   Abatacept
E   Rituximab
F   Efalizumab
G   Infliximab
H   Ustekinumab
I   Denosumab

For each scenario below, choose the most appropriate answer from the list above. Each option may be used once, more than once or not at all.

1   A 46-year-old man with long-standing SLE is seen by his rheumatologist. He had previously been treated with corticosteroids, but has now developed end-organ involvement of his kidneys, lungs and heart.

2   A 56-year-old woman is seen in the rheumatology outpatient clinic. She has long-standing rheumatoid arthritis, which despite treatment with metho-trexate has become more severe. The rheumatologist decides that a CTL4-immunoglobulin fusion protein may help.

3   A 56-year-old man who is undergoing kidney transplant surgery is given medi-cation to prevent allograft rejection. The drug prevents guanine synthesis to induce immunosuppression.

4   A 58-year-old woman who suffers from rheumatoid arthritis is seen by her rheumatologist. She has been taking long-term disease modifying anti-rheumatic drugs, but her condition has recently worsened. As a result the doctor prescribes a TNF-α inhibitor.

5   A 56 year old with known systemic lupus erythematosus has been treated with long-term steroids. The patient presents to a rheumatologist with back pain and a DEXA scan confirms osteoporosis.

9. Nephritic disorders

A   Minimal change disease
B   Wegener's granulomatosis
C   Microscopic polyangitis
D   Lupus nephritis
E   IgA nephropathy
F   Membranoproliferative glomerulonephritis
G   Rapidly progressive glomerulonephritis
H   Post-streptococcal glomerulonephritis
I   Goodpasture's syndrome

For each scenario below, choose the most appropriate answer from the list above. Each option may be used once, more than once or not at all.

1 A 50-year-old woman presents to accident and emergency with haematuria. Blood tests demonstrate deranged renal function and further tests reveal the presence of circulating cANCA antibodies. The patient is noted to have a saddle-shaped nose.

2 A 24-year-old man presents to his GP with a few days' history of blood in his urine. Urinary investigations reveal the presence of proteinuria, red and white cell casts and dysmorphic red cells. The patient's notes state that he was diagnosed with pharyngitis in the previous week. Blood tests reveal a raised IgA level.

3 A 25-year-old man presents to his GP with symptoms and signs of nephritic syndrome. The patient had a sore throat 2 weeks previously. Blood tests reveal anti-streptolysin titre is high, while IgA levels are normal.

4 A 65-year-old man with known renal failure is transferred to the renal team by the accident and emergency department with worsening renal function. A renal biopsy is taken which demonstrates the presence of crescents on histology; immunofluorescence staining of IgG/C3 reveals a granular pattern. The man is very ill with suggestions that he may require a renal transplant.

5 A 3-year-old boy is seen by the GP after his mother noticed swelling of his legs. A week previously the boy had been stung by a bee. Urine dipstick reveals the presence of proteinuria, while blood tests show hypoalbuminaemia and hyper-lipidaemia.

10. Diagnostic immunology

A Histocompatibility testing
B Immunofluorescence
C Latex fixation test
D Radioallergosorbent test
E Patch testing

F Kveim test
G Skin prick test
H Western blot
I Direct antiglobulin test

For each scenario below, choose the most appropriate answer from the list above. Each option may be used once, more than once or not at all.

1 A 39-year-old homosexual man presents to accident and emergency with shortness of breath and a dry cough. A chest X-ray shows widespread pulmonary opacification. PCR confirms the diagnosis of *Pneumocystis pneumoniae* infection. A test is ordered to confirm the underlying diagnosis.

2 A 45-year-old man presents to accident and emergency with worsening shortness of breath. Examination findings are consistent with pulmonary fibrosis. Chest X-ray demonstrates the presence of bihilar lymphadenopathy. Erythema nodosum is observed on the patient's shins.

3   A 50-year-old man with known SLE develops jaundice. On examination he is found to have conjunctival pallor and is short of breath. Blood tests reveal an elevated unconjugated bilirubin level.

4   A 12-year-old girl is referred to a paediatrician after suffering with allergies to a number of foods including peanuts and eggs. Her mother wants to check if she is allergic to any other foods, inhalants or specific materials, so that she can be prevented from coming into contact with potential allergens.

5   A 5-year-old boy presents to accident and emergency with purpura on his legs and buttocks, joint pain and abdominal pain. The boy's mother states that the child had suffered from a sore throat approximately 1 week previously. The doctor would like to perform an investigation to make sure of the diagnosis.

ANSWERS

1. Immunodeficiency (1)

ANSWERS: 1) B 2) A 3) G 4) E 5) H

Severe combined immunodeficiency (SCID; B) causes defects in both T cells and B cells. The most common subtypes can be categorized into an X-linked disease (mutation of IL-2 receptor) or an autosomal recessive condition (mutation of adenosine deaminase gene which leads to a build-up of toxins and hence compromised proliferation of lymphocytes). Characteristically, there is hypoplasia and atrophy of the thymus and mucosa-associated lymphoid tissue (MALT). Clinical features include diarrhoea, failure to thrive and skin disease (graft-versus-host induced, secondary to transplacental maternal T cells or blood transfusion-related caused by donor T cells).

Kostmann syndrome (severe congenital neutropenia; A) is a congenital neutropenia as a result of failure of neutrophil maturation. This results in a very low neutrophil count (less than 500/µL indicates severe neutropenia) and no pus formation. Kostmann syndrome is usually detected soon after birth. Presenting features may be non-specific in infants, including fever, irritability and infection. The nitro-blue-tetrazolium (NBT) test can help with diagnosis; the liquid turns blue due to the normal presence of NADPH. In Kostmann syndrome, NBT test is positive and therefore normal.

Bruton's agammaglobulinaemia (G) is an X-linked disease that presents in childhood. It is caused by a mutation of the *BTK* gene, which expresses a tyrosine kinase. This mutation inhibits B-cell maturation and therefore B-cell and immunoglobulin levels are diminished. Blood tests will reveal a normal T-cell count, but diminished B-cell count as well as IgA, IgM and IgG levels. Plasma cells will also be absent from the bone marrow and lymphatics.

Protein-losing enteropathy (E) is defined as the severe loss of proteins via the gastrointestinal tract. The underlying pathophysiology may relate to mucosal disease, lymphatic obstruction or cell death leading to increased permeability to proteins. If more proteins are lost than synthesized in the body, hypoproteinaemia will result. Causes include Crohn's disease, coeliac disease and rarely, Menetrier's disease. Hypoproteinaemia secondary to such conditions results in fewer immunoglobulins being formed which diminishes the adaptive immune response.

Di George's syndrome (H) is caused by an embryological abnormality in the third and fourth branchial arches (pharyngeal pouches) due to a

22q11 deletion. The result is an absent or hypoplastic thymus, as well as a deficiency in T cells. There is a reduction or absence of CD4+ and CD8+ T cells as well as decreased production of IgG and IgA. B cell and IgM levels are normal. The features of Di George's syndrome can be remembered by the mnemonic 'CATCH': cardiac abnormalities, atresia (oesophageal), thymic aplasia, cleft palate and hypocalcaemia.

Hyper IgM syndrome (C) is caused by a mutation in the CD40 ligand on T cells leading to impaired communication with B cells. B cells are unable to class-switch and therefore only produce IgM (leading to increased levels in the blood) and patients are deficient in IgA, IgG and IgE.

In leukocyte adhesion deficiency (LAD; D) neutrophils are formed but cannot exit the blood stream due to a deficit in leukocyte adhesion molecules resulting in reduced neutrophil chemotaxis. The neutrophil count is very high due to persistence in the blood stream. NBT test is positive.

Cyclic neutropenia (F) is an autosomal dominant condition caused by a mutation in the neutrophil elastase gene (*ELA2*). Neutropenia occurs every 3 weeks and lasts approximately 6 days at a time.

AIDS (I) is characterized by a reduced CD4+ T-cell count. AIDS patients are at greater risk of developing opportunistic infections such as *Pneumocystis jerovicci*.

2. Immunodeficiency (2)

ANSWERS: 1) H 2) B 3) F 4) D 5) A

Wiskott–Aldrich syndrome (WAS; H) is an X-linked condition which is caused by a mutation in the *WASp* gene; the WAS protein is expressed in developing haematopoietic stem cells. WAS is linked to the development of lymphomas, thrombocytopenia and eczema. Clinical features include easy bruising, nose bleeds and gastrointestinal bleeds secondary to thrombocytopenia. Recurrent bacterial infections also result. Blood tests reveal a reduced IgM level and raised IgA and IgE levels. IgG levels may be normal, reduced or elevated.

Common variable immunodeficiency (CVID; B) presents in adulthood. A mutation of MHC III causes aberrant class switching, increasing the risk of lymphoma and granulomas. Patients with CVID also have a predisposition to developing autoimmune diseases. Recurrent infections caused by *Haemophilus influenzae* and *Streptococcus pneumoniae* are common. Clinical sequelae include bronchiectasis and sinusitis. Blood tests reveal a reduced B-cell count, a normal/reduced IgM level and decreased levels of IgA, IgG and IgE.

Chronic granulomatous disease (F) is an X-linked disorder causing deficiency of NADPH oxidase. As a result, neutrophils cannot produce the respiratory burst required to clear pathogens. The disease is characterized by chronic inflammation with non-caseating granulomas. Clinical features include recurrent skin infections (bacterial) as well as recurrent fungal infections. The disease is usually detected by the age of 5 and is diagnosed using the nitro-blue-tetrazolium (NBT) test, which remains colourless due to NADPH deficiency (if NADPH is present the solution turns blue). The patient will have a normal neutrophil count as there is no defect in neutrophil production.

Bare lymphocyte syndrome (D) is caused by either deficiency in MHC I (type 1; all T cells become CD4+ T cells) or MHC II (type 2; all T cells become CD8+ T cells). Clinical manifestations include sclerosing cholangitis with hepatomegaly and jaundice.

Selective IgA deficiency (**F**): IgA specifically provides mucosal immunity, primarily to the respiratory and gastrointestinal systems. Selective IgA deficiency results from a genetic inability to produce IgA and is characterized by recurrent mild respiratory and gastrointestinal infections. Patients with selective IgA deficiency are also at risk of anaphylaxis to blood transfusions due to the presence of donor IgA. This occurs especially after a second transfusion; antibodies having been created against IgA during the primary transfusion. Selective IgA deficiency is also linked to autoimmune diseases such as rheumatoid arthritis, systemic lupus erythematosus and coeliac disease.

Nephrotic syndrome (C) is characterized by renal dysfunction leading to large amounts of protein leaking from the blood to the urine. Consequently, immunoglobulins will be lost as they are passed into the urine, leading to increased risk of infection by encapsulated bacteria.

Sickle cell anaemia (E) leads to hyposplenism; poor spleen function predisposes to encapsulated bacterial infections, for example *Streptococcus pneumoniae*. Such patients are therefore required to take necessary vaccinations and antibiotic prophylaxis.

Reticular dysgenesis (G) is characterized by the absolute deficiency in both granulocytes and lymphocytes, leading to severe sepsis only a few days after birth.

Interferon-gamma receptor deficiency (I) leads to the reduced activation of macrophages and consequently, granulomas cannot form. This results in increased susceptibility to intracellular infections such as *Mycobacterium tuberculosis* and *Salmonella* spp.

3. Transplantation

ANSWERS: 1) A 2) F 3) C 4) B 5) D

HLA-matching (tissue typing; A) is a preventative method of limiting the risk of organ transplant rejection. It is impractical to match all HLA loci and hence tissue typing focuses on major HLA antigens such as HLA-A and HLA-B. HLA-DR is also now routinely typed due to its role in activating recipient's T-helper cells. HLA-matching greatly reduces the chance of hyperacute rejection caused by the presence of pre-formed antibodies against the graft. Pre-formed antibodies may occur as a result of previous blood transfusion or pregnancy.

OKT3 (muromonab-CD3; F) is a mouse monoclonal antibody targeted at the human CD3 molecule used to treat rejection episodes in patients who have undergone allograft transplantation. Administration of the antibody efficiently clears T cells from the recipient's circulation, T cells being the major mediator of acute organ rejection. Primary indications include the acute corticosteroid-resistant rejection of renal, heart and liver transplants. Anaphylaxis can result given a murine protein is introduced to the recipient. OKT3 can also bind to CD3 on T cells, stimulating the release of TNF-α and IFN-γ causing cytokine release syndrome, which if severe, can be fatal.

Cyclosporine A (C) is an important immunosuppressive agent in the organ transplant arena, which inhibits the protein phosphatase calcineurin. This in turn inhibits IL-2 secretion from T cells, a cytokine which stimulates T cell proliferation. Another proposed mechanism of action involves the stimulation of TGF-β production. TGF-β is a growth-inhibitory cytokine, the production of T cells is reduced, hence minimizing organ rejection. Adverse effects include nephrotoxicity, hepatotoxicity, diarrhoea and pancreatitis. On examination, patients taking cyclosporine A may have gum hyperplasia.

Corticosteroids (B) are used as an immunosuppressive agent in both the prevention and treatment of transplant rejection. Corticosteroids inhibit phospholipase A2 thereby blocking prostaglandin formation as well as a series of inflammatory mediators. The immunosuppressive effects of corticosteroids are numerous and include reducing the number of circulating B cells, inhibiting monocyte trafficking, inhibiting T-cell proliferation and reducing the expression of a number of cytokines, for example, IL-1, IL-2 and TNF-α. Prednisolone is used prophylactically before transplantation to prevent rejection; methylprednisolone is used in the treatment of rejection. Side effects are frequent, however, and include osteoporosis, diabetes mellitus and hypertension.

Azathioprine (D) is an antimetabolite agent used in immunosuppressive therapy. Azathioprine is metabolized into 6-mercaptopurine (6-MP), a purine analogue that prevents DNA synthesis, thereby inhibiting the proliferation of cells; lymphocytes are most affected. Antigen presenting cells present non-self proteins (from the allograft) to T cells which in turn produce IL-2 to stimulate T-cell proliferation. However, 6-MP inhibits this proliferation and so the reaction between T cells and the allograft is minimized. Important side effects include hepatotoxicity, hypersensitivity reactions and myelosuppression.

Sirolimus (rapamycin; E) inhibits T-cell proliferation by binding to FK-binding protein-1A (FKBP-1A). Its advantage lies in its low nephrotoxicity in comparison to other immunosuppressive agents.

Tacrolimus (H) is a calcineurin inhibitor that inhibits T-cell proliferation by binding to FKBP-1A. In contrast to sirolimus, which affects T-lymphocyte clonal proliferation, tacrolimus targets T-cell activation.

IL-2 receptor antibody (daclizumab; G) targets the CD25 of IL-2 receptors expressed on the surface of activated T cells. It is especially used in kidney transplant patients to prevent organ rejection.

Anti-lymphocyte globulin (ATG; I) is used in the treatment of allograft rejection. Lymphocytes are injected into horses or rabbits most commonly, to produce anti-lymphocyte antibodies which are subsequently separated and purified.

4. Autoimmune antibodies (1)

ANSWERS: 1) D 2) A 3) C 4) E 5) I

Anti-cyclic citrullinated protein (anti-CCP; D) antibody is associated with rheumatoid arthritis. The antibody is directed at the filament aggregating protein, filaggrin. Rheumatoid arthritis is a chronic systemic autoimmune disease that results in a symmetrical deforming polyarthritis. Clinical features include deformities of the hands (Boutonierre's deformity, swan-neck deformity, Z-thumb and ulnar deviation of the fingers). The proximal interphalangeal joints are affected more than the distal interphalangeal joints. Extra-articular manifestations include pulmonary fibrosis, pericardial effusion, rheumatoid nodules and splenomegaly (Felty's syndrome). Rheumatoid factor is another antibody measured in the investigation of rheumatoid arthritis, but is less sensitive and specific in comparison to anti-CCP.

Anti-smooth muscle (A) antibody (anti-SMA) suggests the diagnosis of autoimmune hepatitis, but can also be present in patients with primary sclerosing cholangitis. Autoimmune hepatitis is characterized by inflammation, hepatocellular necrosis, fibrosis, with cirrhosis in severe cases. Diagnosis requires histological confirmation together with the presence of autoantibodies which may either be non-organ or liver-specific. Autoimmune hepatitis is classified into two major groups depending on the autoantibody present: type 1 is defined by the presence of anti-SMA and/or anti-nuclear antibody, whilst type 2 is characterized by the presence of anti-liver/kidney microsomal-1 antibody (anti-LKM-1).

Anti-Jo1 (C) antibody is present in patients with dermatomyositis. Dermatomyositis is characterized by autoimmune inflammation of muscle fibres and skin. Clinical features include a heliotrope rash around the eyes, Gottron's papules on the dorsum of finger joints as well as weakness of the proximal limb muscles which causes difficulty in climbing stairs and rising from a chair. Dermatomyositis is commonly associated with SLE and scleroderma. The presence of anti-Jo1 in dermatomyositis typically suggests interstitial pulmonary involvement. Blood tests reveal an increased ESR and raised creatine kinase level.

Anti-centromere (E) antibody is associated with limited systemic scleroderma (CREST syndrome). CREST syndrome is characterized by calcinosis, Reynaud's syndrome, oesophageal dysmotility, sclerodactyly and telangiectasia. The pathophysiology is defined by endothelial injury and chronic fibrosis (orchestrated by PDGF and TGF-β). Blood investigations will reveal a raised ESR, anaemia and hypergammaglobulinaemia. Anti-centromere antibodies detected in the presence of primary biliary cirrhosis indicate portal hypertension.

Anti-topoisomerase (I) antibody is characteristic of diffuse systemic scleroderma. Diffuse systemic scleroderma shares some features of limited systemic scleroderma, however, it is more aggressive in its course, affecting large areas of the skin as well as involving the kidneys, heart and lungs. The pathogenesis of diffuse systemic scleroderma is similar to that of limited systemic scleroderma. The presence of anti-topoisomerase antibodies in diffuse systemic sclerosis is associated with pulmonary interstitial fibrosis.

p-ANCA (perinuclear anti-neutrophil cytoplasmic antibodies; B) is a feature of Churg–Strauss syndrome, a medium and small-vessel autoimmune vasculitis. Blood vessels of the lungs, gastrointestinal system and peripheral nerves are most commonly affected.

Anti-double stranded DNA (F) antibodies are characteristic of systemic lupus erythematosus; levels may be used to monitor disease activity.

Anti-parietal cell (G) antibodies are a feature of pernicious anaemia and lead to parietal cell loss and hence reduced intrinsic factor production; this causes reduced vitamin B_{12} absorption.

Anti-thyroid stimulating hormone (anti-TSH; H) antibodies are found in Graves' disease. Anti-TSH antibodies bind to TSH receptors on the thyroid gland stimulating production of thyroxine.

5. Autoimmune antibodies (2)

ANSWERS: 1) F 2) A 3) E 4) B 5) I

Anti-Ro (anti-SS-A; F) and Anti-La (anti-SS-B) antibodies are present in approximately 50 per cent of patients with Sjögren's syndrome, as well as a lower proportion of patients with systemic lupus erythematosus. Sjögren's syndrome is characterized by the destruction of the epithelial cells of exocrine glands. Salivary gland biopsy reveals an infiltrate of T and B cells; CD4+ T cells are most prominent. Clinical features include dryness of the eyes (confirmed by Schirmer's test) and mouth, parotid swelling, fatigue, arthralgia and myalgia. Blood tests will demonstrate a raised ESR and occasionally a mild anaemia.

Anti-mitochondrial (A) antibodies are associated with primary biliary cirrhosis (PBC), and are immunoglobulins against mitochondria in cells of the liver. PBC is an autoimmune disease of unknown cause characterized by lymphocytic destruction of the bile canaliculi of the liver; build-up of bile leads to fibrosis and eventually cirrhosis. Clinical features include pruritis (increased bile acids in circulation) as well as the effects of reduced absorption of fat soluble vitamins (vitamin D, osteomalacia; vitamin K, bruising; vitamin A, blindness).

Anti-glutamic acid decarboxylase (anti-GAD; E) antibody is present in patients with type 1 diabetes mellitus (T1DM). The pathogenesis of T1DM involves the autoimmune destruction of β-cells in the islets of Langerhans in the pancreas. β-Cells are the primary storage site for insulin in the body, and so destruction of these cells leads to diminished insulin release and hyperglycaemia. GAD is an enzyme responsible for the conversion of glutamate to GABA; GABA is the neurotransmitter involved in the release of insulin from β-cells. Presenting features of T1DM include polyuria, polydipsia and weight loss.

c-ANCA (cytoplasmic anti-neutrophil cytoplasmic antibodies; B) are common in patients with Wegener's granulamatosis, a vasculitic disease that is in severe cases life threatening. c-ANCA is directed towards proteinase 3 (PR3) within the neutrophil cytoplasm. Wegner's granulamatosis primarily affects the nose (saddle-nose deformity due to perforated septum; epistaxis), lungs (pulmonary haemorrhage) and kidneys (glomerulonephritis). Due to its fulminant course, patients require life-long immunosuppression, usually with corticosteroids.

Anti-endomysium (I) is characteristic of coeliac disease, autoimmune disease of the small intestine that results from an immune reaction to gliadin (peptide found in wheat, barley and rye). The endomysium is in fact related to muscle fibres; although muscle fibres are not affected in coeliac disease, anti-endomysial antibodies are useful in the diagnosis of coeliac disease. Clinical features include diarrhoea, abdominal pain and mouth ulcers. Other autoantibodies that are used in the diagnosis of coeliac disease are anti-tissue transglutaminase antibody and anti-gliadin antibodies.

Anti-cardiolipin (C) antibody, a form of anti-mitochondrial antibody, is a feature of several diseases including antiphospholipid syndrome, systemic lupus erythematosus and syphilis

Anti-robinucleoprotein (anti-RNP; D) is associated with mixed connective tissue disease (MCTD), an overlap syndrome which has features of various connective tissue disorders combined.

Anti-nuclear (G) antibody is directed against the cell nucleus in several autoimmune diseases. It is indicative of systemic lupus erythematosus but also occurs in Sjögren's syndrome, autoimmune hepatitis and dermatopolymyositis.

Anti-intrinsic factor (H) is characteristic of pernicious anaemia. Intrinsic factor (produced by gastric parietal cells) is physiologically essential for the absorption of vitamin B_{12}.

6. Hypersensitivity (1)

ANSWERS: 1) I 2) B 3) G 4) E 5) H

Pancreatic β-cell proteins (I) are the antigenic target for cytotoxic CD8+ T cells in type 1 diabetes mellitus (T1DM). T1DM is a type IV hypersensitivity reaction since it is T-cell mediated; the pathogenesis involves the destruction of β-cells in the islets of Langerhans in the pancreas by CD8+ T cells. β-cells are the storage site for insulin in the body, and so destruction of these cells leads to diminished insulin release and hyperglycaemia. Presenting features of T1DM include polyuria, polydipsia and weight loss. Antibodies to glutamate decarboxylase (GAD) as well as islet cells may also circulate in T1DM patients.

Ingestion of nuts (B) can lead to a type I hypersensitivity, characterized by a strong CD4+ Th2 response which causes release of IL-4 and IL-13. This causes B cells to produce IgE, which in turn binds to Fc receptors on mast cells. On re-exposure to the allergen the IgE on mast cells cross-links, with resultant mast cell degranulation (release of histamine and tryptases) and arachidonic acid metabolism (producing leukotrienes and prostaglandins). Clinical features include erythema, rhinitis, urticaria, angio-oedema, bronchoconstriction and in severe cases anaphylactic shock.

Chronic exposure to mouldy hay (G) is the cause of farmer's lung, an example of an extrinsic allergic alveolitis. Actinomycetes are the most common pathogen found in hay dust, which are subsequently inhaled. Inhalation over prolonged periods of time leads to immune complex formation as antibodies combine with the inhaled allergen (type III hypersensitivity reaction); the immune complexes are deposited in the walls of the alveoli. Chronic exposure leads to pulmonary fibrosis, with associated shortness of breath, cyanosis and cor pulmonale.

Type IV collagen (E), is the target of soluble IgG in Goodpasture's disease (type II hypersensitivity reaction). Type IV collagen is present in the glomerular basement membrane and lung basement membrane. Pulmonary features include cough, dyspnoea and haemoptysis; renal features include haematuria, acute renal failure and nephrotic syndrome. Investigations reveal the presence of anti-type IV collagen antibodies in the circulation; immunofluorescence will show linear deposition of IgG along the glomerular basement membrane.

Grass pollen (H) may cause allergic rhinitis via a type I hypersensitivity reaction. The allergen triggers IgE production, which bind to the cell surface of mast cells and basophils. On repeated exposure to pollen, the mast cells degranulate, releasing histamine as well as other mediators. This results in the characteristic features of allergic rhinitis such as a runny nose, sneezing, itchiness, watery eyes and nasal congestion.

The TSH receptor (A) is a target for soluble anti-TSH antibodies in Graves' disease, a type II hypersensitivity reaction.

DNA (C) is the target of circulating anti-double stranded DNA antibodies in systemic lupus erythematosus; it is therefore an example of a type III hypersensitivity reaction.

Nickel (D) is a hapten and binds with skin proteins. It is detected by Langerhan's antigen presenting cells in the skin causing a type IV hypersensitivity reaction in contact dermatitis.

Chlamydia trachomatis (F) may trigger a type III hypersensitivity reaction causing a reactive arthritis. As this phenomenon is autoimmune, synovial fluid cultures are negative.

7. Hypersensitivity (2)

ANSWERS: 1) F 2) C 3) D 4) B 5) E

Allergy to peanuts (F) causes a spectrum of clinical manifestations, from mild food allergy to severe anaphylaxis. The underlying pathogenesis is the binding of the allergen to IgE causing mast cell degranulation and histamine release (a potent vasodilator and bronchoconstrictor). In anaphylaxis, this release of histamine occurs throughout the body, leading to the clinical features of shortness of breath, wheeze, swollen lips and signs of shock. Anaphylaxis is a medical emergency and requires prompt administration of intramuscular adrenaline and urgent transfer to a hospital.

Myelin basic protein (C) and proteolipid protein are oligodendrocyte proteins implicated in the pathogenesis of multiple sclerosis. Multiple sclerosis (MS) is a demyelinating disease in which the myelin sheaths surrounding neurons of the brain and spinal cord are destroyed. Associated with the disease process is the antigenic stimulation of CD4+ T cells which in turn activate CD8+ cytotoxic T cells and macrophages; these are directed at oligodendrocyte proteins (type IV hypersensitivity reaction) causing destruction of oligodendrocytes and myelin. Clinical features of MS include optic neuritis, urinary/bowel incontinence, weakness of the arms/legs and dysphagia.

Rhesus antigens (D) are found on the surface of erythrocytes. The rhesus (Rh) blood group system is clinically the most important after the ABO system; the most commonly used Rh antigen is the D antigen, signifying whether a patient is Rh positive or negative. Antibodies directed against the Rh antigen results in autoimmune haemolytic anaemia (AIHA; type II hypersensitivity reaction). Most commonly the cause is idiopathic, however, chronic lymphocytic leukaemia, systemic lupus erythematosus and drugs (methyldopa and penicillin) can trigger AIHA. Direct antiglobulin test is positive.

HBsAg (B) may be associated with the development of polyarteritis nodosa (PAN), a vasculitis of small and medium sized vessels. Immune complexes (type III hypersensitivity reaction) are deposited within such vessels leading to fibrinoid necrosis and neutrophil infiltration; as a result the vessel walls weaken and there is aneurysm development. Investigations will reveal a raised ESR, CRP and immunoglobulin level. pANCA is also associated with PAN. Angiogram will reveal multiple aneurysms. Corticosteroids and cytotoxic agents are required to control disease progression.

Glycoprotein IIb–IIIa (E) on the surface of platelets is the target for IgG autoantibodies (type II hypersensitivity reaction) in autoimmune thrombocytopenic purpura (AITP). IgG directed at platelets makes them more susceptible to destruction by splenic macrophages and as a result the platelet count in affected individuals will be very low. Symptoms depend upon the platelet count: <20 000/μL causes bleeding of the gums and epistaxis for example; <10 000/μL may cause spontaneous bleeding. Secondary causes of AITP include systemic lupus erythematosus and antiphospholipid syndrome.

Stony fruits (A) are associated with oral allergy syndrome (type I hypersensitivity reaction; OAS). In patients sensitized to pollen, IgE cross-reacts with a food substance (usually stony fruit) which has been ingested causing release of histamine from mast cells resulting in local inflammation.

Proteins in antiserum (G) are the cause of serum sickness, a self-limiting condition that occurs when antiserum derived from a non-human animal source is injected intravenously, resulting in immune complex hypersensitivity (type III hypersensitivity reaction).

Synovial membrane antigens (H) are the target for T cells in rheumatoid arthritis (type IV hypersensitivity reaction).

The acetylcholine receptor (I) is the target for autoantibodies in myasthenia gravis (type II hypersensitivity reaction).

8. Immune-based therapies

ANSWERS: 1) A 2) D 3) B 4) G 5) I

Cyclophosphamide (A) is an alkylating agent, attaching an alkyl group to the guanine base of DNA. This causes damage to the DNA structure and therefore prevents cell replication; cyclophosphamide affects B-cell replication more than T cells. Indications include multisystem connective tissue disease and vasculitis such as systemic lupus erythematosus and Wegner's granulomatosis. Cyclophosphamide also has a role in treating cancers such as leukaemia and lymphoma. Complications of therapy include bone marrow suppression, hair loss and it has carcinogenic properties which may cause transitional cell carcinoma of the bladder.

Abatacept (D) is a CTLA4–immunoglobulin fusion protein indicated in the treatment of rheumatoid arthritis (disease which has been resistant to treatment with disease modifying drugs). Abatacept prevents antigen presenting cells from delivering a co-stimulatory signal to T cells in order to activate them; this is achieved by abatacept binding with high affinity to the B7 protein (CD80 and CD86) on the cell surface of APCs. Side effects include increased risk of infection from TB, hepatitis B virus and hepatitis C virus.

Mycophenolate mofetil (B) is the prodrug of mycophenolic acid which inhibits inosine monophosphate dehydrogenase (IMPDH), an enzyme required in guanine synthesis; impaired guanine synthesis reduces the proliferation of both T and B cells, but T cells are affected to a greater extent. Mycophenolate mofetil is indicated as an immunosuppressive agent in transplant patients as well as an alternative to cyclophosphamide in the treatment of autoimmune diseases and vasculitides. Side effects include bone marrow suppression (particularly low white blood cells and platelets) as well as herpes virus reactivation.

Infliximab (G) is a TNF-α antagonist used in the treatment of rheumatoid arthritis, ankylosing spondylitis, Crohn's disease and psoriasis. Infliximab has a high affinity for TNF-α but does not bind to TNF-β. TNF-α has the physiological role of inducing pro-inflammatory cytokines as well as promoting leukocyte migration and endothelial adhesion. Toxicity may result in reduced protection against infection from TB, hepatitis B virus and hepatitis C virus, a lupus-like condition, demyelination and malignancy.

Denosumab (I) is an antibody directed towards the RANK ligand in bones. Osteoblasts are responsible for bone formation, whilst osteoclasts (which contain the cell surface receptor RANK) break down bone. Inhibition of RANK by denosumab therefore inhibits osteoclast function and differentiation, thereby preventing the breakdown of bone. Denosumab is indicated in the treatment of osteoporosis but is also used in the management of multiple myeloma and bone metastases. Toxicity can predispose to respiratory and urinary tract infections.

Basiliximab (C) is an antibody directed towards IL-2α receptor (CD25) which causes reduction in T-cell proliferation. It is used as a prophylactic treatment of allograft rejection.

Rituximab (E) is a CD20 monoclonal antibody which causes reduced proliferation of B cells. It is indicated in the treatment of lymphoma, rheumatoid arthritis and systemic lupus erythematosus.

Efalizumab (F) is an antibody against CD11a on T cells; it inhibits the migration of T cells. It is indicated in the treatment of psoriasis.

Ustekinumab (H) is an antibody to the p40 subunit of IL-12 and IL-23 thereby preventing T-cell and natural-killer cell activation. It is used in the treatment of psoriatic arthritis.

9. Nephritic disorders

ANSWERS: 1) B 2) E 3) H 4) G 5) A

Wegener's granulamatosis (B) is a systemic vasculitis characterized clinically by epistaxis, haemoptysis and haematuria. Wegener's granulomatosis is defined by the presence of cytoplasmic anti-neutrophil cytoplasmic antibodies (cANCA). c-ANCA is directed towards proteinase 3 (PR3), an enzyme normally present within the cytoplasm of neutrophils. It is proposed that an infection is the trigger for the disease, which causes circulating neutrophils to become adherent to the endothelium and upregulation of PR3 on the cell surface. Vasculitis is mediated by both direct effect of PR3 on the endothelium as well as cANCA–PR3 immune complex deposition.

IgA nephropathy (Berger's disease; E) is the most common cause of glomerunephritis in the developed world. The condition occurs after a gastrointestinal or upper respiratory infection; potential offenders are postulated to include *Haemophilus influenzae*, hepatitis B virus and cytomegalovirus. Antigenic targets for IgA are thought to include collagen, fibronectin and laminin. Characteristically there is mesangial proliferation with deposition of IgA together with alternative pathway factors C3 and properdin. Blood tests will reveal a raised IgA level. Henoch–Schonlein purpura has a similar pathogenesis to IgA nephropathy but presents in children and has extra-renal clinical features.

Post-streptococcal glomerulonephritis (H) is usually caused by a preceding group A β haemolytic streptococcus pharyngitis. Anti-streptolysin O titre (ASOT) will be raised. Pathological hallmarks of post-streptococcal glomerulonephritis include diffuse hypercellularity and diffuse swelling of the mesangium and glomerular capillaries. Influx of neutrophils and macrophages may reveal crescent formation on histology. Direct immunofluorescence reveals the sub-epithelial deposition of IgG and C3. The condition usually subsides with supportive treatment, including antibiotic therapy to combat the outstanding infection.

Rapidly progressive glomerulonephritis (RPGN; G) is the most aggressive of all glomerulonephritides, which may cause end-stage renal failure over a period of days. The three sub-types include immune complex disease, pauci-immune disease and anti-glomerular basement membrane disease, all of which demonstrate crescent formation on biopsy (proliferation of macrophages and parietal epithelial cells). Immunofluoresence of IgG/C3 distinguishes between the three sub-types: immune complex disease is characterized by granular staining, pauci-immune disease shows absent/scant staining, while anti-glomerular basement membrane disease demonstrates linear staining.

Minimal change disease (A) is the most common cause of nephrotic syndrome in children. Triggers include a recent allergic reaction such as a bee sting (type I hypersensitivity reaction). Histological characteristics of renal biopsy specimens include a lack of structural change visible on light microscopy, while electron microscopy will demonstrate podocyte effacement. Steroids are the primary treatment modality, which lead to remission of disease in the vast majority of cases.

Microscopic polyangitis (C) is a small vessel vasculitis affecting the arterioles, venules and capillaries. This vasculitis is associated with focal necrotizing glomerulonephritis as well as the presence of perinuclear ANCA (p-ANCA) in the circulation directed towards cytoplasmic myeloperoxidase.

Lupus nephritis (D) is characterized by the deposition of IgG, IgM, IgA and C3 in the sub-endothelial segment of the glomerular basement membrane and in the mesangium.

Membranoproliferative glomerulonephritis (F) is defined by mesangial cell proliferation with thickening of the capillaries. Two types exist: type 1 in which there is classical and alternative complement pathway activation and type 2 that is associated with only alternative pathway activation.

Goodpasture's syndrome (I) is characterized by the presence of anti-glomerular basement membrane proteins, specifically targeting type IV collagen. Pulmonary features include cough, dyspnoea and haemoptysis; renal features include haematuria, acute renal failure and nephrotic syndrome.

10. Diagnostic immunology

ANSWERS: 1) H – 2) F – 3) I – 4) G – 5) B

Western blot (H) is a technique used to detect specific proteins in a patient's serum; it is used in the confirmatory HIV test to detect specific antibodies to HIV. The first step is to separate native proteins by gel electrophoresis. The proteins are subsequently transferred to a membrane on which specific antibodies present in the serum may bind to HIV proteins produced using recombinant DNA. Unbound antibodies are washed away. Enzyme-linked antibodies are then added; these determine to which protein the subject has antibodies.

Kveim test (F) is an investigation used to diagnose sarcoidosis. A sample of spleen from a patient with known sarcoid is injected intradermally into a suspected patient. A positive test is evidenced by the presence of non-caseating granuloma formation on biopsy of the site, 4–6 weeks after the initial injection. Although not used in the UK due to infection concerns (especially bovine spongiform encephalopathy), it is still available in many countries.

Direct antiglobulin test (DAT; I) also known as direct Coombs test, is the investigation of choice for the diagnosis of autoimmune haemolytic anaemia (AIHA). Causes of AIHA include lymphoproliferative disorders, drugs (penicillin) and autoimmune diseases (SLE). The test involves the separation of RBCs from the serum which is subsequently incubated with anti-human globulin. In the case of AIHA, the anti-human globulin will agglutinate the RBCs, which is visualized as clumping of the cells.

Skin prick test (G) is the gold standard for investigating such type I hypersensitivity reactions. The test involves a few drops of purified allergen being pricked onto the skin. Allergens which are tested for include foods, dust mites, pollen and dust. A positive test is indicated by wheal formation, caused by cross-linking of IgE on the mast cell surface leading to histamine release.

Immunofluorescence (B) is an immunological technique used in conjunction with fluorescence microscope. Fluorophores (fluorescent chemical compounds) attached to specific antibodies are directed at antigens found within a biological specimen, most commonly a biopsy sample, to visualize patterns of staining. For example, in Henoch–Schönlein purpura, anti-IgA antibody will demonstrate IgA deposits in the capillary walls of the specimen. Immunofluorescence may be direct (use of a single antibody bound to a single fluorophore) or indirect (secondary antibody carrying the fluorophore binds to the primary antibody).

Histocompatibility testing (A) is a preventative method of limiting the risk of organ transplant rejection. Major HLA antigens such as HLA-A and HLA-B are matched between donor and recipient.

Latex fixation test (C) is an agglutination technique used in the detection of antibodies. It is used in the detection of rheumatoid factor.

Radioallergosorbent test (D) is a radioimmunoassay test for a variety of potential allergens. The test involves the use of radio-labelled anti-human IgE; the antibody is added, which attaches to the IgE bound to the insoluble allergen.

Patch testing (E) is a useful test to determine the causative allergen in contact dermatitis. A patch is prepared with small amounts of allergens; a positive test may be demonstrated by a spectrum of responses, from faint erythema to the presence of bullae.

SECTION 6: IMMUNOLOGY SBAs

Questions

Answers

QUESTIONS

1. Innate immunity (1): Physical barriers

A 10-year-old boy is seen by a paediatrician after suffering recurrent chest infections. His mother reports purulent sputum production and cough for the previous 2 years. Genetic testing reveals the child has a ΔF508 mutation on chromosome 7. Which physical barrier to infection is most likely to be affected by the child's condition?

A   Skin
B   Gastric acid
C   Mucociliary clearance
D   Tears
E   Gut flora

2. Innate immunity (2): Complement investigations

A 62-year-old woman sees her GP for a regular check-up. On examination, she has notable deformities of her hands, including swan-neck and Boutonniere deformities of her fingers. Blood tests reveal a raised CRP. Which of the following investigation results will most likely feature?

A   Reduced AH50 and normal CH50
B   Reduced C1 inhibitor
C   Reduced C3 and C4
D   Reduced C3 and normal C4
E   High CH50

3. Innate immunity (3): Cellular response

A 25-year-old woman, who has a history of allergy to nuts, is taken to accident and emergency after eating a dessert containing peanuts. She has an evident wheeze with an increased respiratory rate, swelling of her lips and itchy skin. Which cell of the innate immune system is most likely to be responsible for her symptoms?

A   Natural-killer cells
B   Dendritic cells
C   Eosinophils
D   Mast cells
E   Neutrophils

4. Adaptive immunity: Antibodies

A 35-year-old man develops diarrhoea with fever and malaise 24 hours after eating a take-away meal. Stool cultures reveal the source of the infection is *Salmonella* spp. Which antibody is responsible for protecting against gastrointestinal infections?

A   IgA
B   IgD
C   IgG
D   IgM
E   IgE

5. Human leukocyte antigen

A 23-year-old man presents to his GP with recent onset diarrhoea, fatigue and weight loss. The patient suggests that his symptoms are worsened after eating bread or rice. Which human leukocyte antigen is most likely to be associated with his disease process?

A   HLA B27
B   HLA DR2
C   HLA DR3
D   HLA DR4
E   HLA DQ2

6. Immune tolerance

A 3-year-old Afro-Caribbean boy is referred to a paediatrician after concerns about his recurrent chest infections. The child's hair slowly fell out and there is evidence of depigmentation of his skin. Blood tests reveal hypocalcaemia and high TSH levels. Which component of the immune tolerance system is likely to be dysfunctional?

A   Regulatory T cell
B   TGF-β
C   Autoimmune regulator
D   Dendritic cells
E   IL-10

7. Mechanisms of autoimmunity

A 34-year-old man presents to his GP with fever, joint pain and a rash on his trunk. On examination, a new murmur is auscultated. Blood investigations reveal a raised anti-streptolysin O titre. What is the most likely mechanism for this disease process?

A   Defective immunoregulation
B   Molecular mimicry
C   T-cell bypass
D   Release of hidden self antigens
E   Cytokines

8. Primary immunodeficiency (1): Phagocyte deficiency

A 2-year-old girl is seen by an infectious disease paediatrician after suffering recurrent infections since she was born. Her neutrophil count is normal. A nitro-blue-tetrazolium (NBT) test is performed, which remains colourless. What is the diagnosis?

A   Kostmann syndrome
B   Cyclic neutropenia
C   Leukocyte adhesion deficiency
D   Chronic granulomatous disease
E   Von Gierke's disease

9. Primary immunodeficiency (2): Complement deficiency

A 29-year-old woman presents to her GP with recent onset joint pain and tired-ness. On examination she has a malar rash. Further blood tests reveal she is anti-nuclear antibody and anti-double stranded DNA positive. Which component of the complement system is she most likely to be deficient in?

A   C3
B   C4
C   C6
D   C9
E   C1 inhibitor

10. Primary immunodeficiency (3): T-cell deficiency

A 4-year-old girl is seen by a paediatrician to investigate possible developmental delay and learning difficulties. Initial blood tests reveal hypocalcaemia, reduced CD4+ and CD8+ T-cell counts as well as deficiency in IgG and IgA. FISH analy-sis reveals the child has a deletion of 22q11. What is the diagnosis?

A   Di George's syndrome
B   Severe combined immunodeficiency
C   Bare lymphocyte syndrome
D   Wiskott–Aldrich syndrome
E   Interferon-gamma receptor deficiency

11. Primary immunodeficiency (4): B-cell deficiency

A 24-year-old man with a history of coeliac disease visits his GP after several bouts of chest and gastrointestinal infections in the past few years. Although the infections are mild, the patient is worried about the cause. What is the diagnosis?

A   Severe combined immunodeficiency
B   Bruton's agammaglobulinaemia
C   Hyper IgM syndrome
D   Selective IgA deficiency
E   Common variable immunodeficiency

12. Secondary immunodeficiency

A 40-year-old man is referred to an infectious disease specialist after he is admitted to hospital with *Pneumocystis jerovicci* pneumonia. On examination the patient also has multiple Kaposi's sarcoma lesions on his chest and abdomen. What is the most likely diagnosis?

A   Inflammatory bowel disease
B   Hyposplenism
C   Nephrotic syndrome
D   AIDS
E   Prematurity

13. Hypersensitivity reactions (1)

A 12-year-old girl has developed a runny nose, itchy eyes and nasal congestion during the summer months for the past 4 years. She is prescribed anti-histamines to help her symptoms. Which of the following cells is responsible for the initial encounter with the allergen?

A   Mast cell
B   B cell
C   Macrophage
D   TH1 cell
E   TH2 cell

14. Hypersensitivity reactions (2)

A 14-year-old girl with a history of eczema presents to accident and emergency with itching and tingling of her lips and tongue. The girl's lips are evidently swollen. All observations are normal. The doctor believes her condition is due to cross-reactivity of allergens. What is the most likely trigger for her allergy?

A   Penicillin
B   Eggs
C   Nickel
D   Dust mite
E   Fruit

15. Hypersensitivity reactions (3)

A 21-year-old woman is at a Thai restaurant, eating her main course when she suddenly develops shortness of breath, wheeze and swelling of her lips. The patient has a known peanut allergy. What is the most appropriate treatment in the first instance?

A   Allergen avoidance
B   Adrenaline
C   Oral anti-histamines
D   Doxepin
E   Nasal steroids

16. Hypersensitivity reactions (4)

A demanding mother takes her 6-year-old son to see the GP. She is concerned by his numerous allergies, including pollen and various foods. She is keen for her son to have allergy testing to determine the substances he is allergic to. Which of the following would be the best test for investigating allergy in this child?

A   Radioallergosorbent test
B   Skin prick test
C   Double-blind challenge
D   Serum tryptase levels
E   Total serum IgE

17. Hypersensitivity reactions (5)

A 56-year-old diabetic man is undergoing a kidney transplant as a result of chronic renal failure. After the operation, the man immediately develops fever and has no urine production. Background checks reveal there was an error in ABO matching of the donor and recipient; the donor's blood group was A, while the recipient's is O. Which of the following immune components is the first to initiate a response in this case?

A   Natural-killer cells
B   C1
C   Neutrophil
D   Mannose binding lectin
E   Macrophages

18. Hypersensitivity reactions (6)

A 54-year-old woman is referred to a dermatologist after developing blisters which she first noticed in her mouth but have now appeared on her right arm. On examination, Nikolsky's sign is positive and immunofluorescent staining demonstrates the presence of acantholytic cells. What is the most likely target for antibodies in this case?

A   Gastric parietal cell
B   Rhesus antigen
C   Acetylcholine receptor
D   Demoglein 1
E   M proteins on group A streptococci

19. Hypersensitivity reactions (7)

A 35-year-old woman presents to her GP with intermittent fatigue and joint pain which began 1 month previously. On examination, the patient has a malar rash on her face. Blood tests reveal anaemia. What is the most likely target for autoantibodies in this disease process?

A   Mouldy hay
B   *Chlamydia trachomatis*
C   DNA
D   Antiserum proteins
E   Hepatitis B virus antigen

20. Hypersensitivity reactions (8)

A 34-year-old woman notices an itchy and desquamating, erythematous rash on her wrist, which has emerged approximately 3 days after wearing a new brace-let. Which cytokine is the first to be released during the initial exposure to the allergen?

A   IL-10
B   IFN-γ
C   IL-2
D   TNF-α
E   IL-12

21. Hypersensitivity reactions (9)

A 56-year-old woman presents to her GP with blurry vision. On examination the woman has some bilateral weakness in her legs. The patient mentions that her vision seems to become more blurry just after she has had a bath. What is the most likely target in this disease process?

A   Pancreatic β-cell proteins
B   Nickel
C   Proteolipid protein
D   Synovial membrane proteins
E   Tuberculin

22. Transplantation and rejection (1)

A 40-year-old diabetic man is to undergo a kidney transplant as a consequence of stage 5 chronic kidney disease. The patient has an identical twin who is willing to donate a kidney, and has been HLA matched at all loci. Which term best describes the type of organ transplant proposed?

A   Autograft
B   Split transplant
C   Allograft
D   Isograft
E   Xenograft

23. Transplantation and rejection (2)

A 45-year-old man, who has blood group O, has undergone a liver transplant secondary to chronic alcoholic liver disease which has led to cirrhosis. One hour after the operation the patient develops a fever and pain in his right upper quadrant. It is soon realized that the donor had blood group B. Which of the following best describes the type of allograft rejection?

A   Hyperacute rejection
B   Acute cellular rejection
C   Chronic rejection
D   Acute vascular rejection
E   Graft-versus-host disease

24. Transplantation and rejection (3)

A 54-year-old man is to undergo a heart transplant as a result of severe heart failure. Prior to the operation the transplant team initiate an immunosuppressive regimen using a drug that inhibits calcinurin. Which of the following drugs is this most likely to be?

A   Cyclosporine A
B   OKT3
C   Azathioprine
D   Corticosteroids
E   Daclizumab

25. Human immunodeficiency virus

A 35-year-old man presents to the GP with fever, lymphadenopathy and a sore throat. Blood tests reveal a leukocytosis and Western blot is positive for HIV infection. Which of the following proteins is responsible for binding to CD4+ T cells to initiate infection?

A   Gag protein
B   gp120
C   gp41
D   Reverse transcriptase
E   CCR5

26. Vaccines

A 13-year-old boy is immunized against an acid-fast bacillus species after a negative Mantoux test. Which term best describes this form of vaccination that has been administered?

A   Live attenuated
B   Inactivated
C   Subunit
D   Conjugated
E   Passive immunity

27. Immune-based therapies (1)

A 3-year-old boy is referred to a paediatrician after experiencing recurrent chest infections. Blood tests demonstrate a reduced B-cell count as well as low IgA, IgM and IgG levels. Genetic testing reveals a defect in the BTK gene. What is the best therapeutic modality for this child?

A   IFN-α
B   IFN-β
C   IFN-γ
D   Intravenous IgG
E   Haematopoietic stem cell transplant

28. Immune-based therapies (2)

A 49-year-old woman with known rheumatoid arthritis is seen in the rheumatology clinic. She has been taking a medication over a long period of time which is used to control proliferation of her white blood cells. The patient explains that she has been feeling tired recently and has suffered with low moods. Routine blood tests reveal she has a macrocytic megaloblastic anaemia.

A   Cyclophosphamide
B   Mycophenolate mofetil
C   Azathioprine
D   Methotrexate
E   Cisplatin

29. Immune-based therapies (3)

A 45-year-old man, who suffers from myasthenia gravis' presents to accident and emergency with difficulty in breathing. Assisted ventilation is administered. Which of the following is the best option for the initial management of the patient's condition?

A   Ciclosporin
B   Tacrolimus
C   Rapamycin
D   Corticosteroids
E   Plasmapheresis

30. Immune-based therapies (4)

A 56-year-old man who is due to undergo a kidney transplant is seen by the transplant surgeon. The surgeon decides the patient should be started on an immunosuppressive agent before the surgery to prevent rejection of the organ. He prescribes a monoclonal antibody directed at the IL-2 receptor. Which drug has been prescribed?

A   Basiliximab
B   Abatacept
C   Rituximab
D   Natalizumab
E   Tocilizumab

31. Immune-based therapies (5)

A 45-year-old woman who has been diagnosed with rheumatoid arthritis is seen by a rheumatologist. The doctor wishes to start the patient on a fully humanized TNF-α monoclonal antibody to prevent progression of the disease.

A   Infliximab
B   Adalimumab
C   Etanercept
D   Ustekinumab
E   Denosumab

32. Rheumatic diseases (1)

A 52-year-old woman presents to her GP with dry eyes and mouth for the past few weeks. Despite using moisturizer the woman also complains of dry skin. The patient has a history of coeliac disease. Which of the following antibodies is most likely to be diagnostic for this patient's condition?

A   Anti-Jo1
B   Anti-cyclic citrullinated protein
C   Anti-centromere
D   Anti-topoisomerase
E   Anti-Ro

33. Rheumatic diseases (2)

A 42-year-old man is referred to the rheumatology outpatient clinic. The patient has been experiencing muscle and joint pain for the past month. On examination a heliotrope rash is observed on the patient's eyelids. Blood tests reveal the patient has circulating anti-nuclear antibodies. Which immunofluorescence staining pattern will be observed in this disease process?

A   Homogeneous
B   Nucleolar
C   Speckled
D   Peripheral
E   Kinetoplast

34. Rheumatic diseases (3)

A 34-year-old woman, diagnosed with *Chlamydia trachomatis* infection 2 weeks previously, sees her GP after experiencing a 1-week history of joint pain and blurry vision. She also complains of a burning sensation when she passes urine. Blood tests reveal a raised CRP and ESR. A joint aspirate of her knee is however sterile. What is the most likely diagnosis?

A   Ankylosing spondylitis
B   Reactive arthritis
C   Enteropathic arthritis
D   Psoriatic arthritis
E   Anterior uveitis

35. Rheumatic diseases (4)

A 54-year-old woman is referred to a rheumatologist. The patient states that she has noticed her fingers becoming very pale on cold days; when she heats her hands against the radiator, she notices her hands becoming red. She mentions that she has also had joint pains in her hands. On inspection, the patient has a small mouth. Which of the following factors is most responsible for fibrosis in this disease process?

A   von Willebrand factor
B   IL-2
C   TGF-β
D   TNF-α
E   Endothelin-1

36. Autoantibodies in type 1 diabetes mellitus

A 12-year-old boy is referred to the paediatric endocrinology outpatient clinic after experiencing recent onset weight loss, tiredness, frequency of urination and thirst. A fasting plasma glucose test reveal a level of 10.1 mmol/L and a diagnosis of type 1 diabetes mellitus is made. Which of the following autoantibodies has tyrosine phosphatase as the target antigen?

A   Islet cell surface antibody
B   Insulin autoantibody
C   Anti-glutamic acid decarboxylase antibody
D   Anti-IA-2 antibody
E   Islet cell antibody

37. Autoimmune thyroid disease

A 40-year-old woman presents to an endocrinologist with weight loss which has occurred over the past month, associated with a tremor, excessive sweating and a sense of feeling warm even on a cool day. On examination, the patient has exophthalmos and an irregularly irregular pulse. Which of the following autoantibodies is most likely to be responsible for the patient's disease process?

A   Anti-TSH receptor (stimulating)
B   Anti-TSH receptor (non-stimulating)
C   Anti-thyroid peroxidase
D   Anti-thyroglobulin
E   Thyroid growth stimulating antibody

38. Autoimmune polyendocrine syndromes

A 10-year-old boy is referred to a paediatrician after experiencing a seizure 1 week previously. Blood tests reveal that the seizure may have occurred secondary to low calcium levels; blood glucose levels are found to be high. The child was already being investigated for ptosis and difficulty with eye movements. What is the most likely diagnosis?

A   Hirata's disease
B   IPEX
C   Kearns–Sayre syndrome
D   POEMS syndrome
E   APECED syndrome type 1

39. Autoantibodies in liver disease

A 6-year-old girl presents to accident and emergency with severe haematemesis, endoscopy revealing the presence of oesophageal varices. Blood tests reveal liver function test derangement and a low level of circulating IgA. Subsequent liver biopsy demonstrates interface hepatitis. Treatment with steroids shows a poor response. Which autoantibody is most likely to be present in this child?

A   Anti-nuclear antibody
B   Anti-smooth muscle antibody
C   Anti-liver kidney microsomal antibody
D   Anti-mitochondrial antibody
E   Anti-HBs antibody

40. Autoimmune gastrointestinal disease

A 24-year-old man is referred to a gastroenterologist following episodes of diarrhoea in the last month. The patient also feels more tired than usual. The man undergoes a colonoscopy and jejunal biopsy results show villous hypertrophy with crypt hyperplasia and an increase in intraepithelial lymphocytes. Which of the following is associated with the greatest predisposition to developing this disease?

A   Dermatitis herpetiformis
B   Vitiligo
C   IgA deficiency
D   HLA DQ8
E   HLA DQ2

41. Skin disease (1)

A 52-year-old Mediterranean woman is referred to the dermatology outpatient clinic as a result of blisters that have developed in her mouth and on her arms. The patient describes the blisters as being very fragile and rupturing easily. Immunological testing reveals the presence of anti-desmoglein 3 antibodies and punch biopsy of a lesion demonstrates the presence of acantholytic cells. What is the most likely diagnosis?

A   Pemphigus foliaceous
B   Pemphigus vulgaris
C   Bullous pemphigoid
D   Epidermolysis bullosa
E   Dermatitis herpetiformis

42. Skin disease (2)

An Afro-Caribbean man with a history of type 1 diabetes mellitus presents to the dermatology outpatient clinic with depigmented areas of his face, arms and legs. On examination the affected areas are completely white. The patient admits that the lesions are leading to low mood. Which of the following is most associated with this disease process?

A   β-Haemolytic streptococcal infection
B   Vancomycin
C   Pregnancy
D   Anti-melanocyte antibodies
E   Multiple myeloma

43. Non-proliferative glomerulonephritis

A 4-year-old boy is referred to a renal physician after his mother noticed swelling of his legs. A week previously the boy had been stung by a bee. Urine dipstick reveals the presence of proteinuria, while blood tests show hypoalbuminaemia and hyperlipidaemia. The child's symptoms rapidly disappear with a course of steroids. What is the most likely diagnosis?

A   Alport syndrome
B   Reflux nephropathy
C   Shunt nephritis
D   Systemic lupus erythematosus
E   Minimal change disease

44. Proliferative glomerulonephritis

A 24-year-old woman is seen by the GP after noticing she is urinating less often as well as seeing some blood when she does pass water. Urine investigations reveal the presence of red cell casts and dysmorphic red blood cells. The patient admits to having had a sore throat 2 weeks previously. Anti-streptolysin O titres are raised. What is the most likely diagnosis?

A   IgA nephropathy
B   Henoch–Schonlein purpura
C   Post-streptococcal glomerulonephritis
D   Membranoproliferative glomerulonephritis
E   Rapidly progressive glomerulonephritis

45. Lupus nephritis

A 44-year-old man with known systemic lupus erythematosus is seen by a renal physician. Initially the patient had proteinuria on a routine urine dipstick. A subsequent renal biopsy demonstrated granular patterned deposition of IgG, IgM, IgA and C3 confined to the mesangium on both light and electron microscopy. Which stage of lupus nephritis is suggested by these findings?

A   Stage I
B   Stage II
C   Stage III
D   Stage IV
E   Stage V

46. Vasculitis

A 53-year-old man presents to accident and emergency with haemoptysis. Blood tests demonstrate deranged renal function and further tests reveal the presence of circulating c-ANCA antibodies. The patient is noted to have a saddle-shaped nose. What is the most likely diagnosis?

A   Cryoglobulinaemia
B   Wegener's granulomatosis
C   Microscopic polyarteritis
D   Polyarteritis nodosa
E   Churg–Strauss syndrome

47. Neurological disease (1)

A 35-year-old builder is referred to a neurologist after experiencing increasing axial rigidity over the previous few weeks; his symptoms are interfering with his work. The patient has a history of type 1 diabetes mellitus and vitiligo. Immunological investigations reveal the presence of circulating anti-glutamic acid decarboxylase antibodies. What is the most likely diagnosis?

A   Myasthenia gravis
B   Multiple sclerosis
C   Acute disseminated encephalomyelitis
D   Lambert–Eaton myasthenic syndrome
E   Stiff man syndrome

48. Neurological disease (2)

A 35-year-old man is transferred to the intensive care unit for ventilator support after suffering an episode of respiratory distress. The patient was admitted 5 days previously after experiencing weakness of his legs. Approximately 2 weeks prior to his admission the man had suffered a bout of gastroenteritis caused by the bacterium *Campylobacter jejuni*. Which of the following is the most likely antigenic target for autoantibodies in this disease process?

A   Ganglioside LM_1
B   Ganglioside GM_1
C   Hu
D   Myelin-associated glycoprotein
E   Purkinje cells

49. Eye disease

A 35-year-old woman is referred to an ophthalmologist after seeing floaters in her right eye. On examination, there is loss of accommodation in the same eye. The patient's notes reveal there had been trauma to the left eye following a car accident 3 weeks previously. It is explained to the patient that she could suffer potential loss of vision if steroid treatment is not commenced urgently. What is the most likely diagnosis?

A   Keratoconjunctivitis sicca
B   Sympathetic ophthalmia
C   Uveitis
D   Keratitis
E   Scleritis

50. Diagnostic immunology

A 52-year-old woman diagnosed with systemic lupus erythematosus develops jaundice and on examination is found to have conjunctival pallor. Blood tests reveal an elevated unconjugated bilirubin. Which of the following is the most useful investigation to determine the diagnosis?

A   Skin prick test
B   Direct antiglobulin test
C   Western blot
D   Immunofluorescence test
E   Patch testing

ANSWERS

Innate immunity (1): Physical barriers

1 C   Physical barriers to infection which form part of the innate immune system provide initial protection against disease-causing organisms. Impaired mucociliary clearance (C) may arise secondary to cystic fibrosis, which is the most likely answer in this scenario. Cystic fibrosis is an autosomal dominant disease which primarily affects the lungs but also the pancreas, liver and gastrointestinal system. The most common mutation is the ΔF508 mutation on chromosome 7, which codes for the cystic fibrosis transmembrane conductance regulator (CFTR). Defective sodium and chloride ion transport across epithelial cells leads to the formation of viscous secretions. In the respiratory tract increased viscous secretions produced by goblet cells cause damage to the cilia, as well as diffuse lung injury, which can result in bronchiectasis. The skin (A) is perhaps the most important physical barrier to infection. Although covered by normal flora, these bacteria are unable to penetrate the numerous layers which make up the skin. However, severe burns which break down this important barrier to infection may allow bacteria to enter the body. Small breaks in the skin that allow a small number of pathogens to enter the body are usually dealt with by other components of the innate immune system. The low pH of gastric acid (B) produced in the stomach destroys most bacteria present in food. Bacteria that reach the large intestines must compete with commensal gut flora (E); extrinsic bacteria are therefore unable to replicate and cannot survive. Tears (D) are produced by the lacrimal glands of the eyes. The lysozyme component reduces the risk of pathogens entering the eye. Keratoconjunctivitis sicca ('dry eye') is a condition that causes reduced production of tears, subsequently increasing the risk of infection.

Innate immunity (2): Complement investigations

2 E   The complement system is composed of the classical, lectin and alternative pathways. These individual pathways culminate in the formation of the membrane attack complex (MAC), which traverses cell surface membranes of pathogens, causing cell lysis. Components of the complement system can be quantified in order to differentiate possible diagnoses. CH50 (total complement activity) measures the level of factors of the classical and final pathways (C1–C9). As complement factors are acute phase proteins, a high CH50 (E) indicates acute or chronic inflammation. Together with the raised CRP and clinical features, this patient is likely to suffer from rheumatoid arthritis. Systemic lupus erythematosus (SLE) is a systemic autoimmune disease characterized by antibody-immune

complex formation and deposition. The classical complement pathway is composed of C1, C2 and C4. Reduced C3 and C4 (C) levels are typical of SLE as a result of complex formation (hence consumption) in an attempt to eliminate immune complexes. C3 and C4 may also be reduced in SLE due to immunodeficiency which predisposes to developing the disease. In membranoproliferative glomerulonephritis (MPGN), anti-nephritic antibodies cause consumption of complement factors, especially C3. As a result, complement profiling reveals a reduced C3 but normal C4 (D); MPGN type III reflects this pattern particularly well.

AH50 is a laboratory investigation to test for abnormalities of the alternative pathway, which involves factors C3, B, D and P. A reduced AH50 and normal CH50 (A) suggest possible deficiency of one or more of the alternative pathway factors; this predisposes to infection by encapsulated bacteria.

Reduced C1 inhibitor (B) levels indicate hereditary angioedema, characterized by facial swelling; in severe cases the airway can become compromised leading to respiratory distress.

Innate immunity (3): Cellular response

3   D   Mast cells (D) are involved in the inflammatory process that occurs in allergy and anaphylaxis (the diagnosis in this case), but also provide a protective function against pathogens. Mast cells are activated by one of three mechanisms: direct injury (toxins or drugs), cross-linking of IgE receptors or by activated complement proteins. Once activated, mast cells release granules containing histamine and heparin. Histamine causes vasodilatation leading to the characteristic features of inflammation (oedema, warmth and redness of the skin). The 'flare and wheal' skin reaction is a feature of histamine release by mast cells. Mast cells play a role in diseases such as asthma, eczema and allergic rhinitis. Anaphylaxis is characterized by systemic degranulation of mast cells leading to life-threatening shock. Natural killer cells (NK cells; A) are responsible for destroying tumour cells and virus-infected cells. NK cells are unique in that they have the ability to kill such cells in the absence of antibodies and major histocompatibility complex. Dendritic cells (B) are antigen-presenting cells (APCs) involved in bridging the gap between the innate and adaptive immune response. Once dendritic cells are activated, they migrate to the lymph nodes to facilitate the adaptive immune system. Eosinophils (C) protect against parasitic infection. Such pathogens stimulate release of granule contents into the extracellular space, which surround the parasite and lead to clearance. Neutrophils (E) are the most common of the granulocytes. Neutrophils are responsible for the innate protection against bacterial pathogens. Stored within neutrophils are a host of bactericidal lysosomes which contain lysozyme,

acid hydrolases and myeloperoxidase. Opsonized pathogens are internalized by neutrophils forming a phagosome. Lysosomal contents enter the phagosome leading to respiratory burst and lysis of the pathogen.

Adaptive immunity: Antibodies

4 A   Antibodies (also known as immunoglobulins) are glycoproteins produced by B cells as part of the adaptive immune system. The basic role of antibodies is to bind to foreign targets, otherwise known as antigens. Antibody functions are numerous and include host defence against pathogens by neutralizing toxins or targeting infective organisms, complement activation and mast cell stimulation. As well as the physiological role of antibodies, they are also used in the diagnosis of infectious diseases by measuring anti-viral and anti-bacterial antibodies. Structurally, antibodies are made up of two heavy chains and two light chains. Each heavy chain and each light chain has a constant region as well as a variable region; the variable regions differ significantly between antibodies and it is this segment that makes antibodies specific to target antigens.

IgA (A) can exist as a monomer or a dimer (joined by a short peptide known as the J chain). Its role is primarily related to the protection of mucosal surfaces via salivary, respiratory, gastrointestinal and lacrimal secretions. IgA is also present in breast milk, providing passive immunity in neonates. IgD (B) is an uncommon immunoglobulin in the body and is found on the cell surface of immature B cells. IgD provides an essential role in lymphocyte activation. IgG (C) is the most abundant antibody and occurs in monomer form in the circulation. The various subclasses of IgG perform different functions, for example IgG2 is important in fighting encapsulated bacteria. IgG also has a role in activating complement proteins. IgM (D) occurs as a pentamer and has a role in the primary response against pathogens. IgE (E) is produced in response to parasitic infections, as well as during type I hypersensitivity reactions where it is involved in mast cell activation.

Human leukocyte antigen

5 E   The human major histocompatibility complex (MHC), otherwise known as human leukocyte antigen (HLA) system, is the collection of genes that relates to immune system function and is located on chromosome 6. The HLA system consists of three major classes: class I (HLA A, B and C), class II (HLA DP, DQ and DR) and class III (complement components). HLAs have a number of roles in immunology including defence against pathogens, transplant rejection and autoimmune disease.

HLA DQ2 (E) represents a risk factor for coeliac disease (HLA DQ8 is also a risk factor but to a lesser extent). The cell surface receptors formed by HLA DQ2 bind with greater affinity to α-gliadin, a protein present in wheat, barley and rye which is responsible for the pathogenesis of coeliac disease. Therefore, receptors formed from HLA DQ2 are more likely to recruit T cells and initiate an autoimmune response compared to other HLAs. HLA B27 (A) is associated with ankylosing spondylitis. The association with HLA B27 suggests the involvement of CD8+ T cells in the pathogenesis of ankylosing spondylitis. HLA DR2 (B) is associated with Goodpasture's syndrome, an autoimmune disease triggered by a type II hypersensitivity reaction. It is characterized by glomerulonephritis and haemoptysis. HLA DR3 (C) is associated with Graves' disease, systemic lupus erythematosus (SLE) and myasthenia gravis. HLA DR4 (D) is associated with type I diabetes mellitus and rheumatoid arthritis; in these diseases, HLA DR4 recruits T cells with subsequent production of islet cell antibodies.

Immune tolerance

6   C   T-cell tolerance is the process by which the body's T cells do not attack self antigens. There are several mechanisms by which this is achieved, including the selection of answers given above. Autoimmune disease is defined as the abnormal response to healthy self components; there is an underlying pathological process which leads to the breakdown of self tolerance. Autoimmune disease may be organ specific (Graves' disease) or non-organ specific (systemic lupus erythematosus).

Central tolerance is the induction of tolerance to self, which is integrated into T-cell development in the thymus, a major site for the maturation of T cells. Within the thymus, T-cell receptors are exposed to self major histocompatibility complexes (MHC). Those binding to these MHCs with some affinity are positively selected, whereas those with no affinity (unable to recognize MHC) are neglected and removed. T cells binding with high affinity are removed by apoptosis, as these cells pose an autoimmune risk. The autoimmune regulator (AIRE; C) is also present within the thymus and presents T-cell receptors with a range of organ-specific antigens. If T-cell receptors bind to such antigens, they swiftly die via apoptosis. Autoimmune polyendocrine syndrome type 1 (APECED; associated with mild immune deficiency, dysfunctional parathyroid gland/adrenal gland, hypothyroidism, gonadal failure, alopecia and vitiligo) results from mutations in the AIRE gene. The child in this scenario has features of APECED.

The mechanisms of central tolerance are, however, not fail-safe, and so peripheral systems exist to remove potential auto-reactive T cells. Regulatory T cells (A) mature in the thymus and are those that express

CD4, CD25 and Foxp3 on the cell surface. Abnormal Foxp3 leads to the development of immunodysregulation polyendocrinopathy enteropathy X-linked syndrome. TGF-β (B) is key in the differentiation of regulatory T cells, while IL-10 (E) has been found to be expressed by regulatory T cells; TGF-β and IL-10 are considered to be anti-proliferative and anti-inflammatory signalling molecules. Dendritic cells (D) can present peripheral T cells with self antigens. Those T cells which react are killed. Aberrant dendritic cells have been linked to the development of autoimmune disease.

Mechanisms of autoimmunity

7   B   Several mechanisms exist by which autoimmune disease can arise. In this case, the patient has presented with post-streptococcal rheumatic fever, for which the pathological mechanism is molecular mimicry (B). Molecular mimicry is the term used to describe the phenomenon whereby pathogens produce antigens that are molecularly very similar to self antigens. The immune response to this pathogenic antigen generates T cells and B cells which are both anti-pathogen and anti-self; this process is known as immunological cross-reactivity. In the case of post-streptococcal rheumatic fever, antibodies to M-proteins present on the surface of group A streptococci cross-react with cardiac myosin; this results in the inflammatory features of rheumatic fever (fever, raised ESR/CRP, leukocytosis, carditis). Defective immunoregulation (A) results in the reduced number or aberrant function of regulatory T cells which bear CD4, CD25 and Foxp3 surface markers. These cells are responsible for maintaining peripheral tolerance. Defective immunoregulation has been associated with thyroid, islet cell and liver autoimmune diseases. T-cell bypass (B) involves the generation of a novel autoantigen epitope. Autoantigens are physiologically internalized by B cells, which are in turn presented to T-helper cells; the B cell is suppressed from producing autoantibodies. If the complex autoantigen is modified, a new epitope is provided for T cells to stimulate antibody production by B cells. Triggers to this modification include drugs and infection, such as *Mycoplasma pneumoniae* inducing autoimmune haemolytic anaemia by modifying erythrocyte surface proteins. Release of 'hidden' self antigens (D) may occur after damage to an organ and causes release of intracellular proteins which have never been exposed to the immune system. This is the case post-myocardial infarction, where release of proteins leads to the generation of autoantibodies against cardiac myocytes (Dressler's syndrome), causing pericarditis. Cytokines (E), such as IL-2, may have an effect on breakdown of immunological tolerance. There is a strong association between IL-2 therapy (solid-organ tumours) and autoimmune thyroid disease.

Primary immunodeficiency (1): Phagocyte deficiency

8 D Chronic granulomatous disease (CGD; D) is an X-linked disorder causing deficiency of NADPH oxidase. As a result, neutrophils cannot produce the respiratory burst required to clear pathogens. The disease is
characterized by chronic inflammation with non-caseating granulomas.
Clinical features include recurrent skin infections (bacterial) as well
as recurrent fungal infections including *Candida* spp. and *Aspergillus*
spp. The disease is usually detected by the age of 5 and is diagnosed
using the nitro-blue-tetrazolium (NBT) test, which remains colourless
due to NADPH deficiency (if NADPH is present the solution turns blue).
The NBT test distinguishes CGD from other phagocyte deficiencies. The
patient will have a normal neutrophil count as there is no defect in
neutrophil production. Treatment involves the use of prophylactic antibiotics and interferon-gamma. Kostmann syndrome (severe congenital
neutropenia; A) is a congenital neutropenia as a result of failure of
neutrophil maturation. This results in a very low neutrophil count and
no pus formation. NBT test is positive. In leukocyte adhesion deficiency
(LAD; C), neutrophils are formed but cannot exit the blood stream
due to a deficit in leukocyte adhesion molecules resulting in reduced
neutrophil chemotaxis. The neutrophil count is very high due to persistence in the blood stream. NBT test is positive. Cyclic neutropenia
(B) is an autosomal dominant condition caused by a mutation in the
neutrophil elastase gene (ELA2). Neutropenia occurs every 3 weeks and
lasts approximately 6 days at a time. Cyclic neutropenia improves after
puberty. Von Gierke's disease (E) is a glycogen storage disease caused
by a deficiency of the enzyme glucose-6-phosphatase. Patients may present with severe hypoglycaemia. Neutropenia is also a manifestation of
the disease.

Primary immunodeficiency (2): Complement deficiency

9 B This patient demonstrates symptoms, signs and diagnostic features consistent with systemic lupus erythematosus (SLE) and is therefore most
likely to have a deficiency of the classical pathway such as C4 deficiency (B). Other possible deficiencies in this pathway include C1q, C1r and
C1s and C2. The classical pathway is responsible for clearing immune
complexes and apoptotic cells; patients who have deficiencies in this
pathway therefore have a greater risk of developing immune complex
disease such as SLE. C3 (A) is a common factor in both the classical
and alternative pathways. Deficiency of C3 leads to recurrent pyogenic
infections as there is no C3b (produced via C3 convertase) available to
opsinize bacteria. C3 deficiency also leads to decreased C3a production,

an anaphylatoxin that mediates inflammation. C6 (C) forms part of the terminal complement pathway, together with C5, C7 and C8, which form the membrane attack complex (MAC) for bacteriolysis. Deficiency of terminal complement pathway factors leads to increased susceptibility to encapsulated bacterial infections, such as *Neisseria gonorrhoea* and *Neisseria meningitides*. While C9 (D) also forms part of the MAC, patients deficient in C9 still retain some ability to clear encapsulated bacterial infection, albeit at a slower rate. Therefore, patients deficient in C9 are usually asymptomatic. C1 inhibitor (E) has the physiological role of inhibiting the kallikrein system and classical pathway. C1 inhibitor deficiency causes increased production of bradykinin and spontaneous activation of the complement pathway; deficiency results in the autosomal dominant condition hereditary angioedema.

Primary immunodeficiency (3): T-cell deficiency

10   A   Di George's syndrome (A) is caused by an embryological abnormality in the third and fourth branchial arches (pharyngeal pouches) due to a 22q11 deletion. The result is an absent or hypoplastic thymus, as well as a deficiency in T cells. There is a reduced level or absence of CD4+ and CD8+ T cells as well as decreased production of IgG and IgA. B-cell and IgM levels are normal. The features of Di George's syndrome can be remembered by the mnemonic 'CATCH': cardiac abnormalities, atresia (oesophageal), thymic aplasia, cleft palate and hypocalcaemia. Two major subtypes of severe combined immunodeficiency (SCID; B) exist, which affect both T and B cells: X-linked disease (mutation of IL-2 receptor) and an autosomal recessive condition (mutation of adenosine deaminase gene which leads to a build-up of toxins and hence compromised proliferation of lymphocytes). Clinical features include diarrhoea, failure to thrive and skin disease (graft-versus-host induced, caused by transplacental maternal T cells, and blood transfusion-related caused by donor T cells). Blood transfusions are contraindicated in patients with SCID. Bare lymphocyte syndrome (C) is caused by either deficiency in MHC I (type 1; all T cells become CD4+ T cells) or MHC II (type 2; all T cells become CD8+ T cells). Clinical manifestations include sclerosing cholangitis with hepatomegaly and jaundice. Wiskott–Aldrich syndrome (WAS; D) is an X-linked condition which is caused by a mutation in the *WASp* gene which leads to lymphocytopenia. WAS is linked to the development of lymphomas, thrombocytopenia and eczema. Interferon-gamma (IFN-gamma) released by T cells induces the activation of macrophages. Therefore, IFN-gamma receptor deficiency (E) leads to the reduced activation of macrophages and so granulomas cannot form, resulting in increased susceptibility to intracellular infections such as *Mycobacterium tuberculosis* and *Salmonella* spp.

Primary immunodeficiency (4): B-cell deficiency

11 D IgA specifically provides mucosal immunity, primarily to the respiratory and gastrointestinal systems. Selective IgA deficiency (D) results from a genetic inability to produce IgA and is characterized by recurrent mild respiratory and gastrointestinal infections. Patients with selective IgA deficiency are also at risk of anaphylaxis to blood transfusions due to the presence of donor IgA. This occurs especially after a second transfusion; antibodies having been created against IgA during the primary transfusion. Selective IgA deficiency is also linked to autoimmune diseases such as rheumatoid arthritis, systemic lupus erythematosus and coeliac disease. The recessive form of severe combined immunodeficiency (SCID; A) is caused by a mutation of the adenosine deaminase gene leading to an accumulation of toxins and therefore compromised proliferation of lymphocytes; CD4+ and CD8+ T-cell levels are decreased. Reduced proliferation of lymphocytes leads to atrophy of the thymus, lymph and mucosa-associated lymphoid tissue. Bruton's agammaglobulinaemia (B) is an X-linked disease that presents in childhood. It is caused by a mutation of the BTK gene, which is a tyrosine kinase. This mutation inhibits B-cell maturation and as a result B-cell and immunoglobulin levels are diminished. Hyper IgM syndrome (C) is an X-linked condition that presents in childhood. It is caused by a mutation in the CD40 ligand on T cells leading to impaired communication with B cells. B cells are unable to class-switch and therefore only produce IgM (leading to increased levels in the blood) and patient are deficient in IgA, IgG and IgE. Patients with hyper IgM syndrome are at risk of *Pneumocystis jerovicci* infection. Common variable immunodeficiency (CVID; E) presents in adulthood. A mutation of MHC III causes aberrant class switching, increasing the risk of lymphoma and granulomas. Clinical features include bronchiectasis and sinusitis. Blood tests reveal a normal IgM level but decreased levels of IgA, IgG and IgE.

Secondary immunodeficiency

12 D Broadly, secondary immunodeficiency can result from either reduced production of immune factors, increased loss or catabolism. Human immunodeficiency virus (HIV) is a double stranded RNA virus that causes AIDS (E). AIDS is characterized by immune dysfunction, the primary defect being a reduced CD4+ T-cell count. AIDS patients are at greater risk of developing opportunistic infections (for example, *Pneumocystis jerovicci* and *Cryptosporidium* spp.) and tumours (Kaposi's sarcoma). Inflammatory bowel disease (IBD; A) is an inflammatory condition of the gastrointestinal tract that may be subdivided into ulcerative colitis (UC; affects the colon) and Crohn's disease (CD; affects anywhere from the mouth to anus). It is mainly CD that causes

protein losing enteropathy as proteins are absorbed in the small bowel. The reduced absorption of proteins in IBD results in fewer immuno-globulins being formed which affects the adaptive immune system response. Hyposplenism (B) may arise due to splenectomy (after trauma) or sickle-cell disease, for example. Poor spleen function or absence of a spleen predisposes to encapsulated bacterial infections, for example *Streptococcus pneumoniae*, *Haemophilus influenzae* and *Neisseria meningitidis*. Such patients are therefore required to take necessary vaccinations and antibiotic prophylaxis. Nephrotic syndrome (C) is characterized by renal dysfunction leading to large amounts of protein leaking from the blood to the urine. Consequently, immunoglobulins will be lost as they are passed into the urine, leading to increased risk of infection by encapsulated bacteria. Prematurity (E) is a cause of secondary immunodeficiency as IgG is transferred across the placenta during the final 2 months of pregnancy. Premature babies will have had less IgG transferred as a fetus. As a result, such babies will be at greater risk of infection before their own immune systems begin to mature (approximately 4 months after birth).

Hypersensitivity reactions (1)

13 C Type I hypersensitivity reactions are mediated by IgE and are associated with allergy and anaphylaxis. The mechanism behind the development of type I hypersensitivity reactions begins with the presentation of the allergen to professional antigen presenting cells. Professional antigen presenting cells include macrophages (C), dendritic cells and B cells. For example, if an allergen is taken up by a macrophage, it is processed intracellularly and peptides are presented via major histocompatibility complex on the cell surface to T cells of the TH2-cell (E) subclass. TH2-cell secrete IL-4, which stimulates B cell (B) proliferation. TH1-cells (D) do not play a role in the pathogenesis of type I hypersensitivity but do contribute to type IV hypersensitivity reactions. B cells in turn produce allergen-specific antibodies of the IgE variety. IgE binds to mast cells (A) via the Fc receptor. During a second exposure, when the allergen encounters the sensitized mast cell, the surface IgE cross-links which leads to an increased intracellular calcium concentration, facilitating the release of pre-formed mediators (histamine, proteases, serotonin and heparin) as well as newly formed lipid mediators (thromboxane, prosta-glandin, leukotriene and platelet activating factor). These mediators correlate with the clinical features of allergic reactions. For example, histamine, leukotrienes and prostaglandins are vasodilators and contribute to the warmth, oedema and redness which are associated with allergic inflammation. Examples of diseases caused by type I hypersensitivity reactions include allergic rhinitis, food allergy and urticaria.

Hypersensitivity reactions (2)

14 E   This patient has signs and symptoms confined to her mouth. Together with the doctor's suspicions regarding the underlying pathogenesis, oral allergy syndrome (OAS) is the most likely diagnosis. OAS occurs secondary to cross-reactivity of antigens inhaled in the mouth, otherwise known as pollen–food allergy. For example, a patient may be sensitized to birch pollen; when pollen is breathed in, IgE is created which cross-reacts with fruit (E) which has been ingested causing release of histamine from mast cells resulting in local inflammation. Known cross-reactants include birch pollen/stone fruits, mugwort pollen/celery and ragweed pollen/melon. All symptoms are confined to the mouth only and include swelling, itching and tingling of the tongue, lips and uvula. There is often a history of atopic disease. Management includes avoiding ingestion of the allergen, anti-histamines and prophylactically carrying an EpiPen in patients who have a history of anaphylaxis. Allergy to penicillin (A) may result in either acute urticaria or in severe cases, anaphylaxis. Acute urticaria lasts for less than 6 weeks, characterized by intermittent rashes which last less than 24 hours at a single site. Systemic IgE activation results in anaphylaxis characterized by swelling of the lips, shortness of breath and signs of shock in severe cases. Eggs (B) are a primary cause of food allergy in children; egg allergy usually resolves by the age of 8 years. Most food allergies are IgE mediated; as some are not, the gold standard to test for food allergies is the double-blind food challenge. Other causes of food allergy include nuts, shellfish, milk and wheat. Nickel (C) causes contact dermatitis, a type IV hypersensitivity reaction. A reaction takes 1–2 days to develop (delayed) leading to desquamation of the skin. As histamines are not involved in type IV reactions, there is no response to anti-histamines. Dust mites (D) cause allergic rhinitis, symptomatically characterized by loss of smell, rhinorrhoea and nasal/eye itchiness.

Hypersensitivity reactions (3)

15 B   This patient is suffering an anaphylactic attack as a result of peanut allergy. Other potential causes of anaphylaxis include penicillin, animal venom and latex. The pathophysiology of anaphylaxis involves IgE binding to the allergen with subsequent systemic release of histamine causing vasodilation and contraction of bronchial smooth muscle. Clinical features include swollen lips, shortness of breath, wheeze and signs of shock. Anaphylaxis is therefore a medical emergency and intramuscular (IM) adrenaline (B) is the primary treatment; many patients who suffer from severe allergy are educated in the use of an EpiPen. IM adrenaline is the best (and life-saving) choice due to its fast acting

vasocontrictive and bronchodilator effects. Non-IgE mediated systemic histamine release by mast cells is known as an anaphylactoid reaction. Causes include opioids, NSAIDs, contrast agents and exercise. Clinical features are similar to anaphylaxis reaction.

As allergies such as allergic rhinitis, oral allergy syndrome and urticaria are IgE mediated causing release of histamine by mast cells, oral anti-histamines (C) are the main-stay treatment for such conditions. Anti-histamines used in allergic disease are H_1 receptor antagonists which negate the effects of histamine. Although effective in treating mild symptoms, oral anti-histamines take longer to have an effect than IM adrenaline. Nasal steroids (E) may also be prescribed to alleviate symptoms of rhinorrhoea, itching and nasal congestion. Patients with known triggers to allergy, such as specific foods, irritants or environmental conditions, are also encouraged to practice allergen avoidance (A) as a conservative measure in managing their symptoms. Doxepin (D) is indicated in the management of chronic urticaria.

Hypersensitivity reactions (4)

16   B   There are a battery of tests available for the investigation of IgE mediated hypersensitivity and the triggers which might be causative of such a reaction. This patient has an allergy to pollen and food: the skin prick test (B) is the gold standard for investigating such type I hypersensitivity reactions. The test involves a few drops of purified allergen being pricked onto the skin. Allergens which are tested for include foods, dust mites, pollen and dust. A positive test is indicated by wheal formation, caused by cross-linking of IgE on the mast cell surface leading to histamine release. Radioallergosorbent test (RAST test; A) is also used to test for a variety of potential allergens. The test involves patient serum being added to a range of insoluble allergens. If antibodies are present to the allergen, these will bind. Radio-labelled anti-human IgE antibody is then added, which binds to the IgE bound to the insoluble allergen. Once the unbound IgE is washed away the radioactivity is measured; the greater the radioactivity the stronger the reaction to the allergen. Radioactivity-based tests have been replaced by enzyme- and fluorescence-based assays. The difficulty with RAST testing is that low IgE levels may be present in the serum which could lead to false negative results. Double-blind challenges (C) are reserved for food allergies where there is some doubt after a skin prick or RAST test. This must be conducted at a centre where necessary equipment is available in case of anaphylaxis. Serum tryptase levels (D) are useful in diagnosing anaphylaxis reaction. Measuring total serum IgE (E) is not very informative in investigating allergy.

Hypersensitivity reactions (5)

17 B   This patient has suffered hyperacute rejection of his graft as a result
        of ABO incompatibility; secondary to a previous sensitizing event, the
        recipient has developed antibodies that have attacked the allograft. This
        is an example of a type II hypersensitivity reaction. Type II hypersen-
        sitivity reactions are IgG and IgM antibody mediated; the antigen is
        fixed to tissues or cell surface. Tissue or organ damage is restricted to
        those areas where the antibody target exists. Binding of the antibody
        to the target antigen causes activation of the classical complement
        pathway, beginning with C1 (B); activation of C1 has a number of
        effects. Fragments C3a and C5a are subsequently generated and attract
        macrophages (E). The final common pathway of complement activation
        involves factors C5–C9 forming the membrane attack complex (MAC)
        which inserts into the target cell membrane, causing lysis. The classical
        pathway also leads to binding of C3b onto the target cell surface mem-
        brane, which causes recruitment of effector cells such as macrophages,
        natural-killer cells (NK cells; A) and neutrophils (C). Effector cells cause
        significant damage by lysing target cells by an antibody-dependent
        cell-mediated cytotoxicity (ADCC) mechanism. Mannose binding lec-
        tin (MBL; D) is part of the lectin complement pathway, which is not
        involved in type II hypersensitivity reactions. Further examples of type
        II hypersensitivity reactions include myasthenia gravis, pemphigus vul-
        garis, haemolytic anaemia and haemolytic disease of the newborn.

Hypersensitivity reactions (6)

18 D   Type II hypersensitivity reactions involve the presence of antibod-
        ies that target antigens fixed to the target cell surface membrane. The
        patient in question has clinical features of pemphigus vulgaris. Such
        features include blistering of the skin and Nikolsky's sign is positive
        (slight rubbing of the skin results in separation of the outermost layer).
        Pemphigus vulgaris results from antibodies directed towards demoglein
        1 (D) and demoglein 3, which are epidermal cadherins of the epidermis.
        Antibodies causing damage to cadherin proteins result in the loss of
        linkages between keratinocytes, hence causing the presence of charac-
        teristic acantholytic cells on biopsy. Gastric-parietal cell (A) antibodies
        are a feature of pernicious anaemia and lead to parietal cell loss and
        hence reduced intrinsic factor production; this causes reduced vitamin
        B_{12} absorption. As a result patients present with vitamin B_{12} deficiency,
        features of which include tiredness (anaemia) as well as sensory or
        motor defects. Rhesus antigens (B) are found on the surface of erythro-
        cytes. As with ABO, the rhesus (Rh) blood group system is a clinically
        important system used for matching in blood transfusions. The most
        commonly used Rh antigen in matching is the D antigen. Antibodies

directed against the Rh antigen result in autoimmune haemolytic anaemia (AIHA). The direct Coombs test, which detects antibodies bound
to the surface of erythrocytes, is positive in AIHA. The acetylcholine
receptor (C) located at the neuromuscular junction is the target for autoantibodies in myasthenia gravis. Myasthenia gravis is a condition which
presents with fatigability of muscles; muscles become fatigued after
periods of movement but recover after rest. In severe cases, muscles of
breathing may become affected, leading to respiratory distress. In post-
streptococcal rheumatic fever, antibodies to M-proteins present on the
surface of group A streptococci (E) cross-react with cardiac myosin; this
results in the inflammatory features of rheumatic fever which include
fever, raised ESR/CRP, leukocytosis and carditis. Rheumatic fever occurs
as a result of molecular mimicry whereby pathogens produce antigens
that are molecularly very similar to self antigens.

Hypersensitivity reactions (7)

19 C   In contrast to type II hypersensitivity reactions, type III hypersensitivity
reactions are characterized by antibodies targeting antigens that are not
fixed to a cell surface. This patient has symptoms and signs characteristic of systemic lupus erythematosus (SLE). SLE is a multisystem disorder
which may manifest in a number of ways, examples of which include
fever, fatigue, loss of appetite, malar rash, mouth ulcers, photosensitiv-
ity, serositis and joint pains. DNA (C) is the target for circulating anti-
double stranded DNA antibodies in SLE. Many of the clinical features
of SLE result from antibody-immune complex deposition. The presence
of anti-Smith antibodies suggests interstitial lung disease involvement.
Chronic exposure to mouldy hay (A) is the cause of farmer's lung, an
example of an extrinsic allergic alveolitis. Actinomycetes are the most
common pathogens found in hay dust, which are subsequently inhaled.
Inhalation over prolonged periods of time leads to immune complex
formation as antibodies combine with the inhaled allergen; the immune
complexes are deposited in the walls of the alveoli. Chronic exposure
leads to pulmonary fibrosis, with associated shortness of breath, cyanosis and cor pulmonale. Antibodies directed at *Chlamydia trachomatis*
(B) may trigger a reactive arthritis (Reiter's syndrome). Clinical features
include arthritis, dysuria, conjunctivitis and uveitis. As this phenomenon is autoimmune, synovial fluid cultures are negative. Proteins in
antiserum (D) are the cause of serum sickness, a self-limiting condition
that occurs when antiserum derived from a non-human animal source
is injected intravenously, resulting in immune complex hypersensitivity. HBsAg (E) may be associated with the development of polyarteritis
nodosa (PAN), a vasculitis of small and medium sized vessels. Immune
complexes are deposited within such vessels leading to fibrinoid necrosis
and neutrophil infiltration; as a result the vessel walls weaken resulting
in the formation of multiple aneurysms.

Hypersensitivity reactions (8)

20 E   Type IV hypersensitivity (delayed type) reactions are those that are mediated by T cells of the immune system. These types of reactions require two exposures to the allergen. During the first encounter, antigen presenting cells such as macrophages engulf the allergen and presents peptides on the cell surface via major histocompatibility complex. CD4+ T cells recognize the peptide and bind to the macrophage. The macrophage then releases IL-12 (E) which leads to the production of memory CD4+ T cells of the TH1 variety. During the second exposure, the macrophage will once again take up the allergen and present peptide to CD4+ T cells. On this occasion however, the sensitized memory T cell releases IFN-γ (B), IL-2 (C) and IL-3 thereby activating macrophages, inducing the production of TNF-α (D); the result is tissue injury and chronic inflammation. As type IV hypersensitivity reactions are cell-mediated, there is a lag time of approximately 48–72 hours before clinical symptoms and signs are visible. IL-10 (E) is not involved in type IV hypersensitivity reactions; IL-10 is produced by TH2 cells which causes inhibition of TH1 cells. As a consequence, IFN-γ would not be produced to activate macrophages and so type IV hypersensitivity would not occur. An example of a disease process caused by type IV hypersensitivity is contact dermatitis occurring secondary to nickel exposure, as is the case in this clinical scenario.

Hypersensitivity reactions (9)

21 C   Type IV hypersensitivity reactions are mediated by T cells and have a delayed onset. Proteolipid protein (C) and myelin basic protein are oligodendrocyte proteins implicated in the pathogenesis of multiple sclerosis (MS). Multiple sclerosis is a demyelinating disease in which the myelin sheaths surrounding neurons of the brain and spinal cord are destroyed. Associated with the disease process is the antigenic stimulation of CD4+ T cells which in turn activate CD8+ cytotoxic T cells and macrophages; these are directed at oligodendrocyte proteins, causing destruction of oligodendrocytes and myelin. Clinical features of MS include optic neuritis, urinary/bowel incontinence, weakness of the arms/legs and dysphagia. Uhthoff's phenomenon describes the worsening of symptoms that occurs after exposure to higher than ambient temperatures. Pancreatic β-cell proteins (A) are the antigenic target for cytotoxic CD8+ T cells in type 1 diabetes mellitus (T1DM). The pathogenesis involves the destruction of β-cells in the islets of Langerhans in the pancreas by CD8+ T cells. β-cells are the storage site for insulin in the body, and so destruction of these cells leads to diminished insulin release and hyperglycaemia. Presenting features of T1DM include polyuria, polydipsia and weight loss. Nickel (B) is a hapten and binds with

skin proteins. It is detected by Langerhan's antigen presenting cells in the skin causing contact dermatitis. This results in a lesion resembling eczema with oedema and scaling. Synovial membrane antigens (D) are the target for T cells in rheumatoid arthritis (RA). RA is defined as a chronic systemic inflammatory disease causing a systemic, inflammatory polyarthritis. The Mantoux test involves the intradermal injection of purified protein derivative tuberculin (E). It is used as a test of previous exposure to *Mycobacterium tuberculosis*. A positive test depends upon a combination of induration size 48–72 hours after the injection, as well as disease risk factors.

Transplantation and rejection (1)

22 D Transplants of organs are indicated in situations where function is lost following end-stage disease. In this case the patient in question has stage 5 chronic kidney disease, also known as end-stage kidney failure, an irreversible pathology. Transplant is the only cure for such a condition. The patient has an identical twin (monozygotic) and hence is genetically very similar. A transplant from the patient's twin is known as an isograft (D); as the two individuals will have a similar genetic profile and the organ has been matched for human leukocyte antigen (HLA), chance of rejection is rare. Allograft (C) transplants are those where the donor is of the same species as the recipient but not identical. As the donor and recipient are genetically different, the organ must be matched in terms of HLA compatibility, as well as ABO blood group. HLA and ABO matching minimizes the risk of organ rejection. The use of immunosuppressive agents is another method of reducing the risk of transplant rejection. An example of a split transplant (B) is a liver that may be divided and shared between two recipients. An autograft (A) is defined as the transplant of tissue to the same patient. Examples include skin grafts and venous graft for use in coronary artery bypass graft (CABG) operations. As the tissue or organ is derived from 'self' there is zero chance of rejection. A xenograft (E) is defined as an organ transplant from one species to another. An example of such a transplant is of a porcine heart valve in an aortic valve replacement which is very successful. However, in general with xenografts, there is a high risk of rejection and disease carried in the animal tissue.

Transplantation and rejection (2)

23 A Patients who are due to undergo a transplant are matched with a donor for human leukocyte antigen (HLA) and ABO blood group. In this case, there has been an error in ABO matching which is a recipe for hyperacute rejection (A). Hyperacute rejection occurs within minutes to hours, and is mediated by pre-formed antibodies against antigens on

the surface of the donor organ. The binding of pre-formed antibodies to the donor organ activates the complement pathway and clotting cascade, leading to thrombosis and ultimately rejection of the donor organ. Acute cellular rejection (B) occurs approximately 1 week after transplantation. It is T-cell mediated (type IV hypersensitivity reaction). In cases where there is HLA-mismatch, antigen presenting cells present peptides that are made of foreign HLA to CD4+ T cells, coordinating an immune response against the donor organ. This involves macrophages, CD8+ T cells, B-cell and pro-inflammatory cytokines (IFN-γ and TNF-α) directed towards the donor organ. Acute vascular rejection (D) may occur with transplant of a xenograft. It is an antibody reaction, which may either be due to a pre-formed antibody (not detected at cross-match) or a new antibody produced by activated B cells. The pathogenesis is similar to hyperacute rejection, but occurs 4–6 days after transplantation. Chronic rejection (C) involves both immune and non-immune reactions; it may occur months to years after transplantation. The pathogenesis involves smooth muscle growth which causes blockage of graft vessel lumens leading to ischaemia and fibrosis. Risk factors include HLA-mismatches, multiple acute rejections, hypertension and hyperlipidaemia. Graft-versus-host disease (GVHD; E) is a complication of allogeneic stem cell transplantation. It occurs when immune cells transferred in the donated stem cells recognize the recipient tissue as foreign causing a graft-versus-host reaction.

Transplantation and rejection (3)

24   A   Cyclosporine A (A) inhibits the protein phosphatase calcineurin. This causes IL-2 secretion from T cells, a cytokine which stimulates T-cell proliferation; the production of T cells is reduced, hence minimizing organ rejection. A common side effect is gum hyperplasia. OKT3 (muromonab-CD3; B) is a mouse monoclonal antibody targeted at the human CD3 molecule used to treat rejection episodes in patients who have undergone allograft transplantation. Administration of the antibody efficiently clears T cells from the recipient's circulation, T cells being the major mediator of acute organ rejection. Primary indications include the acute corticosteroid-resistant rejection of renal, heart and liver transplants. Anaphylaxis is a major potential adverse effect of using murine proteins. Azathioprine (C) is an antimetabolite agent used in immunosuppressive therapy. Azathioprine is metabolized into 6-mercaptopurine (6-MP), a purine analogue that prevents DNA synthesis, thereby inhibiting the proliferation of cells; lymphocytes are most affected. Antigen presenting cells present non-self proteins (from the allograft) to T cells which in turn produce IL-2 to stimulate T-cell proliferation. However, 6-MP inhibits this proliferation and so reaction between T cells and the allograft is minimized. Corticosteroids (D) are

used as an immunosuppressive agent in both the prevention and treatment of transplant rejection. Corticosteroids inhibit phospholipase A2 thereby blocking prostaglandin formation as well as a series of inflammatory mediators. The immunosuppressive effects of corticosteroids are numerous and include reducing the number of circulating B cells, inhibiting monocyte trafficking, inhibiting T-cell proliferation and reducing the expression of a number of cytokines, for example, IL-1, IL-2 and TNF-α. Prednisolone is used prophylactically before transplantation to prevent rejection; methylprednisolone is used in the treatment of rejection. IL-2 receptor antibody (daclizumab; E) targets the CD25 of IL-2 receptors expressed on the surface of activated T cells. It is especially used in kidney transplant patients to prevent organ rejection. Common side effects of all immunosuppressants include increased risk of infections, hepatotoxicity and malignancy.

Human immunodeficiency virus

25 B The human immunodeficiency virus (HIV) is a spherical virus with a lipid envelope. Risk factors for transmission include anal intercourse, infected blood products, intravenous drug use and vertical transmission. Structurally, HIV consists of a core, capsid and envelope. The first step in HIV infection involves binding of the envelope glycoprotein gp120 (B) to the CXCR4 receptor on the cell surface of the CD4+ T cell. Once bound the HIV envelope undergoes structural change allowing the glycoprotein gp41 (C) to penetrate the CD4+ T-cell wall to stabilize the attachment. Once bound, HIV can inject viral RNA and replicating enzymes, including reverse transcriptase (D), integrase and protease, into the target cell. The RNA undergoes reverse transcription via reverse transcriptase to form cDNA, which is integrated into the host DNA by integrase. CD4+ cell death occurs by one of three mechanisms. The infected CD4+ T cells may be killed by cytotoxic CD8+ T cells; budding of HIV may cause CD4+ T cells to burst; infected CD4+ T cells may fuse with uninfected CD4+ T cells forming giant cells (syncytia) that balloon and die. The Gag protein (A) provides infrastructural support for HIV. HIV may also bind to macrophages via the cell surface receptor CCR5 (E). Macrophages infected by HIV are not destroyed but are used as replicating reservoirs as well as a means of gaining entry to the central nervous system as macrophages are able to cross the blood–brain barrier. HIV infection may progress to acquired immunodeficiency syndrome (AIDS) which is defined by a CD4+ count less than 200 cells/μL of blood or an AIDS-defining illness, for example infection by *Mycobacterium avium intracellulare, Candia albicans oesophagutus* and toxoplasmosis. Patients with AIDS are also at increased risk of developing Kaposi's sarcoma, non-Hodgkin's lymphoma and cervical cancer.

Vaccines

26 A The boy in this case has had a Mantoux test to determine if he has a latent tuberculosis (TB) infection. The test is negative and hence he can be given the Bacillus Calmette–Guèrin (BCG) vaccine to provide immunity against TB. The BCG vaccine is a live attenuated (A) vaccination, prepared using a weakened live bovine tuberculosis bacillus. Other examples of live attenuated vaccines include polio (Sabin), MMR and typhoid. Live attenuated vaccines provide long-term immunity and protection against a number of reactive strains; they do not require boosters or adjuvants as such vaccines trigger a sufficiently strong immune response. Live attenuated vaccines are contraindicated in immunocompromised patients. In inactivated (B) vaccines pathogens are destroyed so they are unable to replicate but retain the ability to induce an immune response. Examples include vaccines against cholera, hepatitis A virus and rabies. Inactivated vaccines are suitable for patients with immunodeficiency but require boosters. Subunit (C) vaccines are characterized by the use of antigenic proteins (not whole organisms) and include hepatitis B virus (recombinant), pneumococcal, diphtheria, tetanus and pertussis vaccines. Conjugated (D) vaccines are those used to immunize against encapsulated bacteria such as influenza, pneumococcus and *Nissseria meningitides*. Passive immunity (E) describes immunity derived from the transfer of immunoglobulin. This form of immunity lasts approximately 3 weeks as the immunoglobulin proteins are broken down within the body. Examples of passive immunity include the use of human rabies immunoglobulin (HRIg) in rabies cases, as well as prophylactic and post-exposure use for hepatitis A infection (must be given within 2 weeks of exposure).

Immune-based therapies (1)

27 D A primary role for immune-based therapies is to boost the immune response to improve protection against infection and malignancy, especially in those who are immunodeficient. Bruton's agammaglobulinaemia is characterized by a mutation of the *BTK* gene, a tyrosine kinase. This mutation leads to inhibition of B-cell maturation and as a consequence B-cell and immunoglobulin levels are diminished. Blood investigations will reveal decreased circulating B cells as well as immunoglobulins. Patients are at risk of recurrent infections, particularly encapsulated bacteria, and must therefore receive passive immunity to protect against such pathogens. Intravenous IgG (D) is not a cure for Bruton's agammaglobulinaemia but prolongs survival. Treatment must be continued throughout life. Intravenous IgG is also used in the treatment of hyper IgM syndrome, common variable immunodeficiency as well as secondary antibody deficiencies. Haematopoietic stem cell transplant (HSCT; E)

involves the transplant of multipotent haematopietic stem cells which may either be autologous (from self) or allogenic (from a donor). In either case, myeloablative techniques are used to destroy the remaining cells of the bone marrow which leads to increased risk of infection throughout the course of the treatment. HSCT is indicated in diseases such as severe combined immunodeficiency (SCID), leukaemia and multiple myeloma.

Interferons are signalling proteins involved in the immune system in response to pathogens and tumour cells. They act via the Janus kinase-STAT (Jak-STAT) pathway to produce further anti-viral, anti-proliferative and immunoregulatory factors. IFN-α (A) is used in the treatment of hepatitis B, hepatitis C, Kaposi's sarcoma and chronic myeloid leukaemia. IFN-β (B) is indicated in the treatment of multiple sclerosis, but its mechanism of action is unknown. IFN-γ (C) is used in the treatment of chronic granulomatous disease, a disease in which phagocytes lack the enzyme NADPH, and hence neutrophils are unable to clear pathogens.

Immune-based therapies (2)

28   D   Anti-proliferative agents broadly inhibit DNA synthesis and thereby interfere with cell proliferation, especially those cells with a high turnover, for example leukocytes. In this case, the side effects suggestive of folate deficiency point to methotrexate (D) as the correct answer. Methotrexate is an anti-metabolite and anti-folate drug indicated for the treatment of cancer as well as autoimmune diseases including rheumatoid arthritis and systemic lupus erythematosus. Methotrexate inhibits dihydrofolate reductase (DHFR), an enzyme involved in the synthesis of the nucleoside thymidine; thymidine is essential for DNA synthesis. As folate is required for the synthesis of purine, production of this base is also disrupted. Ultimately, proliferation of leukocytes is interrupted. Side effects include those of folate deficiency (macrocytic megaloblastic anaemia, loss of appetite, tiredness, weakness and depression). The low white cell count that results predisposes to infection; this is an adverse effect of all anti-proliferative drugs. Cyclophosphamide (A) is an alkylating agent, attaching an alkyl group to the guanine base of DNA. This causes damage to the DNA structure and therefore prevents cell replication; cyclophosphamide affects B-cell replication more than T cells. Complications of therapy include bone marrow suppression, hair loss and carcinogenic properties that may cause transitional cell carcinoma of the bladder. Mycophenolate mofetil (B) is the pro-drug of mycophenolic acid which inhibits inosine monophosphate dehydrogenase (IMPDH), an enzyme required in guanine synthesis; impaired guanine synthesis reduces the proliferation of both T and B cells, but T cells are affected to a greater extent. Side effects include bone marrow suppression (particularly low white blood cells and platelets). Azathioprine

(C) is metabolized in the liver to 6-mercaptopurine which causes the inhibition of purine synthesis and preferentially inhibits T-cell activation and proliferation. A proportion of the population have a thiopurine methyltransferase (TPMT) polymorphism, rendering them unable to metabolize azathioprine; patients therefore have a predisposition to azathioprine toxicity. Cisplatin (E) is a chemotherapeutic agent which cross-links with DNA and interferes with cell proliferation. Side effects include nephrotoxicity, neurotoxicity and ototoxicity.

Immune-based therapies (3)

29 E   The patient in question has symptoms and signs suggestive of severe myasthenia gravis (myasthenic crisis), typified by paralysis of the respiratory muscles requiring ventilator assistance. The best treatment in this scenario is plasmapheresis (E), a method of rapidly removing circulating anti-acetylcholine receptor antibodies from the circulation; effects last only for a short period. The patient's own plasma is treated to remove immunoglobulins, and then reinfused. Other indications for plasmapheresis include Goodpasture's syndrome (anti-glomerular basement membrane proteins).

Pharmacological treatment of myasthenia gravis primary involves the use of acetylcholinesterase inhibitors. However, immunosuppressive agents, such as corticosteroids (D), also have a role. Corticosteroids inhibit phospholipase A2, thereby blocking prostaglandin formation as well as a spectrum of inflammatory mediators. The immunosuppressive effects of corticosteroids are numerous and include reducing the number of circulating B cells, inhibiting monocyte trafficking, inhibiting T-cell proliferation and reducing the expression of a number of cytokines, for example, IL-1, IL-2 and TNF-α. Prednisolone is used prophylactically before transplantation to prevent rejection; methylprednisolone is used in the treatment of rejection. Side effects are frequent, however, and include osteoporosis, diabetes mellitus and hypertension.

Inhibitors of cell signalling which have been used in the management of myasthenia gravis include ciclosporin (A). Ciclosporin inhibits the protein phosphatase calcineurin. This in turn inhibits IL-2 secretion from T cells, a cytokine which stimulates T-cell proliferation. Adverse effects include nephrotoxicity, hepatotoxicity, diarrhoea and pancreatitis. Side effects of cyclosporine use include gum hyperplasia. Other inhibitors of cell signalling, although not indicated in myasethenia gravis management, include tacrolimus (B) and rapamycin (sirolimus; C). Tacrolimus is a calcineurin inhibitor that inhibits T-cell proliferation by binding to FK-binding protein-1A (FKBP-1A), ultimately preventing T-cell activation. Rapamycin inhibits T-cell proliferation by binding to FKBP-1A. Its advantage lies in its low nephrotoxicity in comparison to other immunosuppressive agents.

Immune-based therapies (4)

30 A Immunosuppressive agents which are directed against cell surface antigens primarily target cluster of differentiation (CD) molecules. Basiliximab (A) is an antibody directed towards IL-2 receptor α chain (CD25) which causes reduction in T-cell proliferation. It is used as prophylactic treatment of allograft rejection, most commonly in patients undergoing kidney transplant. Adverse effects include increased risk of infection as well as a long-term risk of malignancy. Abatacept (B) is a CTLA4–immunoglobulin fusion protein indicated in the treatment of rheumatoid arthritis, which has been resistant to treatment with disease modifying drugs (DMARDs). Abatacept prevents antigen presenting cells from delivering a co-stimulatory signal to T cells in order to promote activation; this is achieved by abatacept binding with high affinity to the B7 protein (CD80 and CD86) on the cell surface of APCs. Side effects include increased risk of infection from TB, hepatitis B virus and hepatitis C virus. Rituximab (C) is a CD20 monoclonal antibody which causes reduced proliferation of B cells. It has a wide spectrum of indications, including treatment of lymphoma, rheumatoid arthritis and systemic lupus erythematosus. Adverse effects of rituximab include increased risk of hepatitis B reactivation and progressive multifocal leukoencephalopathy (PML). Natalizumab (D) is a monoclonal antibody against α4-integrin, an adhesion receptor which mediates the migration of T cells from the circulation to target organs; natalizumab prevents this migration. It is used in the treatment of multiple sclerosis (reduced T-cell migration to the central nervous system by influencing endothelial cells expressing VCAM1) and Crohn's disease (reduced interaction of MADCAM1 and α4-integrin at sites of inflammation in the gastrointestinal tract). Tocilizumab (E) is a monoclonal IL-6 receptor antibody, indicated in Castleman's disease and rheumatoid arthritis. IL-6 is a pro-inflammatory cytokine which promotes the immune response; inhibition thereby reduces macrophage, neutrophil, T-cell and B-cell activation. Tocilizumab is hepatotoxic and raises serum cholesterol; liver function tests and cholesterol must be monitored regularly.

Immune-based therapies (5)

31 B Immunosuppressive agents may be directed at specific cytokines to modify the pathogenesis of certain disease processes. Adalimumab (B) is a fully human monoclonal antibody to TNF-α. TNF-α has the physiological role of inducing pro-inflammatory cytokines as well as promoting leukocyte migration and endothelial adhesion. Adalimumab has a large number of indications, including rheumatoid arthritis, ankylosing spondylitis and Crohn's disease. Infliximab (A) is a mouse-human chimeric TNF-α antagonist indicated in similar conditions to

adalimumab. Infliximab has a high affinity for TNF-α. Toxicity may result in reduced protection against infection from TB, hepatitis B virus and hepatitis C virus, a lupus-like condition, demyelination and malignancy. Etanercept (C) is also a TNF-α monoclonal antibody, which is a fusion protein between the TNF-receptor 2 and Fc portion of IgG1. Potential adverse effects include increased risk of infection, demyelination and malignancy.

Ustekinumab (D) is an antibody to the p40 subunit of Il-12 and IL-23, thereby preventing T-cell and natural-killer cell activation. It is used in the treatment of psoriatic arthritis. Denosumab (E) is an antibody directed towards the RANK ligand in bones. Osteoblasts are responsible for bone formation, whilst osteoclasts (which contain the cell surface receptor RANK) break down bone. Inhibition of RANK by denosumab therefore inhibits osteoclast function and differentiation, thereby preventing the breakdown of bone. Denosumab is indicated in the treatment of osteoporosis but is also used in the management of multiple myeloma and bone metastases. Toxicity can predispose to respiratory and urinary tract infections.

Rheumatic diseases (1)

32   E   This patient has presented with generalized dryness, a characteristic clinical feature of Sjögren's syndrome. Autoimmune destruction of the epithelial cells of exocrine glands causes such features, including dryness of the eyes (confirmed by Schirmer's test) and mouth; other clinical symptoms and signs include parotid swelling, fatigue, arthralgia and myalgia. Anti-Ro (anti-SS-A; E) and Anti-La (anti-SS-B) antibodies are present in approximately 50 per cent of patients with Sjögren's syndrome, as well as a lower proportion of patients with systemic lupus erythematosus. Blood tests will demonstrate a raised ESR and occasionally a mild anaemia. Anti-Jo1 (A) antibody is present in patients with dermatomyositis. Dermatomyositis is characterized by autoimmune inflammation of muscle fibres and skin. Clinical features include a heliotrope rash around the eyes, Gottron's papules on the dorsum of finger joints, as well as weakness of the proximal limb muscles which causes difficulty in climbing stairs and rising from a chair. Blood tests reveal a raised creatine kinase level. Anti-cyclic citrullinated protein (anti-CCP; B) antibody is associated with rheumatoid arthritis. The antibody is directed at the filament aggregating protein, filaggrin. Rheumatoid arthritis is a chronic systemic autoimmune disease that results in a symmetrical deforming polyarthritis. Clinical features include deformities of the hands (Boutonierre's deformity, swan-neck deformity, Z-thumb and ulnar deviation of the fingers). Extra-articular manifestations include pulmonary fibrosis, pericardial effusion, rheumatoid nodules and splenomegaly (Felty's syndrome). Anti-centromere (C) antibody is

associated with limited systemic scleroderma (CREST syndrome). CREST syndrome is characterized by calcinosis, Reynaud's syndrome, oesophageal dysmotility, sclerodactyly and telangiectasia. Blood investigations will reveal a raised ESR, anaemia and hypergammaglobulinaemia. Anti-topoisomerase (D) antibody is characteristic of diffuse systemic scleroderma. Diffuse systemic scleroderma shares some features of limited systemic scleroderma, however, it is more aggressive in its course, affecting large areas of the skin as well as involving the kidneys, heart and lungs.

Rheumatic diseases (2)

33 C Anti-nuclear antibodies (ANA) are directed at the cell nucleus and are present in a number of rheumatic autoimmune diseases. Indirect immunofluorescence is an immunological technique that can be used to help determine the ANA in question. In this scenario, the patient has signs and symptoms suggestive of dermatomyositis. Dermatomyositis is characterized by the presence of anti-Jo-1 antibodies, which will demonstrate a speckled (C) pattern on immunofluorescence. Dermatomyositis (and polymyositis) are inflammatory diseases of the peripheral skeletal muscles. The disease is associated with HLA DR3 and DR52. Clinical features include weakness of the proximal muscles of the arms and legs; on direct questioning there may be difficulty climbing stairs for example. Dermatological manifestations include the presence of a heliotrope on the eyelids and Gottron's papules. Dermatomyositis is associated with increased risk of lung, ovary, breast and stomach cancer. Other antibodies which demonstrate a speckled appearance on immunofluorescence include anti-Smith (SLE), anti-RNP (mixed connective tissue disease) and anti-Ro (Sjögren's disease). A homogeneous pattern (A) is consistent with the presence of anti-histone antibodies, characteristic of drug-induced SLE. A nucleolar (B) pattern is indicative of anti-RNA polymerase, which suggests underlying systemic sclerosis. A peripheral (D) pattern on immunofluorescence is found in the presence of anti-double stranded DNA (dsDNA) antibodies in SLE. Kinetoplasts (E) are the mitochondria found in *Crithidialuciliae*, a non-pathogenic haemoflagellate, and may be used as a substrate for pure dsDNA in the diagnosis of SLE.

Rheumatic diseases (3)

34 B The seronegative spondyloarthritides are a collection of inflammatory conditions which are rheumatoid factor negative. Other features common to this group of diseases include the association with HLA B27, involvement of the spine and sacroiliac joints and tendency to enthesitis (inflammation at the site of attachment of tendons to bones).

This patient has symptoms, signs and investigative features suggestive of reactive arthritis (B). The term 'reactive' in the disease name is
given due to the disease being preceded by infection (in this case by
Chlamydia trachomatis). Other predisposing infections include *Shigella*,
Yersinia and *Campylobacter* spp. Reactive arthritis is also known as
Reiter's syndrome, which is defined by the triad of uveitis, urethritis and
arthritis ('can't see, pee or bend their knee'). The arthritis will typically
be transient and dactylitis may be a feature. Patients may also develop
constitutional symptoms such as fever, fatigue and weight loss. Blood
tests will reveal a raised ESR and CRP, while joint aspirate will be sterile. Ankylosing spondylitis (AS; A) is a chronic inflammatory condition
involving the spine and sacroiliac joints; approximately 95 per cent of
patients are HLA B27 positive. It is believed the underlying autoimmune
pathogenesis occurs as a result of molecular mimicry. Characteristically,
stiffness of the joints is relieved by exercise. Acute iritis is common in
AS patients. Vertebral syndesmophytes are a feature on imaging of the
spine. Enteropathic arthritis (C) is associated with inflammatory bowel
disease. Psoriatic arthritis (D) occurs in conjunction with psoriasis, primarily affecting the distal interphalyngeal joints and spine. Anterior
uveitis (E) causes redness of the eye, photophobia, excessive lacrima-
tion and blurred vision. It is often associated with other seronegative
spondylarthropathies.

Rheumatic diseases (4)

35 C   Systemic sclerosis is a chronic, inflammatory condition characterized
by fibrosis of the skin, blood vessels and internal organs. It can be
classified into a form that has major skin involvement (diffuse systemic
sclerosis) and a form in which skin involvement is limited to the distal
limbs and face (limited systemic sclerosis; CREST). CREST is defined by
calcinosis, Raynaud's phenomenon, oesophageal dysmotility, sclerodactyly and telangiectasia and is associated with the presence of circulating anti-centromere antibodies. Given the absence of diffuse cutaneous
manifestations and combined with the symptoms and signs, the diagnosis is limited systemic sclerosis. TNF-β (C) is central to the pathogenesis of limited systemic sclerosis. Together with platelet-derived growth
factor (PDGF), TNF-β, produced by macrophages and T cells (IL-2 (B)
produced by CD4+ T cells induces further proliferation of T cells),
stimulate collagen production by fibroblasts. Collagen is deposited in
the extracellular matrix of the skin, oesophagus, alveoli of the lungs,
myocardium of the heart, liver and blood vessels; the pro-fibrotic state
correlates with the clinical features of limited systemic sclerosis.

In the early phase of the disease, activated T cells and TNF-α (D) cause
damage to endothelial cells. Endothelial disruption causes binding of
von Willebrand factor (vWF; A), with consequent platelet aggregation

and release of PDGF. Endothelin-1 (E) is a potent vasoconstrictor, the increased release of which contributes to Raynaud's phenomenon as well as systemic sclerosis-associated pulmonary hypertension.

Autoantibodies in type 1 diabetes mellitus

36   D   Type 1 diabetes mellitus (T1DM) is a hyperglycaemic state caused by autoimmune destruction of the β-cells in the islets of Langerhans of the pancreas. The β-cells are responsible for the production of insulin. The underlying pathogenesis of T1DM relates to T-cell mediated damage of β-cells. The presence of glucose in the urine leads to the symptom of polyuria (glucose is a potent osmolyte attracting water to enter the renal tubules via osmosis). Polydipsia, weight loss and thirst are other characteristic clinical features. An overnight fasting plasma glucose level of above 7.0 mmol/L is diagnostic of diabetes. Another investigative test which can be used is the oral glucose tolerance test. T1DM affects men and women equally and usually presents in the pubertal years. T1DM is strongly associated with HLA DR3 and DR4 alleles.

A number of autoantibodies are implicated in the disease process of T1DM. In this case autoantibodies to tyrosine phosphatase have been detected. Two antibodies to tyrosine phosphatase are present in T1DM: anti-IA-2 antibodies (D) and anti-phogrin antibodies. Tyrosine phosphatase autoantibodies are found in approximately 75 per cent of patients with T1DM. Islet cell surface antibodies (A) are found less frequently in patients with T1DM. However, they are more specific for pancreatic β-cells than tyrosine phosphatase autoantibodies and bind to components of the surface of islet cells. Islet cell antibodies (ICA; E) are directed to components of the islet cell cytoplasm. Patients with T1DM may also have antibodies direct at insulin, or so called insulin auto-antibodies (B). Anti-glutamic acid decarboxylase antibody (anti-GAD antibody; C) is not β-cell specific but is present in a high proportion of T1DM patients. GAD is an enzyme responsible for the conversion of glutamate to GABA; GABA is the neurotransmitter involved in the release of insulin from β-cells.

Autoimmune thyroid disease

37   A   Thyroid disease can be classified as hyperthyroidism (increased thyroid activity) or hypothyroidism (reduced thyroid activity). Autoimmune thyroid disease may be split into Graves' disease (hyperthyroidism) and Hashimoto's thyroiditis (hypothyroidism), each with characteristic clinical and immunological features. The patient in this scenario has clinical features suggestive of Graves' disease. Such symptoms include unintentional weight loss, tremor, excessive sweating, heat intolerance, palpitations and diarrhoea. Signs suggestive of Graves' disease are a

goitre, proximal myopathy, brisk reflexes, tachycardia, atrial fibrillation, pre-tibial myxoedema, ophthalmopathy and exophthalmos. Graves'
disease is defined by the presence of stimulating anti-TSH receptor (A)
antibodies, which bind to the TSH receptor, inducing production of
thyroxine. The pathophysiology behind exophthalmos is thought to be
due to similar receptors to TSH receptor in the extra-ocular muscles, to
which stimulatory anti-TSH antibodies bind, causing protrusion of the
eyes. Isotope scanning will demonstrate diffuse uptake. Thyroid growth
stimulating antibodies (E) are also found in patients with Graves' disease but to a far lesser extent. They induce growth of thyroid follicles.

Hashimoto's thyroiditis is a chronic autoimmune disease, characterized
by thyroid under-activity. Features of hypothyroidism include weight
gain, cold intolerance, constipation, hoarse voice and menstrual abnormalities. Signs indicative of hypothyroidism are slow reflexes, bradycardia and an enlarged, nodular goitre. The two major antibodies found
in Hashimoto's thyroiditis patients are anti-thyroid peroxidase (C) and
anti-thyroglobulin (D); thyroid peroxidase is an enzyme required in the
iodination of thyroglobulin. Non-stimulatory anti-TSH receptor (B) antibodies are a feature of primary hypothyroidism.

Autoimmune polyendocrine syndromes

38   C   The autoimmune polyendocrine syndromes are a group of conditions
characterized by autoimmune disease affecting numerous endocrine
(and non-endocrine) organs. This child has symptoms, signs and investigative features consistent with Kearns–Sayre syndrome (oculocranio-
somatic disease; C). Kearns–Sayre syndrome is a myopathic disease
caused by deletions of mitochondrial DNA. Initially, the disease process
affects the eyelid and extra-ocular muscles leading to ptosis and difficulty with eye movement. Pigmentary retinopathy is another feature,
causing diffuse pigmentation of the retina. Other clinical manifestations
of Kearns–Sayre syndrome are proximal muscle weakness, cardiac con-
duction defects, hearing loss and cerebellar ataxia. Endocrine system
effects include: hypoparathyroidism (causing hypocalcaemia), primary
gonadal failure, diabetes mellitus and hypopituitarism. Hirata's disease
(insulin autoimmune syndrome; A), in contrast to Kearne–Sayre syndrome, is defined by fasting hypoglycaemia as well as autoantibodies to
serum insulin. It is most prevalent in Japan (third most common cause
of hypoglycaemia) but extremely rare in other countries. IPEX (B) is
otherwise known as immunodysregulation polyendocrinopathy enteropathy X-linked syndrome and is caused by dysfunctional regulatory
T cells (as a result of abnormal FoxP3), ultimately predisposing to autoimmune disease. The condition manifests with diabetes mellitus, eczema
and enteropathy. POEMS syndrome (D) is the acronym given to the
following collection of clinical features: polyneuropathy/papilledoema/

pulmonary disease, organomegaly/oedema, endocrinopathy, M-protein (usually IgG or IgM) and skin abnormalities (hyperpigmentation and hypertrichosis). APECED syndrome type 1 (autoimmune polyendocrine syndrome type 1; E) is associated with mild immune deficiency, dysfunctional parathyroid gland/adrenal gland, hypothyroidism, gonadal failure, alopecia and vitiligo) and results from mutations in the AIRE gene, a key player in central tolerance.

Autoantibodies in liver disease

39   C   This patient is most likely to have autoimmune hepatitis (AIH) given the biopsy findings of interface hepatitis, which is typical of the disease. AIH is a disease of unknown aetiology characterized by inflammation, hepatocellular necrosis and fibrosis, which may ultimately lead to cirrhosis and liver failure. Diagnosis is based on a combination of histological and antibody evidence. Patients will commonly have a history of other autoimmune disease. In this case, the patient is most likely to have AIH type 2 due to the early age of diagnosis (more common in paediatric population) and poor steroid response. AIH type 2 is characterized by the presence of anti-liver kidney microsomal antibodies (C). AIH type 2 also has an association with IgA deficiency. A diagnosis of AIH type 1 is suggested by the presence of anti-nuclear antibodies (A) and anti-smooth muscle antibodies (B). AIH type 2 may be diagnosed in patients from 10 years of age to elderly patients. The disease course is less severe than type 2 and responds well to steroid therapy. There is also a third type of AIH which is characterized by the presence of anti-soluble liver antigen antibodies.

Anti-mitochondrial antibodies (D) are present in patients with primary biliary cirrhosis (PBC), a chronic liver disease characterized by the destruction of intrahepatic bile ducts. Patients with PBC often have raised IgM levels. The presence of anti-HBs (E) antibody would suggest hepatitis B virus (HBV) infection. Anti-HBs antibodies are a marker of acquired immune status.

Autoimmune gastrointestinal disease

40   E   Coeliac disease (gluten-induced enteropathy) is an autoimmune condition triggered by gluten intolerance. It is specifically prolamins that induce the immune response; examples of prolamins include gliadin in wheat, hordein in barley and secalin in rye. It has been found that it is the α-gliadin portion of gluten that is implicated in the pathogenesis. Gliadin is resistant to degradation by gastrointestinal enzymes and subsequently translocates across the intestinal barrier. Within the lamina propria, gliadin is deamidated to glutamic acid via the action of transglutaminase. This creates a negative charge which,

in genetically susceptible individuals, is able to bind to HLA DQ2 (E) on the surface of antigen presenting cells with high affinity. Patients with the HLA DQ8 (D) allele are also susceptible to developing coeliac disease but to a far lesser extent. The peptide is presented to T-helper cells which activate plasma cells to produce antibodies (anti-gliadin, anti-endomysial and anti-tissue transglutaminase antibodies), as well as lymphocytes such as natural-killer cells and macrophages, which in turn release IFN-γ, IL-4 and TNF-α causing enterocyte damage. Disease is characterized histologically by villous atrophy, crypt hyperplasia and an intraepithelial infiltrate of lymphocytes. Clinical features include abdominal pain, diarrhoea, steatorrhoea, as well as symptoms and signs of nutrient deficiencies.

Coeliac disease is also strongly associated with dermatitis herpetiformis (A), a dermatological condition characterized by sub-epidermal deposits of IgA. Coeliac disease may exist in conjunction with other autoimmune diseases such as vitiligo (B), systemic lupus erythematosus and/or type 1 diabetes mellitus. Patients with IgA deficiency are also at increased risk of developing coeliac disease (C) compared to those who are not deficient; IgA deficiency increases the difficulty of serological testing.

Skin disease (1)

41 B   Autoimmune skin disorders are characterized by autoantibodies directed at components of the epidermis, basement membrane zone and dermis. This patient has presented with a blistering condition (bullous disease). The fact that anti-desmoglein 3 antibodies have been detected, together with the histological finding of acantholysis, point to pemphigus vulgaris (B) as the correct diagnosis. Pemphigus vulgaris is more prevalent in the Mediterranean population. Direct immunofluorescence reveals intercellular epidermal IgG and C3 deposition, while indirect immunofluorescence demonstrates intercellular IgG. Skin histology shows the presence of acantholytic cells, which is defined as the separation of keratinocytes caused by loss of intercellular cadherin connections. Clinical features include blisters appearing in the mouth and skin, which are very friable. Unaffected skin becomes increasingly fragile and exfoliation of such areas occurs with light rubbing (Nikolsky sign positive). High dose steroids (with or without immunosuppressive agents such as azathioprine) is the mainstay treatment.

Pemphigus foliaceous (A) is characterized by immunological and histological findings similar to pemphigus vulgaris. However, it is desmoglein 1 which is the target for autoantibodies, and the clinical course is far less severe in the case of pemphigus foliaceous. Autoantibodies to components of hemidesmosomes of the basement membrane zone are associated with bullous pemphigoid (C). Indirect immunofluorescence demonstrates a linear pattern of IgG and C3 at the basement membrane zone. Clinical features include generalized blisters on the skin which are very itchy. Epidermolysis bullosa (D) is caused by autoantibodies to type VII collagen, which forms anchors between the layers of the skin; as a result, bullae are usually induced by trauma. Dermatitis herpetiformis (A) is characterized by vesicles located on extensor surfaces. Immunological studies reveal deposits of IgA at the dermal papillae. Dermatitis herpetiformis is associated with coeliac disease, and anti-gliadin and anti-endomysial antibodies may be present in the circulation.

Skin disease (2)

42 D This patient has presented with skin depigmentation, lesions appearing completely white; the most likely diagnosis is vitiligo. It is associated with autoimmune disease, including type 1 diabetes, pernicious anaemia and Addison's disease. Vitiligo is also a common feature in patients with autoimmune polyendocrine syndromes. The pathogenesis of vitiligo involves the autoimmune destruction of melanocytes, which are responsible for the production of the pigment melanin; anti-melanocyte antibodies (D) are found in patients with vitiligo. As a result, histology of affected areas will reveal an absence of melanocytes. Other causes of hypopigmentation (which are usually generalized) include albinism and phenylketonuria.

Psoriasis is a chronic skin condition characterized by pink/salmon plaques covered in silvery scales which occur primarily over the extensor surfaces of the body as well as the scalp. Other clinical features include pitting of the nail beds and onycholysis. Auspitz's sign relates to the disease and is defined by pin-point bleeding when psoriatic plaques are peeled away. Triggers for disease are thought to include β-haemolytic streptococcal infection (A), trauma, drugs and UV radiation. The pathogenesis of psoriasis involves the migration of neutrophils and T cells from the dermis to the epidermis, which induce skin cell proliferation. Vancomycin (B) is associated with linear IgA bullous dermatosis (LABD), characterized by linear deposition of IgA on direct immunofluorescence. Pemphigoid gestationis is a bullous disorder associated with pregnancy (C). Bullae appear in the second or third trimester of pregnancy, which are characterized by itchiness; the condition tends to resolve post-partum. Multiple myeloma (E), as well as other lymphoproliferative disorders, is associated with paraneoplastic pemphigus.

Non-proliferative glomerulonephritis

43 E The non-proliferative glomerulonephritides are characterized by a lack of hypercellularity of the glomeruli. This group of conditions cause nephrotic syndrome, as this child has presented with, defined by the

classical triad of hypoalbuminaemia, proteinuria (greater than 3.5 g) and oedema. Hyperlipidaemia and lipiduria may also be present. The pathogenesis of nephrotic syndrome begins with immune damage to the glomerulus which subsequently becomes leaky; proteinuria arises leading to hypoalbuminaemia. Hypoalbuminaemia consequently causes reduction in oncotic pressure and hence oedema ensues. In an attempt to maintain oncotic pressure the liver compensates by increasing lipid production; those are lost through the leaky glomeruli (lipiduria). The most common cause of nephrotic syndrome in children is minimal change disease (E), which is the correct answer in this scenario due to the recent allergic reaction (bee sting; type I hypersensitivity reaction) as well as the strong response to steroid treatment, which leads to remission of disease in the vast majority of cases. Histological characteristics of renal biopsy specimens include a lack of structural change visible on light microscopy, while electron microscopy will demonstrate podocyte effacement.

Focal segmental glomerulonephritis (FSGN) is another cause of nephrotic syndrome, characterized histologically by focal sclerosis of glomeruli. Immunofluorescence will reveal the presence of IgM and C3 deposition in affected areas. Patients will usually present with some degree of renal impairment. FSGN may be idiopathic or occur secondary to conditions such as Alport syndrome (A) and reflux nephropathy (B). Alport syndrome is a hereditary syndrome (mutation of $\alpha 4$ chain of type IV collagen) associated with glomerulonephritis, end-stage kidney disease and hearing loss. Reflux nephropathy results from vesico-ureteric reflux due to chronic pyelonephritis.

Membranous glomerulonephritis most commonly occurs in adults, and demonstrates a thickened glomerular basement membrane and spike/dome protrusions on histology. Direct immunofluorescence reveals the presence of sub-epithelial granular deposits of IgG and C3. Causes of membranous glomerulonephritis include infections, neoplasia, drugs and connective tissue disease, for example systemic lupus erythematosus (D). Patients with hydrocephalus who have a cerebral shunt *in situ* are prone to shunt nephritis (C), a cause of membranous glomerulonephritis. The pathogenesis involves the increased risk of long-term bacterial infection, leading to immune complex deposition in the glomeruli.

Proliferative glomerulonephritis

44   C   Proliferative glomerulonephritides is characterized by an increased number of cells in the glomerulus. This group of diseases usually present with nephritic syndrome, defined by the presence of haematuria, red cell casts, dysmorphic red cells, oliguria and hypertension.

Proteinuria and oedema may also be present. Immune damage to the glomerular vessels results in severe inflammation, allowing red cells to pass into the tubule; in the process these red cells experience mechanical damage while passing through the inflamed vessels and as a result are dysmorphic. Cells of the distal convoluted tubule and collecting duct secrete a glycoprotein called Tamm–Horsefell protein which sticks red cells together forming cylindrical red cell casts. The patient in this scenario has features of nephrotic syndrome; the history of a sore throat preceding the new symptoms, combined with the raised anti-streptolysin O titre, suggests a streptococcal infection. Post-streptococcal glomerulonephritis (C) is usually caused by a preceding infection (most commonly group A β haemolytic streptococci). Pathological hallmarks of post-streptococcal glomerulonephritis include diffuse hypercellularity and diffuse swelling of the mesangium and glomerular capillaries. Direct immunofluorescence reveals the subepithelial deposition of IgG and C3. The condition usually subsides with supportive treatment.

IgA nephropathy (Berger's disease; A) is the most common cause of glomerulonephritis in the developed world. Characteristically there is mesangial deposition of IgA. The condition occurs a few days after a gastrointestinal or upper respiratory infection, especially caused by *Haemophilus influenzae*. Henoch–Schönlein purpura (HSP; B) is a small vessel vasculitis in which IgA and C3 are deposited in blood vessels, leading to systemic clinical effects. In contrast to IgA nephropathy, which tends to affect adults, HSP has a greater prevalence in children.

Membranoproliferative glomerulonephritis (D) is defined by mesangial cell proliferation with thickening of the capillaries. Two types exist: type 1 in which there is classical and alternative complement pathway activation and type 2 which is associated with only alternative pathway activation.

Rapid progressive glomerulonephritis (RPGN; E) is the most aggressive of all glomerulonephritides, and may cause end-stage renal failure over a period of days. The three sub-types include immune complex disease, pauci-immune disease and anti-glomerular basement membrane disease, all of which demonstrate the crescent sign on biopsy (proliferation of macrophages and parietal epithelial cells).

Lupus nephritis

45 B Systemic lupus erythematosus (SLE) is a multisystem autoimmune condition characterized by the presence of anti-nuclear antibodies; glomerunephritis is a common complication of the disease process, also known as lupus nephritis. Generally, lupus nephritis is characterized by the deposition of IgG, IgM, IgA and C3 in the sub-endothelial segment

of the glomerular basement membrane and in the mesangium. However, the disease can be more accurately classified based on the pathological features, which is a useful tool for monitoring disease and assessing severity. The classification is as follows:

Stage	Light microscopy	Electron microscopy and immunofluorescence
Stage I (minimal mesangial lupus nephritis)	No changes to glomeruli	Mesangial immune deposits
Stage II (mesangial proliferative lupus nephritis)	Changes confined to mesangium	Mesangial immune deposits
Stage III (focal lupus nephritis)	Focal, segmental or glomerulonephritis involving <50 per cent of all glomeruli	Subendothelial and mesangial immune deposits
Stage IV (diffuse proliferative nephritis)	Focal, segmental or glomerulonephritis involving >50 per cent of all glomeruli	Subendothelial immune deposits
Stage V (membranous lupus nephritis)	Glomerular sclerosis involving >90 per cent of glomeruli, fibrosis and tubular atrophy	Subepithelial and intramembranous immune deposits

From the above classification, it is clear that the biopsy investigation points to stage II (B) as the correct answer. The stage of disease is also consistent with the clinical features. Stage II suggests mild disease with haematuria or proteinuria; supportive treatment is warranted. Stage I (A) is characterized by mild proteinuria. Stage III (C) suggests mild-to-moderate disease which may be accompanied by worsening renal function tests. Stage IV (D) suggests moderate–severe disease; the patient may have hypertension, reflecting renal disease, worsening renal function tests and active SLE. Stage V (E) is characterized by the presence of nephrotic syndrome.

Vasculitis

46 B   The vasculitides are a group of conditions that are characterized by inflammation within blood vessels leading to systemic clinical manifestations. The vasculitides are classified based on the size of vessel affected; renal disease is usually caused by either small or intermediate vessel vasculitides. The patient in this scenario has presented with epistaxis, haemoptysis and is positive for cytoplasmic anti-neutrophil cytoplasmic antibody (c-ANCA); these features point to Wegener's granulomatosis as the correct answer (B). The antibody, c-ANCA, is central to the pathogenesis, and is directed towards proteinase 3 (PR3), an enzyme normally present within the cytoplasm of neutrophils. It is proposed that an infection is the trigger for the disease, which causes circulating neutrophils

to become adherent to the endothelium; in the process PR3 is upregulated on the neutrophil cell surface as well as being released into the blood vessel lumen. c-ANCA present in the circulation binds to the cell surface PR3 on neutrophils preventing them from migrating through the endothelium. Vasculitis is caused by both direct effect of PR3 on the endothelium as well as c-ANCA–PR3 immune complex deposition. Cryoglobulinaemia (A) is defined by the presence of cryoglobulins in the circulation; these are immunoglobulins that precipitate at low temperatures. Secondary causes include connective tissue diseases and lymphoproliferative conditions. It is, however, unknown why such immunoglobulins are formed in the first instance. When precipitation does occur at cold temperatures, the immunoglobulins adhere to vessel walls, leading to complement activation, neutrophil recruitment and, consequently, vessel damage. Microscopic polyangitis (C) is a small vessel vasculitis affecting the arterioles, venules and capillaries. This vasculitis is associated with focal necrotizing glomerulonephritis as well as the presence of perinuclear ANCA in the circulation (directed towards cytoplasmic myeloperoxidase). Polyarteritis nodosa (PAN; D) is a vasculitis of small and medium-sized vessels associated with hepatitis B infection. Immune complexes (type III hypersensitivity reaction) are deposited within such vessels leading to fibrinoid necrosis and neutrophil infiltration; as a result the vessel walls weaken and there is aneurysm development. PAN is associated with the presence of p-ANCA antibodies. Angiogram will reveal multiple aneurysms. Churg–Strauss syndrome (E) is a medium-and small-vessel autoimmune vasculitis. Blood vessels of the lungs, gastrointestinal system and peripheral nerves are most commonly affected. There is an association with p-ANCA antibodies.

Neurological disease (1)

47   E   The patient in question has presented with axial rigidity/stiffness associated with a history of autoimmune disease and circulating anti-glutamic acid decarboxylase antibodies (anti-GAD), which point to stiff man syndrome (SMS; E) as the correct answer. SMS is a very rare neurological condition which is poorly understood. Clinical features include progressive axial and abdominal wall stiffness. It is strongly associated with the presence of anti-GAD antibodies. However, only a small minority of type 1 diabetes mellitus patients suffer with SMS, suggesting that anti-GAD antibodies do not tell the whole story in terms of aetiology. However, SMS does occur in patients who suffer from other autoimmune diseases including thyroid disease, pernicious anaemia and type 1 diabetes mellitus. Myasthenia gravis (A) is characterized by autoantibodies directed towards the acetylcholine receptor located at the neuromuscular junction. Myasthenia gravis is a condition which presents

with fatigability of muscles; muscles become fatigued after periods of movement but recover after rest. In severe cases, muscles of breathing may become affected, leading to respiratory distress. The presence of a thymus and treatment with D-penicillamine for rheumatoid arthritis are associated with the development of myasthenia gravis. Lambert–Eaton myasthenic syndrome (LEMS; D) is defined by proximal muscle weakness, which is improved by muscle contraction, loss of tendon reflexes and autonomic nervous system dysfunction. Leg involvement is greater than that of myasthenia gravis. It is considered a paraneoplastic syndrome due to its association with small cell lung cancer. LEMS is caused by autoantibodies that target the voltage-gated calcium channels of the pre-synaptic membrane. The pathogenesis of multiple sclerosis (MS; B) is mediated by T cells. Proteolipid protein and myelin basic protein are oligodendrocyte proteins implicated in the pathogenesis of MS.

MS is a demyelinating disease in which the myelin sheaths surrounding neurons of the brain and spinal cord are destroyed. Clinical features of MS include optic neuritis, urinary/bowel incontinence, weakness of the arms/legs and dysphagia. Uhthoff's phenomenon describes the worsening of symptoms that occurs after exposure to higher than ambient temperatures. Acute disseminated encephalomyelitis (ADEM; C) is a demyelinating condition that follows vaccination or infection. Clinical features include fever, headache and reduced consciousness; focal signs include optic neuritis, cranial nerve palsies and seizures. Most cases are followed by recovery within a few months.

Neurological disease (2)

48   A   Several polyneuropathies have an underlying immune component, characterized by the presence of autoantibodies targeted at components of the nervous system. In this scenario, the patient has experienced weakness following a gastrointestinal infection, now complicated by respiratory involvement. The most likely diagnosis is Guillain–Barrè syndrome (GBS), for which ganglioside LM_1 (A) is the implicated target for autoantibodies. GBS is a symmetrical inflammatory polyneuropathy that begins in the legs and ascends to involve motor neurons of the arms, face and finally those supplying muscles of respiration. GBS usually follows an infection, most frequently after viral infection such as cytomegalovirus or bacterial gastroenteritis caused by *Campylobacter jejuni*. The pathogenesis involves cross-reactivity between antibodies against the pathogen and components of peripheral nerve myelin components, such as ganglioside LM_1. Other potential myelin targets include P_2 protein and galactocerebroside. Amyotrophic lateral sclerosis (ALS) is a sub-type of motor neuron disease characterized by loss of neurons in the motor cortex as well as anterior horn of the spinal

cord; it is therefore associated with both upper and lower motor signs. The pathogenesis of ALS has been suggested to be due to antibodies to the ganglioside GM_1 (B). Paraneoplastic subacute sensory neuropathy (PSSN) is associated with malignancies such as small cell lung cancer. Antibodies are directed at Hu (C) proteins which are a constituent part of peripheral nerves. Paraneoplastic cerebellar degeneration is associated with antibodies to Purkinje cells (E) of the central nervous system. The pathogenesis is thought to be secondary to cross-reactivity between antibodies to tumour cells and antigens present on cerebellar Purkinje cells. Paraprotein-associated polyneuropathy is typified by the presence of antibodies that target myelin-associated glycoprotein (MAG; D).

Eye disease

49 B Immune disorders of the eye can be classified according to the anatomical site of disease: cornea, sclera/episclera, uvea and retina. This patient presents with floaters and loss of accommodation in her right eye, several weeks after experiencing trauma to her left eye. The most likely diagnosis is therefore sympathetic ophthalmia (B), a granulomatous CD4+ T-cell mediated disease. The trigger for the disease is trauma to the damaged eye. The eye is an immunoprivileged site and is therefore, under normal circumstances, protected from possible autoimmune attack. Trauma to the eye breaks such tolerance, and there is consequently increased photoreceptor antigen presentation to immune cells, triggering cytokine release and recruitment of CD4+ T cells. These CD4+ cells soon encounter the same antigen presented at normal levels in the healthy eye, leading to a break in tolerance. Activated T cells cause ocular damage which may, in severe cases, lead to blindness.

Immune diseases of the cornea include keratoconjunctivits sicca (A) and keratitis (D). Keratoconjunctivits sicca is a feature of Sjögren's syndrome when present with a dry mouth and rheumatoid arthritis. It is caused by autoimmune destruction of the lacrimal glands, which leads to dry eyes which may predispose to infection. Schirmer test can be used to formally diagnose the condition. Keratitis may be caused by herpes simplex viral infection; this leads to recurrent bouts of keratitis.

Diseases of the sclera include scleritis (E), which occurs as a result of chronic inflammatory conditions such as connective tissue diseases (ankylosing spondylitis, systemic lupus erythematosus and rheumatoid arthritis), as well as type IV hypersensitivity reactions. Episcleritis is also an immune disease of the sclera which is a self-limiting condition.

Uveitis (C) is defined as inflammation of the uveal tract, which occurs either as an idiopathic disease, or secondary to chronic inflammatory conditions as with scleritis, including inflammatory bowel disease.

Diagnostic immunology

50 B   The patient in question has signs and blood test results consistent
with haemolysis; together with the known diagnosis of systemic lupus
erythematosus (SLE), this points to autoimmune haemolytic anaemia
(AIHA) as a likely diagnosis. AIHA is caused by autoantibodies that
bind to red blood cells (RBCs) leading to destruction in the spleen. AIHA
can be classified as either 'warm' or 'cold' depending on the temperature at which antibodies bind to RBCs. Warm AIHA is IgG mediated,
which bind to RBCs at 37°C; causes include lymphoproliferative disorders, drugs (penicillin) and autoimmune diseases (SLE). Cold AIHA is
IgM mediated, which bind to RBCs at temperatures less than 4°C; this
phenomenon usually occurs after an infection by mycoplasma or EBV.
Direct antiglobulin test (DAT; B), also known as direct Coombs test, is
the investigation of choice for the diagnosis of AIHA. The test involves
the separation of RBCs from the serum which is subsequently incubated
with anti-human globulin. In the case of AIHA, the anti-human globulin will agglutinate the RBCs, which is visualized as clumping of the
cells. Skin prick test (A) is the gold standard for investigating allergy.
The test involves a few drops of purified allergen being pricked onto
the skin. Allergens which are tested for include foods, dust mites, pollen
and dust. A positive test is indicated by wheal formation. Western blot
(C) is a technique used to detect specific protein in a patient's serum; it
is used in the confirmatory HIV test to detect specific antibodies to HIV.
Immunofluorescence (D) is an immunological technique used in conjunction with fluorescence microscopy. Fluorophores (fluorescent chemical compounds) attached to specific antibodies are directed at antigens
found within a biological specimen, most commonly a biopsy sample, to
visualize patterns of staining. Patch testing (E) is a useful test to determine the causative allergen in contact dermatitis. A patch is prepared
with small amounts of allergens; a positive test may be demonstrated by
a spectrum of responses, from faint erythema to the presence of bullae.

SECTION 7: MICROBIOLOGY EMQs

Questions

Answers

QUESTIONS

1. Respiratory tract infections

A	*Streptococcus pneumoniae*	F	*Chlamydia pneumoniae*
B	*Moraxella catarrhalis*	G	*Mycobacterium tuberculosis*
C	*Haemophilus influenzae*	H	*Pneumocystis jirovecii*
D	*Legionella pneumophila*	I	*Staphylococcus aureus*
E	*Mycoplasma pneumonia*		

For each scenario below, choose the most appropriate answer from the list above. Each option may be used once, more than once or not at all.

1 A 25-year-old man with a history of recurrent chest infections presents to an infectious disease specialist. A subsequent chest X-ray demonstrates widespread pulmonary infiltrates. A sputum stain using Gomori's methenamine silver reveals characteristic cysts.

2 A 54-year-old woman admitted to the respiratory ward is found to have right sided consolidation on chest X-ray. Histological examination reveals Gram-positive cocci arranged in pairs.

3 A 65-year-old woman is brought into accident and emergency with severe respiratory distress. The patient's history revealed that she had been seen by her GP due to a viral infection 2 weeks previously. Histological examination reveals Gram-positive cocci arranged in clusters.

4 A 40-year-old HIV positive man is seen by his GP. The patient admits a 4-week history of cough. The GP requests acid-fast staining of the patient's sputum.

5 A 36-year-old engineer presents to his GP with a 1-week history of headache, myalgia and cough. Blood tests reveal hyponatraemia. A urinary antigen test is found to be positive.

2. Gastrointestinal infections

A	*Vibrio cholerae*	F	Shigellae
B	*Staphylococcus aureus*	G	*Campylobacter jejuni*
C	Enterobacteriaecae	H	*Giardia lamblia*
D	*Listeria monocytogenes*	I	*Entamoeba histolytica*
E	*Salmonella enteritidis*		

For each scenario below, choose the most appropriate answer from the list above. Each option may be used once, more than once or not at all.

1 A 34-year-old HIV-positive woman is seen in the GP clinic due to 3 days of diarrhoea, headaches and fever. History reveals the patient had recently drunk unpasteurized milk. The causative organism is found to be β-haemolytic with tumbling motility.

2 A 10-year-old girl has just returned from a summer swimming camp at Lake Windermere. She presents to accident and emergency with bloody diarrhoea and abdominal pain. Blood tests reveal anaemia and thrombocytopenia.

3 An 18-year-old on his gap year in India suddenly develops severe watery diarrhoea. Microscopy of his stool reveals no leukocytes but rods with fast movements.

4 A 25-year-old homosexual man presents to his GP with a 3-day history of foul smelling, non-bloody diarrhoea, with abdominal cramps and flatulence. Stool microscopy reveals pear-shaped organisms.

5 A 35-year-old woman presents to accident and emergency with fever, diarrhoea and signs of shock. Her husband mentions that she had attended a work colleague's barbeque the previous day. The consultant believes superantigens are responsible for the patient's condition.

3. Central nervous system infections

A   *Neisseria meningitides*
B   Herpes simplex virus-2
C   *Leptospira interrogans*
D   *Listeria monocytogenes*
E   *Cryptococcus neoformans*

F   *Escherichia coli*
G   *Streptococcus pneumoniae*
H   *Borrelia burgdorferi*
I   *Mycobacterium tuberculosis*

For each scenario below, choose the most appropriate answer from the list above. Each option may be used once, more than once or not at all.

1 A 45-year-old man presents to his GP with a 2-month history of headache. After a CT scan demonstrates an opacity, a lumbar puncture is performed and cerebrospinal fluid (CSF) analysis reveals a protein level of 4.5 g/L (0.15–0.4), lymphocyte count 345 (1–5) and glucose 4.0 mmol/L (2.2–3.3).

2 A 26-year-old man has recently returned to the UK from a year of working in Africa where he was taking part in a charity farming project. He presents to accident and emergency with signs of meningism. A serological microscopic agglutination test is positive.

3 A 19-year-old woman who has recently started university is brought to accident and emergency with a headache and a spreading non-blanching rash. Gram-stain of a blood sample reveals the presence of Gram-negative diplococci.

4 A 46-year-old man with a history of HIV presents to accident and emergency with neck stiffness, fever and severe photophobia. Examination of the CSF with India ink reveals yeast cells surrounded by halos.

5   A 35-year-old woman presents to her infectious disease specialist due to recur-
     rent episodes of meningitis. During her last presentation CSF analysis reveals
     a protein level of 0.8 g/L (0.15–0.4), lymphocyte count 290 (0–5) and glucose
     2.2 mmol/L (2.2–3.3).

4. Sexually transmitted infections

A	*Treponema pallidum*	F	*Chlamydia trachomatis*
B	*Klebsiella granulomatis*	G	Bacterial vaginosis
C	*Neiserria gonorrhoeae*	H	*Haemophilus ducreyi*
D	*Trichomonas vaginalis*	I	Herpes simplex virus 2
E	*Candidia albicans*		

For each scenario below, choose the most appropriate answer from the list above.
Each option may be used once, more than once or not at all.

1   A 28-year-old woman sees her GP complaining of fever, lower abdominal pain
     and painful intercourse. Vaginal swabs are sent for a nucleic acid amplification
     test which reveal sexually transmitted bacteria that can also cause lymphogran-
     uloma venereum.

2   A 68-year-old man presents to his GP with a gumma on his nose. On examina-
     tion, the patient is found to have pupils that accommodate to light but do not
     react. The man admits to unprotected sexual intercourse during his youth.

3   A 35-year-old man presents to an infectious disease specialist with a painful
     penile ulcer and associated unilateral lymphadenopathy of the inguinal nodes. A
     swab of the ulcer is cultured on chocolate agar.

4   A 28-year-old woman sees her GP complaining of fever, lower abdominal pain
     and painful intercourse. A vaginal swab is taken and subsequent Gram-staining
     reveals Gram-negative diplococci.

5   A 35-year-old woman presents to her GP with a 2-week history of a fishy
     odorous vaginal discharge, which occurs especially after sexual intercourse.
     Microscopy of the discharge reveals clue cells.

5. Anti-microbials

A	Amoxicillin	F	Cefotaxime
B	Doxycycline	G	Vancomycin
C	Co-amoxiclav IV	H	Trimethoprim
D	Meropenam	I	Flucloxacillin
E	Chloramphenicol		

For each scenario below, choose the most appropriate answer from the list above.
Each option may be used once, more than once or not at all.

1   A 54-year-old man presents to his GP with a 1-week history of fever, cough and fatigue. On examination his respiratory rate is 20 breaths per minute and he is normotensive. Subsequent chest X-ray reveals right lower lobe consolidation.

2   A 38-year-old man presents to accident and emergency with an inflamed and swollen right leg. He mentions that he had cut the same leg 2 days previously playing football. A swab of the area isolates *Staphylococcus aureus*.

3   A 34-year-old woman presents to her GP with lower abdominal pain and dysuria. A dipstick of her urine reveals the presence of protein, white cells and nitrites.

4   A 56-year-old man is being cared for on the surgical ward after excision of a segment of his bowel after being diagnosed with colorectal carcinoma. The following day the surgical wound site is found to be inflamed. The patient has a fever and his blood pressure is slowly declining. Blood cultures reveal Gram-positive cocci arranged in clusters that are resistant to β-lactam antibiotics.

5   An 18-year-old woman student presents to accident and emergency with headache, neck stiffness and photophobia. CT scan reveals no raised intracranial pressure. Gram-negative diploccoci are visualized on Gram-staining of the patient's CSF.

6. Viral infections

A	Human immunodeficiency virus (HIV)	E	Hepatitis D virus
B	Epstein–Barr virus (EBV)	F	Varicella zoster virus
C	Hepatitis B virus	G	Hepatitis C virus
D	Cytomegalovirus (CMV)	H	Human herpes virus 8
		I	Influenza virus

For each scenario below, choose the most appropriate answer from the list above. Each option may be used once, more than once or not at all.

1   A 38-year-old man presents to his GP with vomiting, mild fever and loss of appetite. He admits to travelling to sub-Saharan Africa 2 months previously. On examination the patient is evidently jaundiced.

2   A 39-year-old homosexual man is referred to the gastroenterology department for an oesophogastroduodenoscopy (OGD) due to recent onset odynophagia. The OGD reveals multiple raised white plaques that can be removed by endoscopic scraping.

3   A 15-year-old girl presents to her GP complaining of a sore throat, fever, fatigue and loss of appetite. A blood film demonstrates atypical lymphocytes and monospot test is positive.

4   A 68-year-old woman presents to her GP after a 3-day history of fever, cough, headache and nasal congestion. The doctor believes her symptoms are due to a virus that binds to sialic acid receptors.

5   A 55-year-old man who is being treated for lung cancer with chemotherapeutic agents sees his oncologist for a routine check-up. There is a rash in a dermatomal pattern on the patient's forehead; the patient complains that there is a burning sensation in the distribution of the rash.

7. Anti-virals

A	Acyclovir	F	Lamivudine
B	Oseltamivir	G	Efivarenz
C	Interferon-α	H	Ritonavir
D	Zidovudine	I	Adamantadine
E	Gancylcovir		

For each scenario below, choose the most appropriate answer from the list above. Each option may be used once, more than once or not at all.

1   A 40-year-old man presents to an infectious disease specialist with a 4-month history of weight loss, fever and malaise. On examination the patient has lymphadenopathy. His CD4 count is found to be 289 copies/μL. The patient is started on lamivudine, ritonavir and one other drug.

2   A 38-year-old intravenous drug user presents to an infectious disease specialist with a 1-week history of fever and malaise; on examination hepatomegaly is noted. The patient is found to be HBeAg positive and is subsequently commenced on lamivudine and one other drug.

3   A 25-year-old man presents to his GP with a 3-day history of fever, cough, body aches and severe headaches. The patient is told to rest and drink plenty of fluids. However, he returns the following week stating his symptoms have not improved and is started on a drug that acts on viral neuraminidase.

4   A 3-year-old girl diagnosed with severe combined immunodeficiency is due to undergo a bone marrow transplant. She is given a drug as prophylaxis against cytomegalovirus infection.

5   A 28-year-old woman presents to her GP with cold sores dotted across her lower lip. She is started on a medication that inhibits DNA polymerase function to speed the healing processes.

8. Fungal infections

A	*Cryptoccus neoformans*	F	*Tinea capitis*
B	*Pityriasis versicolour*	G	*Sporothrix schenckii*
C	*Aspergillus flavus*	H	*Tinea corporis*
D	*Histoplasma capsulatum*	I	*Candida albicans*
E	*Phialophora verrucosa*		

For each scenario below, choose the most appropriate answer from the list above. Each option may be used once, more than once or not at all.

1   A 38-year-old man with known HIV presents to his GP with a 1-week history of white coloured creamy deposits inside his mouth. The patient is prescribed an oral nystatin wash.

2   A 45-year-old man with known HIV presents to accident and emergency with headache, nausea, confusion and fever. Investigation of the patient's CSF with India ink stain reveals yeast cells surrounded by a halo.

3   A 35-year-old woman presents to her GP with hyperpigmented spots on her back. Scrapings of the affected areas reveal a 'spaghetti with meatballs' appearance under the microscope.

4   A 48-year-old HIV positive man who has recently migrated from sub-Saharan Africa presents to accident and emergency with chest pain, shortness of breath, fever and cough. A chest X-ray demonstrates a spherical opacity in the upper left lung field.

5   A 32-year-old gardener presents to his GP with small raised lesions on his left arm. He remembers working in a garden a few days previously which had been swamped with rose-thorns.

9. Zoonoses

A	Psittacosis	F	*Mycobacterium marinium*
B	Rabies	G	Lyme disease
C	Brucellosis	H	Cat scratch disease
D	Q fever	I	Rocky mountain spotted fever
E	Leptospirosis		

For each scenario below, choose the most appropriate answer from the list above. Each option may be used once, more than once or not at all.

1   A 45-year-old man has returned to the UK from a holiday to France. A week later he presents with flu-like symptoms, drenching sweats, a recurring fever and is beginning to complain of a lower back pain. He admits to have brought back some local cheeses on visits to regional farms.

2   A 36-year-old man presents to his GP with a painful right knee. He states that he visited the Prairie regions of Canada a month previous to this episode and states that his wife had mentioned there was a red rash on his back; on examination a target shaped rash is observed.

3   A 38-year-old sewage worker presents to his GP with 1-week history of flu-like symptoms with diarrhoea. A microscopic agglutination test reveals the diagnosis.

4   A 48-year-old man presents to his GP with flu-like symptoms. On examination the patient has a maculopapular rash on his trunk. The patient also shows an area where a vague bite mark is visible.

5   A 34-year-old bird handler presents to his GP with a few days' history of fever, mild cough and myalgia. The patient states that his shop had recently taken a new shipment of parrots from Central America. Giemsa staining of the patient's sputum reveals cytoplasmic inclusions.

10. Neonatal and childhood infections

A	Rubella	F	*Listeria monocytogenes*
B	Syphilis	G	Cytomegalovirus
C	Measles	H	*Haemophilus influenzae*
D	Hepatitis B	I	HIV
E	Mumps		

For each scenario below, choose the most appropriate answer from the list above. Each option may be used once, more than once or not at all.

1   A 10-year-old boy is brought to see the GP by his mother as he has recently developed parotid swelling associated with a fever. Blood tests reveal a raised amylase level. The boy's mother reveals that his immunization schedule is not complete as they were living in Tunisia at the time.

2   A 3-week-old baby develops vomiting and is feeding poorly. On examination he has a reduced level of consciousness and an arched back. Analysis of the CSF reveals the presence of Gram-positive rods.

3   A 3-year-old girl presents to the GP with a cough, fever and runny nose. On examination, the child has white spots scattered on the buccal mucosa. Her mother admits that she denied her child a certain vaccine due to scares presented by the media.

4   A 4-year-old boy presents to accident and emergency with a reduced level of consciousness, headache and neck stiffness. Analysis of the CSF reveals the presence of Gram-negative rods. The child's mother reveals that his immunization record is not complete as they have only migrated from Ethiopia recently.

5   An 8-month old girl is seen by a paediatrician due to concerns about developmental delay. On examination cataracts are noted in both eyes. Echocardiography reveals a patent ductus arteriosus.

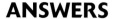

ANSWERS

1. Respiratory tract infections

ANSWERS: 1) H 2) A 3) I 4) G 5) D

Pneumocystis jirovecii (H) is a yeast-like fungus that primarily affects immunocompromised patients such as those with HIV. Pneumocystis pneumonia may be the presenting feature of HIV and patients with a CD4 count less than 200 cells/μL are particularly susceptible. Clinically, *Pneumocystis jirovecii* infection presents with fever, non-productive cough, weight loss and night sweats. Chest X-ray may show signs of diffuse bilateral pulmonary infiltrates. Definitive diagnosis involves histological examination of sputum or bronchio-alveolar lavage fluid. Gomori's methenamine silver stain reveals 'flying saucer' shaped cysts on microscopy.

Streptococcus pneumoniae (pneumococci; A) are α-haemolytic Gram-positive cocci arranged in pairs (diploccoci). As *Streptococcus pneumoniae* are capsulated bacteria, the Quelling reaction in which pneumococci are mixed with anti-serum and methylene blue causes the capsule to swell can be visualized under the microscope. Optochin-sensitivity also differentiates pneumococcus from *Streptococcus viridans* (also α-haemolytic), which is optochin-insensitve. Clinically, lobar consolidation is visible on X-ray, which represents a collection of pus, bacteria and exudate in the alveoli.

Staphylococcus aureus (I) are β-haemolytic Gram-positive cocci arranged in grape-like clusters. All staphylococci are also catalase positive, whereas streptococci are catalase negative. Clinically, *S. aureus* can cause consolidation, cavitations of the lungs and empyema (pus in the pleural space). *Staphylococcus aureus* has a number of virulence factors including anti-immune proteins (haemolysins, leukocidins and penicillinase) as well as tissue break-down proteins (hyaluronidase, staphylokinase and protease).

Mycobacterium tuberculosis (G) is an acid-fast bacillus which is transmitted via aerosol droplets. Clinical manifestations include fever, cough (with possible haemoptysis), weight loss and night sweats. Tuberculosis is highly prevalent in HIV patients due to impaired cell-mediated immunity. Chest X-ray reveals bihilar lymphadenopathy. Most commonly, Ziehl–Neelson staining is performed on a sputum sample demonstrating acid-fast bacilli, but auramine–rhodamine staining can also be used. *Mycobacterium tuberculosis*, however, take approximately 6 weeks to culture, and hence faster polymerase chain reaction diagnostic tests are being developed.

Legionella pneumophila (D) is an aerobic Gram-negative rod which causes an atypical pneumonia. It primarily affects those who work with air-conditioning units and can lead to milder Pontiac fever or more severe Legionnaire's disease. Clinical features of legionellosis are non-specific and may include headache, myalgia, confusion, rhabdomyolysis and abdominal pain. Blood chemistry may reveal hyponatraemia, hypophosphataemia and/or deranged liver enzymes. Diagnosis involves culture of respiratory secretions on buffered charcoal yeast extract agar, although a rapid urinary antigen test can also be used.

Moraxella catarrhalis (B) are aerobic Gram-negative diploccoci. This bacterium is particularly problematic in patients with chronic lung disease and causes exacerbations of chronic obstructive pulmonary disorder (COPD). Other targets of infection include ears, eyes and central nervous system.

Haemophilus influenzae (C) are Gram-negative bacilli that cause influenza (flu) outbreaks annually. Chocolate agar is used as a culture medium. Further oxidase and catalase tests are positive.

Mycoplasma pneumoniae (E) are obligate intracellular bacteria which cause an atypical pneumonia or a mild bronchitis. A cold-agglutinin test can be used for the diagnosis. In rare cases, infection may lead to Stevenson–Johnson syndrome.

Chlamydia pneumoniae (F) are obligate intracellular bacteria which cause an atypical pneumonia. Less commonly, this infection can cause meningoencephalitis, arthritis, myocarditis and/or Guillain–Barré syndrome.

2. Gastrointestinal infections

ANSWERS: 1) D 2) C 3) A 4) H 5) B

Listeria monocytogenes (D) is a β-haemolytic anaerobic Gram-positive rod that may cause outbreaks of non-invasive gastroenteritis. Sources include refrigerated food and unpasteurized dairy products. Clinical features of listeria infection include watery diarrhoea, abdominal cramps, headaches and fever, but minimal vomiting. Listeria demonstrates 'tumbling motility' as a result of flagellar-driven movements. Neonates and immunocompromised patients are particularly susceptible. Invasive infection can cause more serious problems in these groups including septicaemia, meningitis and encephalitis.

Escherichia coli (C) is a Gram-negative rod-shaped bacterium that is a common cause of traveller's diarrhoea in those returning from abroad. Transmission occurs via food and water that become contaminated with human faeces, as can swimming in contaminated lakes. Enterohaemorrhagic *E. coli* infection (serotype O157:H7) can lead to haemolytic uraemic syndrome (HUS), characterized by haemolytic anaemia, acute renal failure (uraemia) and a low platelet count (thrombocytopenia). Other diarrhoea-causing strains of *E. coli* include enterotoxigenic, enteropathogenic and enteroinvasive forms.

Vibrio cholerae (A) are comma-shaped oxidase positive bacteria, causing profuse watery diarrhoea containing no inflammatory cells on microscopy. Transmission occurs via the faecal-oral route. *Vibrio cholerae* colonizes the small intestinal section of the gut and secretes enterotoxin containing subunits A (active) and B (binding). B subunit binds to GM1 ganglioside on the intestinal epithelial cells. Intracellularly, there is activation of cAMP by A subunit, which causes active secretion of sodium and chloride ions; as a consequence water is lost due to the osmotic pull of NaCl.

Giardia lamblia (H) is a pear-shaped trophozite containing two nuclei, four flagellae and a suction disc. Transmission occurs via ingestion of a cyst from faecally contaminated water and food. Trophozites attach to the duodenum but do not invade. Instead, protein absorption is inhibited, drawing water into the lumen of the gastrointestinal tract. *G. lamblia* must be considered in travellers, hikers and homosexual men. Clinically, foul smelling non-bloody steatorrhoea is produced, with stool containing cysts visible on microscopy.

Staphylococcus aureus (B) are β-haemolytic Gram-positive cocci arranged in grape-like clusters. In the gastrointestinal tract, *S. aureus* produces the exotoxin TSST-1, which acts as a superantigen causing non-specific activation of T cells and subsequent release of IL-1, IL-2 and TNF-α. A massive non-specific immune response follows causing shock and multiple organ failure. Enterotoxin produced by bacteria causes vomiting and diarrhoea 12–24 hours after the culprit food has been consumed.

Salmonella typhi (E) infection, also known as enteric fever, multiplies in the Peyer's patches of the small intestine. Clinical features include slow onset fever, constipation and splenomegaly. Rose spots are pathognomonic.

Shigellae (F) are non-motile, non-hydrogen sulphide producers. The bacteria cause dysentery via invasion of mucosal cells of distal ileum and colon as well as the production of an enterotoxin, known as Shiga toxin.

Campylobacter jejuni (G) are oxidase positive, non-motile bacteria. Transmission occurs via the faecal–oral route, generally due to contamination by dog faecal matter, causing a watery, foul smelling diarrhoea. Complications include Guillain–Barré syndrome and Reiter's syndrome.

Entamoeba histolytica (I) is a motile trophozite. Ingestion of the cysts leads to colonization of caecum and colon, which may cause a 'flask-shaped' ulcer to develop. Clinical features involve dysentery, chronic weight loss and liver abscess formation.

3. Central nervous system infections

ANSWERS: 1) I 2) C 3) A 4) E 5) B

Mycobacterium tuberculosis (I) may lead to a subacute or chronic meningitis. Symptoms are non-specific, including fever, headache and confusion. Focal signs may be present as a result of a cerebral granuloma. A tuberculous granuloma that occurs in the cortex of the brain, subsequently rupturing into the subarachnoid space, is termed a Rich focus. Diagnosis of tuberculous meningitis involves a lumbar puncture; the CSF appears colourless and characteristically has high protein, low glucose and raised lymphocyte levels. Nucleic acid amplification tests as well as imaging studies (CT and MRI) can be useful in the diagnostic work-up.

Leptospira interrogans (C) causes leptospirosis (also known as Weil's syndrome). Transmission occurs via contact with animals. Leptospira are thin aerobic spirochaetes that are tightly coiled. The first stage of infection is known as the leptospiramic phase, during which the patient suffers non-specific symptoms such as fever, headache, malaise and photophobia. In the second immune phase, IgM antibodies have formed and meningitis, liver damage (causing jaundice) and renal failure may develop. CSF examination will reveal a raised white cell count. The microscopic agglutination test is considered the gold standard for diagnosing leptospirosis.

Neisseria meningitides (meningococcus; A) is a Gram-negative diplococcus. Infants aged 6 months to 2 years are most at risk as well as large numbers of adults living in close quarters. Virulence factors include its capsule (antiphagocytic), endotoxin (lipopolysaccharide causes haemorrhage from blood vessels resulting in characteristic petechiae in meningococcaemia) and IgA1 protease (destroys IgA). *Neisseria meningitides* can lead to meningitis (headache, photophobia and neck stiffness) and meningococcaemia (signs of sepsis with spreading petechial rash). *Neisseria meningitides* is grown best on Thayer–Martin VCN media (only allows *Neisseria* species to grow).

Cryptococcus neoformans (E) is a polysaccharide encapsulated yeast that causes a subacute or chronic meningoencephalitis. It is transmitted by inhalation (the source of which is pigeon droppings). *Cryptococcus neoformans* is usually asymptomatic, but can be pathogenic in immunocompromised patients such as those with HIV. As well as meningitis, *C. neoformans* can also cause pneumonia, skin ulcers and bone lesions. Diagnosis is made by examination of CSF; India ink staining reveals yeast cells with a surrounding halo. Cryptococcal antigen test is, however, a more sensitive test.

Herpes simplex virus *2* (HSV-2; B) is the most common cause of viral meningitis of all the herpes family. HSV-2 is transmitted via sexual contact or via the mother during birth. The virus infects mucosal epithelial cells or lymphocytes; retrograde transport occurs from peripheral nerves to ganglion. Viral causes of meningitis can be diagnosed on examination of CSF; it appears colourless, with a raised lymphocyte level, moderately raised protein and normal glucose concentration. Recurrent aseptic meningitis (Mollaret's meningitis) can be caused by both HSV-1 and HSV-2.

Listeria monocytogenes (D) is a Gram-positive bacillus. Infection usually occurs in neonates, the immunocompromised and elderly. Manifestations include meningitis, encephalitits, pneumonia and septicaemia

Escherichia coli (F) is a Gram-negative bacillus. The K1 antigen of the bacterium as well as a lack of circulating IgM are responsible for severe meningitis in neonates.

Streptococcus pneumoniae (G) is a Gram-positive α-haemolytic diplococcus. It is the most common cause of meningitis in adults together with *N. meningitides*.

Borrelia burgdorferi (H) is a Gram-negative zoonotic spirochaete that causes Lyme disease. In the late stages of disease the patient will experience arthritis, peripheral neuropathy and/or encephalopathy.

4. Sexually transmitted infections

ANSWERS: 1) F 2) A 3) H 4) C 5) G

Chlamydia trachomatis (F) is a small Gram-negative obligate intracellular bacterium, causing the sexually transmitted infection chlamydiosis. It has an affinity towards columnar epithelia that line mucous membranes. Serovars D–K cause genital chlamydiosis (as well as opthalmia neonatorum) resulting in dyspareunia, dysuria and vaginal/penile discharge. Serovars L1, L2 and L3 cause lymphogranuloma venereum, defined by a painless papule or ulcer on the genitals which heals spontaneously; the bacteria migrate along regional lymph nodes leading to lymphadenopathy.

Treponema pallidum (A) causes syphilis. Syphilis has three clinical stages: primary, secondary and tertiary. Primary syphilis is defined by a firm painless chancre that appears approximately 1 month after sexual contact and resolves within a few weeks. Secondary syphilis is a bacteri aemic stage during which a widespread rash forms with lymphadenopathy. Tertiary syphilis occurs decades after the primary infection and involves multiple organs: gummatous lesions on skin and bone, aneurysm of the aortic arch, peripheral neuropathy, tabes dorsalis and Argyll–Robertson pupils.

Haemophilus ducreyi (H) is a Gram-negative coccobacillus that causes a tropical ulcer disease (chancroid) and is contracted by sexual transmission. Chancroid is characterized by a painful genital ulcer that leads to unilateral painful swollen inguinal lymph nodes. Infected lymph nodes may rupture releasing pus. The differential diagnosis for genital ulcers includes syphilis (painless ulcer with bilateral painless lymphadenopathy), herpes simplex virus 1 and 2 (vesicles that eventually break down) and lymphogranuloma venereum (slowly developing painless inguinal lymph nodes). *Haemophilus ducreyi* can be cultured on chocolate agar.

Neiserria gonorrhoeae (gonococcus; C) is an intracellular Gram-negative diplococcus that causes gonorrhoea. Virulence factors allow gonococci to evade phagocytosis and adhere to the non-ciliated epithelium of the fallopian tubes. In both men and women *N. gonorrhoeae* causes urethritis which presents with dysuria and purulent discharge (with associated dyspareunia in women). Long-term complications include pelvic inflammatory disease in women and epididymitis, prostititis as well as urethral stricture in men. Systemic invasion of bacteria causes pericarditis, endocarditis, meningitis and/or septic arthritis. Diagnosis involves Gram stain and culture on Thayer–Martin VCN medium, or PCR.

Bacterial vaginosis (BV; G) is caused by an imbalance in the naturally occurring bacterial flora of the vagina and is a condition associated with sexual activity (not transmitted). A 'fishy' smelling white–cream vaginal discharge is characteristically produced. Diagnosis involves obtaining vaginal swabs. A litmus test will indicate loss of acidity with a pH greater than 4.5 (normal vaginal pH = 3.8–4.2). If a sample of the discharge is visualized under a microscope with sodium chloride, clue cells will be seen.

Klebsiella granulomatis (B) is a Gram-positive rod that causes the ulcerating sexually transmitted infection donovanosis. It is diagnosed using giemsa stain of biopsy, which reveals Donovan bodies.

Trichomonas vaginalis (D) is a flagellated protozoan that causes vaginal discharge and urethritis in humans. It is otherwise asymptomatic and can be diagnosed by wet preparation microscopy, culture or PCR.

Candida albicans (E) is a fungal infection that causes candidiasis (thrush). Superficially, infection causes redness, itching and discharge from the vagina. In immunocompromised patients, infection can involve the oesophagus as well as causing candidaemia.

Herpes simplex virus 2 (HSV-2; I) causes genital herpes. Infection causes fluid-filled blisters to form over the genital area.

5. Anti-microbials

ANSWERS: 1) A 2) I 3) H 4) G 5) F

Amoxicillin (A) is a β-lactam antibiotic which inhibits enzymes responsible for cell wall synthesis, leading to osmotic lysis of the bacteria. As a result, β-lactams are ineffective against bacteria that lack cell walls such as *Mycoplasma* spp. and *Chlamydia* spp. In this case, amoxicillin is the best choice antibiotic to treat mild community acquired pneumonia. It is also useful in the treatment of urinary tract infection (UTI), *Listeria* meningitis, endocarditis prophylaxis and protection against *Streptococcus pneumoniae* in asplenic patients. Major side effects can be divided into allergic (anaphylaxis) and non-allergic (Steven–Johnson syndrome) consequences.

Flucloxacillin (I) is a β-lactam antibiotic that is especially effective against Gram-positive bacteria that produce β-lactamase, for example *S. aureus*. Just like amoxicillin, flucloxacillin inhibits cell wall synthesis. Indications for its use include staphylococcal skin infections such as cellulitis (in this case), folliculitis and mastitis as well as pneumonia (adjunct), osteomyelitis, septic arthritis, endocarditis and prophylaxis in surgery. A rare side effect of flucloxacillin is cholestatic jaundice which may develop weeks after treatment is stopped.

Trimethoprim (H) is an inhibitor of folate metabolism; it impairs synthesis of DNA by interfering with folic acid metabolism. It is used in the treatment of uncomplicated UTIs. Trimethoprim should be used with caution in patients with megaloblastic anaemia due to its interaction with folate. Side effects of trimethoprim include thrombocytopenia, megaloblastic anaemia and hyperkalaemia (via antagonism of sodium channels in the distal convoluted tubule of nephrons). Trimethoprim combined with another folate inhibitor, sulphamethoxazole, forms co-trimoxazole, which is used in the treatment of *Pneumocystis jirovecii* infection.

Vancomycin (G) is the drug of choice in cases of methicillin-resistant *Staphylococcus aureus* infections (MRSA). Vancomycin is a glycopeptide antibiotic that inhibits cell wall synthesis. It is too large to traverse the cell wall of Gram-negative bacteria and hence is primarily targeted to Gram-positive bacteria. Side effects include renal failure, ototoxicity, blood disorders, rash and anaphylaxis. Due to the potential side effects, serum drug levels must be monitored. Vancomycin is also a second-line antibiotic in the treatment of *Clostridium difficile* infection.

Cefotaxime (F) is a third generation cephalosporin and is the drug of choice in treating *Neisseria meningitidis*, which is the most common cause of meningitis in the UK. Cefotaxime is a β-lactam antibiotic and therefore inhibits cell wall synthesis. If meningitis is suspected in the community, the patient should be started on benzyl-penicillin until they are transferred to a secondary care unit. Cefotaxime is also useful in the treatment of pyelonephritis, sepsis secondary to hospital acquired pneumonia and soft tissue infections.

Doxycycline (B) is a tetracycline antibiotic that interferes with protein synthesis by binding to the 30S ribosomal subunit. It is used in COPD exacerbations, sexually transmitted infections (gonorrhoea and chlamydia) and acne.

Co-amoxiclav IV (augmentin; C) is the combination of amoxicillin and clavulinic acid (β-lactamase inhibitor). It is usually prescribed when β-lactamase-producing strains are suspected and other treatment has failed.

Meropenem (D) is a broad-spectrum carbapenem antibiotic which is used in the management of severely sick patients, usually in intensive care. It is resistant to β-lactamase, including extended spectrum β-lactamase producing bacteria.

Chloramphenicol (E) acts on 50S ribosomes to inhibit protein synthesis. It is used in cases of Rocky Mountain spotted fever. Side effects include aplastic anaemia.

6. Viral infections

ANSWERS: 1) C 2) A 3) B 4) I 5) F

Hepatitis B virus (HBV; C) is a double-stranded DNA virus that is prevalent in sub-Saharan Africa. It is transmitted via sexual contact, contaminated blood products, intravenous drug use as well as vertical transfer from mother to child during child birth. The virus has an incubation period of 2–6 months with 80 per cent of infections remaining acute and 20 per cent becoming chronic with risk of cirrhosis and hepatocellular carcinoma. HBV antigens include HBsAg (surface antigen), HBcAg (core antigen) and HBeAg (soluble antigen).

Human immunodeficiency virus (HIV; A) possesses single-stranded RNA as well as enzymes (reverse transcriptase, integrase and protease) in its core. HIV is transmitted via sexual intercourse, blood products, intravenous drug use and vertically from mother to child. HIV infects CD4+ T cells; within the cell the RNA undergoes reverse transcription to make DNA which is integrated into the host DNA; the virus then becomes latent or buds to infect further. AIDS (CD4+ count <200) defining illnesses include bacterial (*Mycobacterium avium-intracellulare*, TB), fungal (*Candida albicans* oesophagitis), protozoal (*Pneumocystis jerovicci*) and viral infections as well as certain cancers (Kaposi's sarcoma).

Epstein–Barr virus (EBV; B) primarily infects B lymphocytes, binding via a complement receptor. Transmission involves person-to-person transfer through close contact. EBV is associated with glandular fever (infectious

mononucleosis) which causes pharyngitis, lymphadenopathy, fever, splenomegaly and hepatomegaly. Rare sequelae include thrombocytopenia
and erythema multiforme. EBV can also cause Hodgkin's lymphoma
(latent reactivation of EBV), Burkitt's lymphoma and nasopharyngeal
cancers. It is diagnosed on blood film (atypical lymphocytes), monospot test (positive heterophil antibody test) and/or EBV antibodies in the
blood.

Influenza virus (I) is part of the orthomyxoviridae group of viruses and
causes epidemics of influenza annually. The influenza virus causes primary pneumonia as well as delayed secondary bacterial pneumonia and
otitis media in immunocompromised patients. It is a spherical virion
with haemagglutinin (HA) and neuraminidase (NA) glycoproteins on the
surface. HA binds to sialic acid receptors present in the upper respiratory tract; viral RNA is subsequently inserted into the host cell and HA is
cleaved by clara cell tryptase. NA cleaves neuraminic acid, a component
of protective mucin; as a result the protective barrier is disrupted expos-
ing sialic acid receptor sites beneath. NA also has a role facilitating the
release of newly formed influenza virions.

Varicella zoster virus (VZV; F) is a droplet-spread herpes virus that
causes chickenpox in children and shingles in adults. Chickenpox is
characterized by fever, malaise and a rash (erythematous base with
fluid top) that spreads over the body. Complications include secondary bacterial infection and encephalitis. VZV remains dormant in
the dorsal root ganglia and may reactivate in states of immunosuppression. The most common symptom is neuralgia which occurs in a
dermatomal distribution; other manifestations include encephalitis,
Guillain–Barré syndrome, facial palsy and progressive outer retinal
necrosis.

Cytomegalovirus (CMV; D) can be transmitted vertically from contaminated blood products and transplant organs (50 per cent risk of infection in seropositive donor and seronegative recipient). It is especially
prevalent in the immunocompromised.

Hepatitis D virus (HDV; E) is a helical single-stranded RNA virus that
requires hepatitis B co-infection. HDV produces an acute-on-chronic
picture in HBV patients and puts them at higher risk of cirrhosis and
subsequent liver failure.

Hepatitis C virus (HCV; G) is a single-stranded RNA virus that is transferred via contaminated blood products and vertically from mother to
child during birth. Twenty per cent remain acute, while 80 per cent
become chronic.

Human herpes virus 8 (HHV-8; H) is transmitted primarily via saliva as
well as semen to a lesser extent. It causes Kaposi's sarcoma, primary
effusion lymphoma and multicentric Castleman's disease.

7. Anti-virals

ANSWERS: 1) D 2) C 3) B 4) E 5) A

Zidovudine (D) is a nucleoside reverse transcriptase inhibitor (NRTI) used in the treatment of HIV/AIDS (as well as prevention of vertical transmission from infected mothers). Treatment is commenced once the CD4 count falls below 350 copies/µL. Zidovudine works by inhibiting the action of the enzyme reverse transcriptase, preventing the conversion of HIV RNA to DNA, which consequently cannot be incorporated into the host DNA. Side effects include anaemia, neutropenia, hepatic and cardiac dysfunction as well as myopathy. The standard treatment regimen involves the use of two nucleoside reverse transcriptase inhibitors (NRTIs) and a non-nucleoside reverse transcriptase inhibitor (NNRTI; Efivarenz) or a protease inhibitor (PI; Ritonavir).

Interferon-α (IFN-α; C) is a protein that is used in the treatment of hepatitis B; it potentiates the immune system to fight active viral infection. IFN-α acts on the JAK-STAT pathway; IFN-α binds to the IFN-α receptor, causing phosphorylation of STAT1 and STAT2, which subsequently form a complex with IRF9 (a transcription factor), leading to the synthesis of anti-viral proteins. A NRTI and IFN-α is the standard treatment for hepatitis B infection. Pegylated-IFN-α is used in the treatment of hepatitis C; similar to IFN-α, the addition of polyethylene glycol increases the half life of the drug.

Oseltamivir (B) is a viral neuraminidase inhibitor used in the treatment of influenza. Osteltamivir is in fact a pro-drug; once metabolized in the liver the active form GS4071 is produced. Once a newly formed influenza virion is produced, the surface viral protein haemagglutinin is bound to sialic acid receptors along the upper respiratory tract. Neuraminidase is normally responsible for cleaving the haemagglutinin–sialic acid receptor bond, hence facilitating the release of newly formed virions. Therefore, inhibiting neuraminidase activity prevents further viral replication.

Gancyclovir (E) is a 2′-deoxyguanosine analogue used in the treatment of cytomegalovirus (CMV) infection. It is the first line drug for the prophylaxis of CMV in bone marrow transplant patients. 2′-deoxyguanosine is phosphorylated to the triphosphate form, which prevents viral DNA polymerase from elongating viral DNA and therefore inhibits CMV replication. Gancyclovir can cause bone marrow toxicity; it may therefore be prescribed together with granulocyte-colony stimulating factor (G-CSF). Gancyclovir is also used in the treatment of human herpes virus 6 (HHV-6) and Epstein–Barr virus infection.

Acyclovir (A) is a guanosine analogue anti-viral drug used primarily in the treatment of herpes simplex virus infections (HSV-1 and HSV-2). It is converted to acyclo-guanosine monophosphate (acyclo-GMP) by viral thymidine kinase. Acyclo-GMP is further phosphorylated to acyclo-guanosine triphosphate (acyclo-GTP). Acyclo-GTP is incorporated into the viral DNA strand, terminating the chain and stopping DNA polymerase from functioning. Aciclovir is also indicated for the treatment of varicella zoster, Epstein–Barr virus and cytomegalovirus infections (with decreasing efficacy).

Lamivudine (F) is an NRTI (analogue of cytidine). It leads to the inhibition of reverse transcriptase and is therefore effective for the treatment of hepatitis B and HIV.

Efavirenz (G) is an NNRTI used in the treatment of HIV. The drug causes inhibition of the reverse transcription enzyme.

Ritonavir (H) is a protease inhibitor used in the management of HIV. Ritonavir inhibits viral assembly by preventing the cleavage of proteins that belong to newly formed virions.

Amantidine (I) is an M2 ion channel inhibitor preventing the uncoating of influenza virions and therefore inhibiting entry into susceptible cells.

8. Fungal infections

ANSWERS: 1) I 2) A 3) B 4) C 5) G

Candida albicans (I) can affect both immunocompetent and immunocompromised hosts. In the immunocompetent host, clinical features range from oral thrush (creamy-white patches with red base over mucous membranes of mouth; treated with nystatin) to vaginitis (vaginal inflammation, pruritis and discharge; speculum examination reveals patches of cottage cheese-like clumps fixed to vaginal wall). In immunocompromised patients, *C. albicans* infection leads to oesophagitis, characterized by odynophagia. Candidaemia can lead to severe flu-like symptoms and can be diagnosed by testing for blood β-D-glucan (a component of fungal cell walls).

Cryptococcus neoformans (A) is an encapsulated yeast that is transmitted via inhaled spores from pigeon droppings. It is usually asymptomatic in most cases. Seventy-five per cent of cases occur in immunocompromised patients, characterized by the development of sub-acute or chronic meningitis. Cryptococcal meningitis is fatal without treatment due to the associated cerebral oedema and brainstem compression. Diagnosis is made by CSF analysis with India ink stain which reveals yeast cells surrounded by a halo (polysaccharide capsule). A cryptococcal antigen test can also be used which offers higher sensitivity.

Pityriasis versicolor (B) is a chronic fungal infection caused by *Malassezia furfur*, characterized by hypopigmentation (in patients with dark skin tones) and hyperpigmentation (in patients with pale skin tones). Spots affect the back, underarm, arms, legs, chest, neck and rarely the face. Microscopic investigation of the *M. furfur* with potassium hydroxide reveals a 'spaghetti with meatballs' appearance. Wood's light may also reveal an orange fluorescence in some cases.

Aspergillus flavus (C) is a fungus that commonly grows on stored grains and can cause a spectrum of disease. Allergic reaction in the airways may cause allergic broncho-pulmonary aspergillosis (ABPA) which occurs due to an IgE mediated type I hypersensitivity reaction leading to bronchospasm and eosinophilia. Infection in pre-formed lung cavities (for example in TB patients) may lead to a fungal ball visible on chest X-ray (aspergilloma). Invasive aspergillosis is a chronic necrotizing infection that may occur in neutropenic patients (chemotherapy) or patients with end stage AIDS (CD4 count <50). Strains may produce the carcinogen aflatoxin, which has a strong association with hepatocellular carcinoma.

Sporothrix schenckii (Rose garderner's disease; G) is a fungus found in soil and plants that causes sporotrichosis. A prick by thorns causes nodular lesions to appear on the surface of the skin. Initially the lesions will be small and painless; left untreated they become ulcerated. Infection may also spread to joints, bone and muscle by this route. Inhalation of spores may lead to pulmonary disease and systemic infection may lead to central nervous system involvement. Treatment options include itraconazole, fluconazole and oral potassium iodide.

Histoplasma capsulatum (D) is a fungus transmitted by inhaled spores; it is highly prevalent in the Mississippi River region. Although mostly subclinical, a minority of infections will proceed to a chronic progressive lung disease.

Phialophora verrucosa (E) is a copper coloured soil saprophyte found on rotting wood that causes chromoblastomycosis. Infection is characterized by a warty lesion resembling a cauliflower.

Tinea capitis (F) is a cutaneous dermatophyte fungal infection of the scalp leading to scaly red lesions with loss of hair. It primarily affects children. Infection is characterized by an expanding ring on the scalp.

Tinea corporis (H) is also known as ringworm. It is a cutaneous dermatophyte fungal infection affecting the trunk, arms and legs. It is identified by raised red rings.

9. Zoonoses

ANSWERS: 1) C 2) G 3) E 4) I 5) A

Brucellosis (C) is a Gram-negative rod-shaped bacterium that is harboured by cattle (*Brucella abortus*), goats (*B. melitensis*), pigs (*B. suis*) and dogs (*B. canis*). *Brucella* spp. are transmitted by inhalation, unpasteurized dairy produce and direct contact with animals. Symptoms include fever, myalgia, arthralgia, tiredness and in chronic cases may be associated with depression. Diagnosis is made by blood culture on Castaneda medium. Complications include granulomatous hepatitis (histology of liver biopsy demonstrates granulomata), endocarditis, oseteomyelitis and thrombocytopenia.

Lyme disease (G) is caused by the spirochaete *Borrelia burgdorferi* which is transmitted by the *Ixodes* ticks harboured by certain species of mice and deer. Initial symptoms include erythema migrans (a spreading annular skin lesion with a characteristic target-shaped appearance), malaise, fever and musculoskeletal pain. Several weeks after the primary infection, the patient may experience neurological (headache, meningitis and Bell's palsy) and cardiac (arrhythmias, myocarditis and pericarditis) effects. Late features include arthralgia and arthritis.

Leptospirosis (Weil's disease; E) is a zoonotic disease caused by *Leptospira interrogans* which is harboured by both wild and domestic animals. It is transmitted via drinking water that has become contaminated with the urine of infected animals; as a result those involved in water-sports and sewage workers are at particular risk. Lyme disease is characterized by an influenza-like disease with/without gastrointestinal symptoms. Diagnosis can be made by ELISA, PCR or microscopic agglutination test (MAT). Long-term complications include hepatitis and renal failure.

Rocky Mountain spotted fever (I) is caused by *Rickettsia* spp. infection, a Gram-negative genus of bacteria, most prevalent in North and South America. It is harboured in small wild rodents and domestic animals (transmitted to humans by ticks). *Rickettsia* bacteria invade the endothelial lining of capillaries causing a vasculitis. Clinical features include headache, fever, myalgia, vomiting and confusion. Late signs include a rash that is maculopapular and/or petechial on the distal parts of the limbs which then spreads to the trunk and face. Rocky Mountain spotted fever may lead to thrombocytopenia, hyponatraemia and/or elevated liver enzymes.

Psittacosis (A) is a zoonotic infectious disease caused by *Chlamydia psittaci* which is contracted from a wide variety of birds (parrots, pigeons and cockatiels to name a few). Human symptoms mainly involve a severe pneumonia (with or without hepatitis). Although the patient may report mild symptoms, the X-ray will generally appear to show severe pathology. Diagnosis is made by visualizing cytoplasmic inclusions on Giemsa or fluorescent antibody stained sputum or biopsy sample.

Rabies (B) is a viral zoonotic infectious disease caused by a bite or scratch, usually from an infected dog or bat. Infection leads to progressive and incurable encephalitis, hydrophobia and muscle spasm. Cerebral Negri bodies (inclusion bodies) are pathognomonic.

Q fever (D) is caused by *Coxiella burnetti*. Transmission occurs by inhalation of aerosols of urine, faeces or amniotic fluid from infected livestock.

Mycobacterium marinium (F) is harboured by fish and is transmitted by a bite or injury from the fin. Infection causes nodules to appear on the elbows, knees and feet.

Cat scratch disease (H) is caused by *Bartonella* spp. bacteria transmitted by bites from cats. Classically, infection results in tender and swollen lymph nodes with headache and backache. Atypically, infection may result in Parinaud's oculoglandular syndrome.

10. Neonatal and childhood infections

ANSWERS: 1) E 2) F 3) C 4) H 5) A

Mumps (E) is spread by droplets in the air which travel via the lungs to parotid tissue and subsequently to distant sites. Clinical features of infection consist of fever, malaise and transient hearing loss. Parotitis is characteristic of mumps infection with unilateral or bilateral swelling and pain on chewing. Plasma amylase levels may be elevated as a result of inflammation of the salivary glands. Complications such as viral meningitis, orchitis/oophoritis, mastitis and arthritis may result from long-standing infection. The MMR vaccine given at 12–18 months has drastically reduced the incidence of mumps.

Listeria monocytogenes (F) is a β-haemolytic anaerobic Gram-positive rod that can cause meningitis in the neonate to 3 months age group. *Listeria monocytogenes* may be transmitted vertically from mother to baby *in utero* (due to the ingestion of infected food by the mother) or during birth (transvaginal transfer). Early signs of meningitis are non-specific in the age group affected (fever, poor feeding, vomiting, seizures and reduced consciousness) whereas late signs include a bulging fontanelle, neck stiffness, opisthotonos (arched back), Brudzinski and Kernig signs positive as well as meningococcaemia.

Measles (C) is a viral respiratory system infection caused by the genus *Morbillivirus*. Infection presents with cough, coryza, conjunctivitis and/or a discrete maculopapular rash. White spots on the buccal mucosa (Koplik spots) are pathognomonic for measles. Complications of measles infection may involve the respiratory (pneumonia and tracheitis) and neurological (febrile convulsions and encephalitis) systems. Subacute sclerosing panencephalitis (SSPE) may occur several years after the primary infection; infection persists in the central nervous system leading to loss of neurological function, dementia and eventually death.

Haemophilus influenzae (H) is a Gram-negative rod shaped bacterium that causes meningitis in children older than 3 months who have not been vaccinated. Other organisms that cause meningitis in older children include *Streptococcus pneumoniae* and *Neisseria meningitidis*. Diagnosis involves culture of the bacteria using chocolate agar, with subsequent Gram-stain and microscopy. Latex particle agglutination and PCR are more sensitive and specific investigative tests. The *Haemophilus influenzae* type B (Hib) vaccine has dramatically reduced Hib-related meningitis; the first dose is given when the child is 8 weeks old.

Rubella (German measles; A) is a viral infection which can be congenital or acquired. Congenital rubella syndrome (CRS) occurs in a developing fetus if the mother has contracted rubella in her first trimester. CRS is characterized by sensorineural deafness, eye abnormalities (cataracts, glaucoma, retinopathy) and congenital heart disease (patent ductus arteriosus). Other associations include microcephaly and developmental delay. Acquired rubella is transmitted via the respiratory route. Characteristically, a rash appears on the face which spreads to the trunk and disappears after a few days.

Hepatitis B (D) may be vertically transmitted from mother to child during childbirth. Mothers who are HBeAg positive are especially at risk of transmitting the virus; infection may become chronic in 20 per cent of cases.

Syphilis (B) can be congenitally transmitted. Symptoms that may develop in the first few years of life include hepatosplenomegaly, rash, fever and neurosyphilis. Long-term complications include saddle-nose deformity, Higoumenakis' sign (unilateral enlargement of the clavicle) and Clutton's joints (symmetrical joint swelling).

Cytomegalovirus (G) may be transmitted in the perinatal period from infected mothers. Presentation may include low birth weight, microcephaly, seizures and/or petechial rash.

HIV (I) transmission may occur *in utero* or during birth. Infected mothers are advised to take Zidovudine during pregnancy; the infant is required to take Zidovudine for 6 weeks following birth.

SECTION 8: MICROBIOLOGY SBAs

Questions

19. Treatment for diarrhoea (1)
20. Treatment for diarrhoea (2)
21. Confusion (1)
22. Confusion (2)
23. Lumbar puncture
24. Abdominal distension
25. Hepatitis C (1)
26. Hepatitis C (2)
27. Lethargy
28. Difficulty swallowing
29. Treatment for a cough (1)
30. Treatment for a cough (2)
31. Muscle weakness
32. Malaria (1)
33. Malaria (2)
34. Malaria (3)
35. Malaria (4)

Answers

QUESTIONS

1. Sputum culture

A 24 year-old Asian man presents with a persistent cough. A sputum sample is taken and cultured on Lowenstein–Jensen medium, appearing as brown, granular colonies after several weeks. The organism implicated is:

A   *Coxiella burnetti*
B   *Streptococcus pneumoniae*
C   *Mycobacterium tuberculosis*
D   *Legionella pneumophilia*
E   *Mycobacterium leprae*

2. Mantoux test

A 24-year-old HIV-positive Asian man presents with a cough. A Mantoux test is performed. After 72 hours, the wheal diameter is measured at 5.8 mm. This indicates:

A   He has never been exposed to TB
B   He has been exposed to TB
C   He has had a BCG vaccination in the past
D   He has latent TB which is now reactivated
E   It is not possible to say

3. Pneumonia (1)

An 18-year-old university student develops a lower lobe pneumonia, with a raised white cell count and CRP. A sputum culture reveals a Gram-positive optochin-sensitive diplococcus. The most likely causative agent is:

A   *Staphylococcus aureus*
B   *Streptococcus viridans*
C   *Mycoplasma pneumoniae*
D   *Streptococcus pneumoniae*
E   *Haemophilus influenzae*

4. Pneumonia (2)

A 58-year-old Caucasian alcoholic man presents to his GP with a history of sudden onset high fever, flu-like symptoms and, thick, blood stained sputum. A chest X-ray is arranged which shows marked upper lobe cavitation. The most likely causative agent is:

A   *Klebsiella pneumoniae*
B   *Mycobacterium tuberculosis*
C   *Staphylococcus aureus*
D   *Moraxella catarrhalis*
E   *Pnemocystis jirovecii*

5. Endocarditis

A 27-year-old intravenous drug user presents with a 2-week history of fevers, weight loss and a systolic murmur. The most likely causative agent is:

A   *Streptococcus viridans*
B   *Candida albicans*
C   *Staphylococcus aureus*
D   *Streptococcus bovis*
E   *Kingella*

6. Anti-virals

A patient with shingles is treated with an anti-viral. The drug used is a guanosine analogue and acts as a substrate for viral thymidine kinase. The most likely drug she has been given is:

A   Foscarnet
B   Lamivudine
C   Cidofovir
D   Acyclovir
E   Ganciclovir

7. Vaccine schedule

According to the UK immunization schedule, which vaccine should be given to a 2-month-old baby who has already received DTaP (diptheria, tetanus, pertussis), IPV (polio) and Hib (*Haemophilus influenzae* type B) vaccines?

A   Pneumococcus
B   MMR
C   Meningitis C
D   BCG
E   Hepatitis B

8. Urinary tract infections

A 24-year-old sexually active woman presents to her GP with dysuria. A urinary tract infection is diagnosed. Which of the following is the most likely causative agent?

A   *Enterobacter*
B   *Escherichia coli*
C   *Klebsiella pneumoniae*
D   *Staphylococcus saphrophyticus*
E   *Proteus mirabilis*

9. Diarrhoea (1)

A 44-year-old woman patient returns from her holiday in India with a 2-day history of watery, offensive diarrhoea, bloating, excessive flatulence and abdominal pain. The GP obtains a stool sample. Microscopy reveals a flagellate pear-shaped protozoan. The most likely organism implicated is:

A   *Bacillus cereus*
B   *Salmonella enteritidis*
C   *Giardia lamblia*
D   *Entamoeba histolytica*
E   *Cryptosporidium parvum*

10. Diarrhoea (2)

A 21-year-old medical student returns from her elective in India with a history of abdominal cramps, vomiting, fevers and profuse, watery stools which she describes as resembling 'rice-water'. The GP obtains a stool sample. Analysis reveals curved, comma shaped organisms that were shown to be oxidase positive. The most likely organism implicated is:

A   Hepatitis A
B   *Clostridium difficile*
C   *Yersinia enterocolitica*
D   *Campylobacter jejuni*
E   *Vibrio cholerae*

11. Protozoal disease

A 35-year-old HIV-positive man presents to his GP complaining of a general feeling of tiredness, weight loss and night sweats. On examination there is hepatosplenomegaly and hyperpigmentation of the skin. The most likely diagnosis is:

A   Visceral leishmaniasis
B   Cutaneous leishmaniasis
C   Mucocutaneous leishmaniasis
D   Malaria
E   Schistosomiasis

12. Investigation of an ulcer

A 22-year-old student presents to accident and emergency with a raised, erythematous, scaly ulcer on his forearm which has not been healing. On examination he is also found to have lymphadenopathy. He gives a history of recently returning from a 2-month trek in the rainforests of South America. Tissue is aspirated from the margin of the ulcer, and the organism is cultured in Novy–MacNeal–Nicolle medium. The organism implicated is:

A   *Toxoplasma gondii*
B   *Treponema pallidum*
C   *Leishmania dovani*
D   *Leishmania major*
E   *Leishmania braziliensis*

13. Fever (1)

A 35 year-old male clothing merchant has returned to the UK 2 weeks ago from a visit home to Syria. A week later he presents with flu-like symptoms, drenching sweats and a recurring fever and is beginning to complain of lower back pain. After further questioning, he mentioned that he worked on a farm during his trip. He is successfully treated with oral doxycycline and gentamicin. What is the most likely diagnosis?

A   Malaria
B   Tuberculosis
C   Influenza
D   Brucellosis
E   Typhoid

14. Fever (2)

A 50-year-old man has returned from hiking a segment of the Appalachian Trail on the Eastern coast of the USA during the summer months. Ten days later he presents to casualty with flu-like illness and a rash showing some central fading. What is the most likely organism implicated?

A   Herpes simplex
B   Epstein–Barr virus
C   *Streptococcus pyogenes*
D   *Treponema pallidum*
E   *Borrelia burgdorferi*

15. Swollen joint (1)

A 26-year-old squash player is admitted with a red, swollen left knee. He reports no history of trauma. On examination he has a temperature of 38°C. A joint aspirate is taken. What is the most likely causative organism?

A   *Neisseria gonorrhoeae*
B   *Staphyloccocus aureus*
C   *Haemophilus influenzae*
D   *Streptococcus viridans*
E   *Chlamydia trachomatis*

16. Swollen joint (2)

A 26-year-old squash player is admitted with a red, swollen left knee. He reports no history of trauma. On examination he has a temperature of 38°C. A joint aspirate is taken which grows Gram-negative diplococci. What is the antibiotic treatment regimen of choice for this patient?

A   Oral flucloxacillin for 4–6 weeks
B   IV flucloxacillin for 4–6 weeks
C   IV flucloxacillin for 2–4 weeks
D   IV flucloxacillin and vancomycin for 6–8 weeks
E   IV cefotaxime for 4–6 weeks

17. Hepatitis B serology (1)

You order hepatitis B serology tests for one of your patients, a 24-year-old man who is an intravenous drug user. The results that come back from the laboratory are as follows:

- HBsAg = positive
- Anti-HBs = negative
- HBeAg = positive
- Anti-HBe = negative
- Anti-HBc IgM = negative
- Anti-HBc IgG = positive

What is the most likely diagnosis based on these results?

A   The patient has chronic hepatitis B infection which is currently highly infectious
B   The patient has chronic hepatitis B infection which is not currently infectious
C   The patient has acute hepatitis B infection which is not currently infectious
D   The patient is immune due to hepatitis B vaccination
E   The patient is immune due to natural infection

18. Hepatitis B serology (2)

You order hepatitis B serology tests for one of your patients, a 24-year-old man who is an intravenous drug user. The results that come back from the laboratory are as follows:

- HBsAg = negative
- Anti-HBs = positive
- HBeAg = negative
- Anti-HBe = negative
- Anti-HBc IgM = negative
- Anti- HBc IgG = negative

What is the most likely diagnosis based on these results?

A   The patient has chronic hepatitis B infection which is currently highly infectious
B   The anti-HBs is a false positive result
C   The patient has a resolved hepatitis B infection
D   The patient is immune due to hepatitis B vaccination
E   The patient is immune due to natural infection

19. Treatment for diarrhoea (1)

A 79-year old woman is admitted to the hospital for treatment of pneumonia and is commenced on intravenous antibiotic therapy. Her respiratory symptoms begin to improve, but 5 days later she develops profuse diarrhoea. The most appropriate treatment is:

A   Oral metronidazole for 7 days
B   Oral metronidazole for 14 days
C   Isolation and treatment with intravenous fluids
D   IV metronidazole for 7 days
E   Oral co-amoxiclav for 7 days

20. Treatment for diarrhoea (2)

A 79-year old woman is admitted to hospital for treatment of pneumonia and is commenced on intravenous antibiotic therapy. Her respiratory symptoms begin to improve, but 5 days later she develops profuse diarrhoea. After treatment with oral metronidazole she shows gradual improvement, but the profuse diarrhoea returns 2 weeks later. The same organism is found to be responsible. The most appropriate course of action is:

A   Oral metronidazole for 7 days
B   Oral metronidazole for 14 days
C   Isolation and treatment with intravenous fluids
D   IV metronidazole for 7 days
E   Oral vancomycin for 14 days

21. Confusion (1)

A 65-year old retired mechanic is brought by his family to his GP due to their concern over his recent increase in confusion. This has occurred rapidly over the past 4 months, and he now struggles to recognize members of his family. His daughter also reports occasionally seeing intermittent, jerky movements of both his arms. The GP organizes a CT scan and dementia screen, which are both found to be normal. Which is the next most useful diagnostic test for the GP to order?

A   MRI brain
B   Electroencephalogram
C   Electrocardiogram
D   Ultrasound scan of both carotids
E   Tonsillar biopsy

22. Confusion (2)

A 61-year-old patient has recently been diagnosed with sporadic CJD. His GP is keen to do a lumbar puncture. Which of the following statements is true regarding this investigation in this situation?

A   The lumbar puncture is used to look for the levels of protein, glucose and polymorphs
B   The lumbar puncture is used to look for the levels of a protein called 14-3-3
C   A lumbar puncture is the most specific test for variant CJD
D   The lumbar puncture is not useful in sporadic CJD, but is an important test in variant CJD
E   A tonsillar biopsy would be a more useful test than a lumbar puncture for sporadic CJD

23. Lumbar puncture

A 16-year-old student complains of a headache of recent onset at school. He is taken to accident and emergency and on examination has a temperature of 37.6°C. A lumbar puncture is performed, and the results are as follows:

- Appearance: Clear fluid
- Protein: 0.82 g/L
- WCC: 90.5×10^7 (>95 per cent lymphocytes)

What is the most likely diagnosis?

A   Subarachnoid haemorrhage
B   Tension headache
C   Bacterial meningitis
D   Viral meningitis
E   Tuberculous meningitis

24. Abdominal distension

A 42-year-old alcoholic is admitted with abdominal distension. The shifting dullness test is positive and he is found to have diffuse abdominal tenderness. His observations are as follows: pulse 115, blood pressure 116/83, temperature 37.9°C. The next best course of action is:

A   Begin therapeutic paracentesis
B   Observe, administer analgesia and closely monitor his vital signs
C   Commence intravenous spironolactone
D   Commence intravenous amoxicillin
E   Commence intravenous cefotaxime

25. Hepatitis C (1)

A 63-year-old asymptomatic housewife is referred to a gastroenterologist after her GP found that she had abnormal liver function tests on a routine blood test. A thorough history reveals that she received a blood transfusion during her pregnancy in 1979. Further tests confirm that she has contracted hepatitis C. She is commenced on a course of anti-viral treatment. Which of the following factors is most significant in influencing her chance of clearing the virus?

A   The length of time between contracting the disease and being diagnosed
B   The route by which she contracted the disease
C   Her liver function test results
D   The virus genotype
E   The level of alpha-feto-protein

26. Hepatitis C (2)

A 63-year-old asymptomatic housewife is referred to a gastroenterologist after her GP found that she had abnormal liver function tests on a routine blood test. A thorough history reveals that she received a blood transfusion during her pregnancy in 1979. The best test to confirm whether the patient has hepatitis C would be:

A   Liver biopsy
B   Anti-hepatitis C antibodies
C   Alanine aminotransferase levels
D   Hepatitis C RNA PCR
E   Viral genotyping

27. Lethargy

A 33-year-old backpacker visits his GP complaining of feeling weak, lethargic and feverish since he returned from his trip to South Africa 3 months previously. He is accompanied by his wife, who reports a change in his behaviour and disturbed sleeping pattern since his return. On examination, his GP discovers that he has enlarged cervical lymph nodes, and there is a small chancre on his forearm that is approximately 2 cm in diameter. The most likely causative organism is:

A   *Plasmodium falciparum*
B   *Trypanosoma brucei gambiense*
C   *Trypanosoma brucei rhodesiense*
D   *Trypanosoma cruzi*
E   *Leishmania infantum*

28. Difficulty swallowing

A 20-year-old student seeks medical attention due to recent difficulty in swallowing, and severe weight loss. A thorough travel history reveals that he returned several months ago from a gap year in Brazil. During his trip he remembers becoming unwell at one point with a fever, diarrhoea, vomiting and swollen eyelids, but this resolved in approximately 3 weeks with no treatment. A chest X-ray is ordered as one of his investigations, and this reveals marked dilatation of his oesophagus. The vector responsible for transmitting this disease is:

A   Tsetse fly
B   Reduviid bug
C   Sandfly
D   *Aedes* mosquito
E   *Ixodes* tick

29. Treatment for a cough (1)

A 46-year-old Somalian woman presents to her GP with a dry cough and weight loss of 5 kg over 3 weeks. She is sent to the hospital, and a chest X-ray reveals cavitating lung lesions. The most appropriate therapy is:

A   Rifampicin and isoniazid for 6 months, ethambutol and pyrazinamide for 2 months
B   Rifampicin and isoniazid for 2 months, ethambutol and pyrazinamide for 6 months
C   Rifampicin and pyrazinamide for 4 months, ethambutol and isoniazid and for 2 months
D   Rifampicin and streptomycin for 4 months, pyrazinamide and ethambutol for 2 months
E   Rifampicin, isoniazid, ethambutol and pyrazinamide for 6 months

30. Treatment for a cough (2)

A 46-year-old Somalian woman presents to her GP with a dry cough and weight loss of 5 kg over 3 weeks. She is sent to the hospital, and a chest X-ray reveals cavitating lung lesions. She is started on a course of anti-tuberculous medication. Which of the following statements about this regimen is true?

A   Liver function tests only need to be checked in those with pre-existing liver disease

B   Ethambutol can cause a peripheral neuropathy

C   Pyridoxine should always be given with isoniazid treatment

D   Rifampicin can cause optic neuritis

E   Ethambutol should be avoided in renal failure

31. Muscle weakness

A 35-year-old banker develops a fever, vomiting and diarrhoea after a barbeque. This resolves within 2 weeks, but he then suddenly develops unilateral facial weakness. This is followed by severe muscle weakness which rapidly spreads over the next 5 days from his feet and legs to his trunk. The most likely diagnosis is:

A   Polio

B   Lyme disease

C   Guillan–Barré syndrome

D   Haemolytic uraemic syndrome

E   Influenza

32. Malaria (1)

A young girl returns from visiting her relatives in India, feeling feverish and with flu-like symptoms. A diagnosis of malaria is suspected. Her fevers started on Monday, regressed for a few days and then returned on Thursday. She was well again over the weekend, and was then brought to the GP the following Monday when her fever had again returned. The most likely causative agent in this case is:

A   *Plasmodium falciparum*

B   *Plasmodium vivax*

C   *Plasmodium ovale*

D   *Plasmodium malariae*

E   *Plasmodium knowlesi*

33. Malaria (2)

A young girl returns from visiting her relatives in India, feeling feverish and with flu-like symptoms. A diagnosis of malaria is suspected. The form of the malaria parasite which invades erythrocytes is known as a:

A   Sporozite
B   Schizont
C   Merozite
D   Hypnozoite
E   Gametocyte

34. Malaria (3)

A 55-year-old housewife returns from visiting her relatives in India, with a high fever and with flu-like symptoms. A diagnosis of uncomplicated falciparum malaria is confirmed. The most appropriate management plan is:

A   Discharge with oral quinine and doxycycline
B   Discharge with oral mefloquine and chloroquine
C   Admit, give IV paracetemol and observe
D   Admit and give IV quinine
E   Admit and give oral quinine and doxycycline

35. Malaria (4)

A 55-year-old housewife returns from visiting her relatives in India, with a high fever and with flu-like symptoms. Thick and thin films are requested, and Maurer's clefts are seen under the microscope. The diagnosis is:

A   *Plasmodium falciparum*
B   *Plasmodium vivax*
C   *Plasmodium ovale*
D   *Plasmodium malariae*
E   *Plasmodium knowlesi*

ANSWERS

Sputum culture

1 C   This gentleman is most likely suffering from *Mycobacterium tuberculosis* which characteristically presents with a persistent cough, haemoptysis, fever, night sweats and weight loss. Lowenstein–Jensen medium is a growth medium used to culture *Mycobacterium* species at 37°C. The most common indication for its use is to culture *Mycobacterium tuberculosis* (C), where it appears as brown coffee-coloured (buff), granular bread crumb-like colonies (rough) which often stick to the bottom of the growth plate and are hard to remove (tough). This is often remembered as 'buff, rough and tough'. It usually takes approximately 4–6 weeks to obtain these visible colonies, an important fact to remember when treating patients. Another characteristic feature is the formation of serpentine rods from chains of cells in smears. There are a few other important points to remember about staining results for *Mycobacterium tuberculosis*. They are classified as acid-fast bacteria, because they are resistant to losing their colour during staining procedures. The Ziehl–Neelson stain is the most common method used to stain this type of bacterium, and they appear bright red against a blue background. The stain contains carbofuchsin, a pink dye which binds to the unique mycolic acids found in the mycobacterium cell wall. Another stain that can be used for acid-fast bacilli is the auramine stain, which also binds to mycolic acids to give a yellow fluorescence.

Mycobacterium leprae (E) is another acid-fast bacillus, responsible for causing leprosy. It can be detected using a skin biopsy or nasal smear, using Fite stain. It has proven difficult to culture on artificial cell media, but instead has been grown on mouse foot pads and nine-banded armadillos. Symptoms of leprosy include hypopigmented skin lesions, nodules and loss of sensation.

Coxiella burnetii (A) causes Q fever, which was first described in abbatoir workers. It is an obligate intracellular Gram-negative bacterium found in farm animals and pets, and is transmitted by aerosol or contact with animal products like milk or faeces. It manifests as flu-like symptoms, but can progress to an atypical pneumonia or less often a granulomatous hepatitis. Typical chest X-ray features include a ground glass appearance. It does not grow on Lowenstein–Jensen medium.

Streptococcus pneumoniae (B) is a Gram-positive coccus causing a lobar pneumonia, and can be differentiated from *Streptococcus viridans* using an optochin test. *Streptococcus pneumoniae* and *viridans* are alpha haemolytic, but *Strep. pneumoniae* are optochin sensitive whilst *Strep.*

viridans are optochin resistant. It also does not grow on Lowenstein–Jensen medium.

Legionella pneumophilia (D) is a Gram-negative bacterium that causes Legionnaire's disease. It typically presents initially with flu-like symptoms, progressing to a productive cough and sometimes diarrhoea and confusion due to hyponatraemia. It can be detected using a urinary antigen test, or by culture on buffered charcoal yeast extract, but not Lowenstein–Jensen medium.

Mantoux test

2 B   The Mantoux test is a diagnostic test for tuberculosis. It consists of an intradermal injection of 0.1 mL of purified protein derivative (PPD) tuberculin, which is a glycerol extract of the bacillus. The diameter of the induration that subsequently forms is read 48–72 hours later, but one also needs to take into account the patient's risk of being infected with TB and of progression to disease if they were infected in interpreting the result. The Centers for Disease Control and Prevention provide the following classification for the skin test:

1   An induration of 5 mm or more is considered positive in:
   • Patients with HIV
   • A recent contact of a person with TB disease
   • People with fibrotic changes on chest radiograph consistent with prior TB
   • Patients with organ transplants
   • People who are immunosuppressed for other reasons (for example taking the equivalent of >15 mg/day of prednisone for 1 month or longer)

2   An induration of 10 mm or more is considered positive in:
   • Recent immigrants (<5 years) from high-prevalence countries
   • Intravenous drug users
   • Residents and employees of high-risk congregate settings
   • Mycobacteriology laboratory personnel
   • Persons with clinical conditions that place them at high risk
   • Children <4 years of age
   • Infants, children, and adolescents exposed to adults in high-risk categories

3   An induration of 15 mm or more is considered positive in any person, including those with no known risk factors for TB

So for the patient in the question, a lower cut off is used to interpret the test as he has HIV. The reasoning behind this is that as he is likely to have a depleted CD4 T-cell count, which are the cells involved in mounting a type IV sensitivity reaction to the injection to produce a positive result; if we were to use the normal cut off of 15 mm there is a chance we would obtain a false negative result for him. A positive result indicates that the person has been exposed to TB (B), which could include previous BCG exposure (C). Whilst (C) could also be correct, the single best answer in this case is (B) as this encompasses both possibilities. Answers (A) and (E) are clearly not correct, as using the above guidelines the result is positive for an HIV patient. Answer (D) could again be possible but it may also be true that his infected state is a result of a *de novo* infection, and not a reactivation of latent TB.

Pneumonia (1)

3 D   It is useful to remember that streptococci can essentially be divided into alpha haemolytic, beta haemolytic and non-haemolytic groups. Alpha haemolytic streptococci can be further divided into *Strep. pneumoniae* (D) and *Strep. viridans* (B) according to their optochin sensitivity (amongst other factors). The beta haemolytic streptococci are further classified according to Lancefield groups A, B, C, F and G. Finally the non-haemolytic streptococci include the enterococci.

Optochin is an antibiotic used to differentiate *Strep. pneumoniae* from other alpha haemolytic streptococci such as *Strep. viridans*. The pneumococcus will typically produce a zone of inhibition around an optochin disc, indicating that it is sensitive to the antibiotic, whereas *Strep. viridans* is resistant to it so its growth will not be affected. This can be remembered using the mnemonic 'OVeR PS' (Optochin – Viridans Resistant, Pneumococci Sensitive). As the organism in the question is optochin sensitive, the answer is (D).

Staphylococcus aureus would not be optochin sensitive, so (A) is not the correct answer. It is a Gram-positive bacterium that obtained its name because of the golden yellow colonies that form when grown on blood agar plates (*aurum* is Latin for gold). *Mycoplasma pneumoniae* (C) generally causes an atypical pneumonia in children and young adults. It is called the 'walking pneumonia' because patients can sometimes continue walking around despite suffering from it, and many are asymptomatic. The clinical features of this pneumonia can on occasion be relatively insignificant compared to the radiological findings. It too is not optochin sensitive so is not the correct answer here. *Haemophilus influenzae* (E) is a Gram-negative bacillus so can be easily eliminated as a potentially correct answer here. Clinically the pneumonia caused by *Haemophilus* is not easily distinguished from that caused by *Strep. pneumoniae*.

Pneumonia (2)

4 A *Klebsiella pneumoniae* (A) is a Gram-negative rod-shaped bacillus that can cause an atypical pneumonia, most frequently in alcoholics. It can result in sudden, severe systemic upset in these patients, and the production of thick, purulent and sometimes blood-stained sputum said to resemble 'red-currant jelly'. Haemoptysis occurs more frequently with *K. pneumoniae* than with *pneumonia* caused by other bacteria. Radiological features can include upper lobe consolidation, with marked cavitation as described in the question. It is more likely to lead to complications such as lung abscesses and empyemas than pneumonias caused by *Strep. pneumoniae*.

Mycobacterium tuberculosis (B) can cause haemoptysis and upper lobe cavitation. Whilst a plausible answer, the indication that the patient is alcoholic, coupled with the characteristic description of thick, blood-stained sputum, is more characteristic of *Klebsiella*. Also note the absence of other typical indicators of tuberculosis such as night sweats, weight loss and Asian ethnicity. Pneumonia caused by *Staphyloccous aureus* (C) can follow an influenza virus infection, and may result in the formation of abscesses. The radiological findings can include extensive cavitation, and thin walled abscesses may break down to give a cystic appearance. Whilst *S. aureus* could potentially lead to the above clinical picture, *Klebsiella* is again more likely to give blood-stained sputum in an alcoholic.

Moraxella catarrhalis (D) is a Gram-negative diplococcus that may cause pneumonia in patients with underlying lung disease such as chronic obstructive pulmonary disease (COPD). It can be implicated in an infective exacerbation of their condition in these patients. It can also lead to laryngitis, otitis media and sinusitis. Given the presumed absence of an underlying lung condition in this patient, it is less likely to be the causative agent than *Klebsiella*.

Pneumocystis jirovecii (E) tends to affect immunocompromised patients, and used to be called pneumocystis pneumonia (PCP). Typical clinical features include severe shortness of breath, dry cough and the presence of bilateral crackles. If you get an HIV patient whose saturations drop on exertion in a question, think about this organism! It does not normally give bilateral cavitation on a chest X-ray, but instead would characteristically show peri-hilar interstitial infiltrates, giving a 'bat's wing' appearance. Histology may reveal classic boat-shaped organisms, and the diagnostic stain used is the silver stain.

Endocarditis

5 C Infective endocarditis can be classified into two broad categories: acute and sub-acute. Acute infective endocarditis is less common, and

the most likely causative agent is *Staphylococcus aureus* (C). It can affect both normal and abnormal valves, and can typically be found in intravenous drug users, such as the patient described. The tricuspid valve is most commonly affected in these cases, which can easily be remembered as this is the first valve that the bacteria will encounter following injection into a vein. Therefore, (C) is the correct answer in this case.

The other category of infective endocarditis is the sub-acute form, which is more common. It is most often caused by *Streptococcus viridans* (A), and usually occurs on damaged valves. Patients typically present with an insidious onset of fevers, night sweats, and weight loss. Other clinical features can result from emboli, such as cerebral emboli causing a stroke, or less commonly recurrent pulmonary emboli in right sided endocarditis. If asked about the signs of endocarditis, steer away from mentioning the rare eponymous signs first! You can remember the signs as rules of two: two signs in the hands include clubbing and splinter haemorrhages, two signs in the abdomen are splenomegaly and microscopic haematuria, and two signs elsewhere can include new or changing heart murmurs and embolic phenomena. Remember that the most common valves to be affected are the aortic and mitral valves.

Fungi such as *Candida albicans* (B) are a much less common cause of endocarditis. They can also be found in intravenous drug users, but this is much less likely than *Staphylococcus aureus*. They can include *Aspergillus* and *Candida* species, and usually cause a sub-acute picture. *Strep. bovis* (D) has also been implicated as a rarer cause of infective endocarditis, and is part of the natural flora of the bowel. If found in a patient with endocarditis, a colonoscopy may be important as its presence is associated with colonic malignancies. The HACEK organisms consist of a Gram-negative group which includes *Haemophilus parainfluenzae*, *Aggregatibacter*, *Cardiobacterium hominis*, *Eikenella corrodens* and *Kingella* (E). They typically result in a culture negative endocarditis. Whilst all of the above answers are possible, the single best answer is *Staphylococcus aureus* because the patient is an intravenous drug user and has developed an acute form of the disease.

Anti-virals

6 D Acyclovir (D) is a guanosine analogue that causes obligate chain termination when it attaches to DNA. It is phosphorylated by the enzyme thymidine kinase found in viruses, which is far more effective than the cellular thymidine kinase for this process. This means that normal cells which are not infected by the virus are not affected as much by

acyclovir, as there is no viral thymidine kinase present. The acyclovir monophosphate which then forms is further phosphorylated to a diphosphate and then to a triphosphate by the cellular thymidine kinase. This triphosphate potently inhibits viral DNA polymerase, leading to chain termination. It is effective against the herpes viruses, for example herpes simplex and herpes zoster which causes shingles.

Foscarnet (A) is a pyrophosphate analogue used for the treatment of CMV, and works by inhibiting viral DNA polymerase via a different mechanism to acyclovir. It can also be used for herpes zoster, but is usually a second line if the infection is resistant to acyclovir. It does not require phosphorylation by viral thymidine kinase. Lamivudine (B) is used for the treatment of hepatitis B and HIV, not shingles. It is a cytidine analogue, and acts as a potent nucleoside analogue reverse transcriptase inhibitor. Cidofovir (C) works by inhibiting viral DNA polymerase, and is used for cytomegalovirus retinitis. It is not dependent on phosphorylation by viral enzymes in the way acyclovir is. Ganciclovir (E) is thought to be the drug of choice for treating cytomegalovirus infections. Unlike acyclovir it is also phosphorylated by uninfected cells, so it is more toxic in comparison.

Vaccine schedule

7   A   The current UK immunization schedule is as follows:

- Two months: Hib/IPV/DTaP/PCV
- Three months: Hib/IPV/DTaP/Men C
- Four months: Hib/IPV/DTaP/PCV/Men C
- Twelve months: Hib/Men C
- Thirteen months: MMR/PCV
- Three years four months old or soon after: MMR/DTaP/IPV
- 13–18 years: Booster Diptheria and tetanus/IPV

DTap stands for diphtheria, tetanus and acellular pertussis, and IPV is the inactivated poliovirus vaccine. This can be challenging to remember but is often asked about in exams. One way of remembering it is this: H = Hib, I = IPV, D = DTaP, P = PCV, **Men** = Men C, M = MMR:

- Two months: H.I.De your little baby Please.
- Three months: the first three as above, but meningitis C instead of PCV
- Four months: all the above
- Twelve months: now we want to H.I.De them from **Men. C**?!
- Thirteen months: MMR/Please!
- Three years four months old or soon after: things are starting to D.I.M now so we need to booster it!
- 13–18 years: I'D like my teenager to go back for a jab!

Urinary tract infections

8 B The most common cause of a urinary tract infection in all groups of patients is *Escherichia coli* (B). Do not be misled by the fact that the patient is a young, sexually active woman. The *E. coli* bacterium is a lactose-fermenting Gram-negative rod. It has various properties that aid its pathogenesis: a flagellum to enable it to move upstream, fimbrae so that it can adhere to the urothelium, and haemolysin to form pores in white blood cells. It also has a protective capsule called the K-antigen. The other lactose fermenting organisms are *Klebsiella* and *Enterobacter*, whilst non-lactose fermenting organisms include *Proteus* and *Pseudomonas*. Lactose fermenting organisms turn MacConkey agar pink, whereas non-lactose fermenters do not. Useful investigations for urinary tract infections can include a urine dipstick to look for nitrites and leukocytes, and urine cultures looking for a bactiuria of greater than 10^5 colony forming units.

Enterobacter (A) is less commonly implicated in urinary tract infections. They are Gram-negative, lactose-fermenting, rod-shaped bacteria. They tend to cause opportunistic infections in immunocompromised hosts, so it is unlikely to be the causative agent here. *Klebsiella* (C) is also a Gram-negative, non-motile, lactose-fermenting organism. Patients that are immunocompromised or have indwelling catheters are at increased risk of *Klebsiella* infections. *Staphylococcus saphrophyticus* (D) is a Gram-positive cause of urinary tract infections. It is the second most common cause of urinary tract infections in young, sexually active women after *E. coli*. It is coagulase positive like other staphylococcal species, but catalase negative unlike *S. aureus*. *Proteus mirabilis* (E) is an example of a non-lactose fermenting bacterium. It is not a likely cause of this patient's UTI, but is more common in young boys and hospitalized patients. It has the ability to split urea into ammonia, which raises the pH of the urine. This predisposes to the formation of phosphate stones, particularly staghorn calculi.

Diarrhoea (1)

9 C *Giardia lamblia* (C) is a flagellated protozoan parasite which causes giardiasis. It attaches to the small bowel wall, but does not invade it. If you can remember this fact, you will find it easier to remember that it interferes with absorption, and so leads to the classic symptoms of weight loss, flatulence, chronic diarrhoea and bloating, as in the patient in this question. Because it does not invade the small bowel wall, the diarrhoea is not bloody but it is watery. Microscopy of a stool sample may show a pear-shaped protozoan. If you imagine a pear making you feel very bloated, you will remember this fact which often crops up in

questions! Very rarely, a string test may be done if other methods to detect the parasites fail but there is still a high index of clinical suspicion. A gelatine capsule attached to a long string is swallowed, with the end of the string remaining outside the mouth and taped to the patient's cheek. It remains in place for about 4–6 hours, before the end is examined under the microscope. Treatment of giardiasis is typically oral metronidazole.

Bacillus cereus (A) causes food poisoning with vomiting and sometimes diarrhoea, usually from re-heated food such as rice. The symptoms appear quite quickly, within a couple of hours of consumption. The bacteria produce spores, which are activated by changes in temperature (such as re-heating or refrigerating food) to produce heat-labile and heat-stabile toxins. The patient in question has no vomiting, no history of eating re-heated food and has unusual symptoms of flatulence and bloating which would not normally be associated with this infection.

Salmonella enteritidis (B) is an important cause of food poisoning, usually from contaminated meat and eggs. Do not confuse this with enteric fevers which are systemic illnesses caused by *Salmonella typhi* and *paratyphi*. The incubation period is 12–48 hours, after which the patient may present with nausea, vomiting and malaise, after which follows abdominal pain and diarrhoea. This can occasionally become bloody. Most cases are self limiting within approximately 3 days. Again the patient in the question does not fit this picture.

Entamoeba histolytica (D) causes amoebic dysentery. Trophozites invade the bowel wall and lead to classical 'flask shaped ulcers', causing bloody diarrhoea. Trophozites can enter the portal vein and lead to liver abscesses too. The entamoeba cysts classically have four nuclei. One way to remember these somewhat obscure facts that appear in exam questions is to picture four runners 'ent-ering' a race, and the winner gets a silver flask!

Cryptosporidium parvum (E) is another parasite that causes acute, watery diarrhoea which is not usually bloody. This is of particular concern in immunocompromised patients, such as those with AIDS, where the severe dehydration can be fatal.

Diarrhoea (2)

10 E *Vibrio cholerae* (E) causes profuse watery diarrhoea and vomiting. It can in fact be one of the most rapidly fatal infectious illnesses if not treated, because of the severe dehydration causing circulatory shock. The bacteria produce a toxin which has an A and a B subunit. It is the A subunit which activates a G protein and results in the production of cAMP, which initiates the secretion of Na^+, K^+, Cl^-, and HCO_3^- into the small intestine lumen. Most people only have a mild illness which simply

resembles other diarrhoeal illnesses. Sometimes, as in this case, the diarrhoea is profuse and is known colloquially as 'rice-water' stools because of its appearance. The diagnosis is predominantly clinical, but if stool culture is performed the classical appearance will be of curved shaped, oxidase-positive organisms. You can remember this as the Cholera Comma! Rehydration therapy forms the mainstay of treatment.

Hepatitis A (A) can cause diarrhoea in travellers to developing countries, but the stools are not 'rice-water', and the organisms would not be demonstrated on microscopy as above. The more common symptoms are flu-like, and for this reason it can be mistaken for influenza. Jaundice can also develop with tender hepatomegaly. Treatment is mainly supportive – there is no specific anti-viral for hepatitis A.

Clostridium difficile (B) is an anaerobic, Gram-positive rod that produces enterotoxins and cytotoxins. It can cause antibiotic-associated diarrhoea. A severe form is known as pseudomembranous colitis, of which a complication is toxic megacolon. Diagnosis is usually by demonstrating the presence of the *Clostridium difficile* toxin in faeces using cell-culture assay or immunoassay.

Enterocolitis caused by *Yersinia enterocolitica* (C) is also characterized by fever, abdominal pain and diarrhoea. It is a Gram-negative rod, so would not result in the comma-shaped organisms found here. It is normally self-limiting.

Campylobacter jejuni (D) is a common cause of gastroenteritis. Whilst vomiting is not a prominent feature, the diarrhoea that occurs can be bloody. Sources can include unpasteurized milk and meat – remember this as the food and drink you might take with you camping! It is a Gram-negative bacterium that is also oxidase positive, but has a corkscrew rather than a comma appearance. Diagnosis is made by stool culture. It is usually self-limiting, but sometimes oral erythromycin is used for treatment.

The oxidase test mentioned in the question is used to determine if bacteria produce a certain type of oxidase enzyme. Important oxidase positive organisms that sometimes appear in questions are: Pseudomonas, Neisseria, Campylobacter, Helicobacter, Moraxella, Vibrio, and Legionella. This can be remembered using the mnemonic: 'Pu.N.C.H. Me Very Lightly!'

Protozoal disease

11 A Leishmaniasis is transmitted by phlebotomine sandflies and occurs in Africa, America and the Middle East. Visceral leishmaniasis (A) is also known as 'Kala-azar', and the most common clinical features include fever and splenomegaly. Hepatomegaly, skin hyperpigmentation and dry warty skin occur less frequently, and bone marrow invasion can result

in pancytopenia. It can be mistaken for malaria, which is dangerous as it can be fatal if left untreated. *L. donovani* and *L. infantum* are thought to cause the disease in Africa, Asia and Europe, whilst *L. chagasi* is implicated in South America.

The most common form of leishmaniasis is called cutaneous leishmaniasis (B), where an itchy papule develops at the bite site and develops into an ulcer with raised edges. Local lymphadenopathy can also occur, but the lesion usually heals within 8 months leaving a depigmented scar. The organisms implicated are *L. major* and *L. tropica*. Mucocutaneous leishmaniasis (C) can produce destructive and disfiguring facial lesions, and so is the most feared form of cutaneous leishmaniasis. It may begin in the same way as the cutaneous form, but years later ulceration can appear in mucous membranes leading to mutilation of those areas. It is most often caused by *L. braziliensis*. A single ulcer caused by *L. major* or *L. tropica* may be left to heal spontaneously, but otherwise the first-line drug for leishmaniasis is a pentavalent antimonial such as sodium stibogluconate.

Malaria (D) can present with non-specific flu-like symptoms, but hyper-pigmentation of the skin is not a feature. Hepatosplenomegaly can occur however, and other clinical features might include malaise, head-ache, vomiting or diarrhoea. Malaria should be considered as the most likely diagnosis in a patient with a fever returning from an endemic area.

Schistosomiasis (E), also known as bilharzia, is transmitted by blood flukes. An itchy rash, known as 'swimmer's itch', may develop at the site where the vectors penetrate the skin. They may then migrate to the liver, causing 'Katayama fever' with clinical features such as fever, rash, myalgia and sometimes hepatosplenomegaly. Following maturation in the liver, the flukes migrate to either mesenteric veins causing intestinal schistosomiasis, or to the urinary tract leading to urinary schistosomiasis. Hepatosplenomegaly can occur, but again the dry warty skin lesions described are not usually a feature.

Investigation of an ulcer

12 D The picture described is consistent with cutaneous leishmaniasis, the most common form of leishmaniasis. An itchy, scaly papule develops at the bite site and develops into a crusty ulcer with raised edges. Local lymphadenopathy can also occur, but the lesion usually heals within 8 months leaving a depigmented scar called an oriental sore. The organisms implicated are *Leishmania major* (D) and *L. tropica*. You can remember this if you picture lots of skin lesions cropping up in travellers from the 'major tropics'! It is found in many countries, ranging from South America to the Middle East. Diagnosis can be by Giemsa staining of slit skin smears, or from tissue aspirated from the ulcer.

The organism can be cultured on Novy–Macneal–Nicolle medium as described in the question.

The other forms of leishmaniasis are visceral and mucocutaneous. Visceral leishmaniasis is also known as 'Kala-azar', and the most common clinical features include fever and splenomegaly. Hepatomegaly, skin hyperpigmentation and dry warty skin occur less frequently. *Leishmania donovani* (C) and *L. infantum* are thought to cause the disease in Africa, Asia and Europe, whilst *L. chagasi* is implicated in South America. Mucocutaneous leishmaniasis can produce destructive and disfiguring facial lesions, and so is the most feared form of cutaneous leishmaniasis. It may begin in the same way as the cutaneous form, but years later ulceration can appear in mucous membranes leading to mutilation of those areas. It is most often caused by *L. braziliensis* (E).

Toxoplasma gondii (A) is a protozoal disease, for which the cat family is the definitive host. It can infect humans by eating undercooked meat or from contact with cat faeces. Like other protozoa they become trophozites in the gut and spread to the brain, eyes and lungs. It would not normally cause an ulcer, and cannot be cultured in Novy–Macneal–Nicolle medium. Most infections are asymptompatic in immunocompetent hosts, but in the immunocompromised or in fetuses affected via pregnant mothers the consequences can be fatal. In AIDS patients it can have neurological manifestations such as cranial nerve palsies, meningo-encephalitis and focal neurological deficits secondary to a space-occupying lesion. In the eyes it can cause chorioretinitis. Characteristically a CT scan may show ring enhancing lesions with surrounding oedema. If you can picture the 'O's in tOxO-plasmosis jumping out at you like rings on a CT scan, you should be able to recall this important diagnostic fact!

Treponema pallidum (B) is the organism responsible for syphilis. The first stage of syphilis presents with a papule which ulcerates to become a painless chancre. This may be associated with regional lymphadenopathy that is also painless. This fact often crops up in exam questions and can be remembered by thinking of the word 'syphilis' corresponding to the 2 **S**s found in painless! This organism also cannot be grown as described, but diagnosis would be by dark ground microscopy or serology of anti-treponemal antibodies.

Fever (1)

13 D The *Brucella* species are Gram-negative, rod shaped, intracellular bacteria that cause a highly contagious zoonosis known as brucellosis (D). The causative agent in cattle is *B. abortis*, but in dogs it is *B. canis*. Infection in cattle can lead to miscarriages, hence the name '*abortis*'. Infection is usually contracted from unsterilized milk, cheese or meat.

Clinical features of brucellosis can include a long history of undulating fevers, arthralgia and myalgia, weight loss, fatigue, lymphadenopathy, sacroilitis and depression. Many cases present as pyrexia of unknown origin. Hepatomegaly and/or splenomegaly can sometimes be found on examination.

You can remember these by picturing an old man called Bruce, walking with a stick due to his back and muscle pain (arthralgia, myalgia, sacroilitis), feeling down (depression), looking thin (anorexia), sweating (fevers), and with lots of protruding lumps (hepatosplenomegaly and lymphadenopathy)! Draw this picture, label it with these features and it will be easier to remember! The most common diagnostic method is serum agglutination for antibodies. Antibiotics that can be used for treatment include doxycylcine and gentamicin for approximately 6 weeks, though streptomycin and rifampicin are other agents that are used. Because the bacteria are intracellular, usually more than one antibiotic is needed and relapse is common.

Whilst tuberculosis (B) can cause drenching sweats, it would not typically cause lower back pain and certainly would not be treated with doxycycline. Do not forget the treatment for TB can be remembered as RIPE: Rifampicin, Isoniazid, Pyrazinamide and Ethambutol. The last two drugs, pyrazinamide and ethambutol, are usually only used for the first 2 months. The features of brucellosis and influenza (C) are not dissimilar, but influenza would usually have an incubation period of 1–4 days. Note also the history of working on a farm: any unusual facts like this are not red herrings, but are usually put in to help guide you to the right answer! Treatment of influenza would not be with doxycycline, but is usually symptomatic.

Typhoid (E) is caused by *Salmonella typhi*, and again can present with non-specific features like brucellosis. However, there are a few unusual clinical features of typhoid that are worth remembering using the mnemonic A.B.C.C.D.E: Abdominal distension, Bradycardia, Cough, Constipation, Diarrhoea and Erythematous rose spots. Antibiotics of choice in the treatment of typhoid are the quinolones such as ciprofloxacin for 2 weeks.

Fever (2)

14 E   *Borrelia burgdorferi* (E) is a Gram-negative bacterium that causes Lyme disease. It is a spirochaete, which is the name for a group of bacteria that are helically coiled in shape. Lyme disease is actually thought to be the most common vector borne disease in England and Wales. It is named after a town called Lyme in Connecticut, where the disease was first seen. The vector is a tick called the *Ixodes* tick, which can be found on deer and rodents.

Lyme disease is a multisystemic disorder which has three main stages: the local stage, disseminated stage and a late stage. The local stage involves a characteristic skin lesion called erythema chronicum migrans, usually appearing 7–10 days after the initial infection. It usually starts off as a red macule or papule, and approximately 1 week later expands to leave a target appearance with an area of central fading. Other symptoms at this stage are usually constitutional, such as a fever and headache. The somewhat unusual features of the next stage can be remembered using the word **PEACH**: Peripheral neuropathy, Erythema chronicum migrans (persists in this stage), Arthritis, Cranial nerve palsies and Heart block. Finally, the late stage can include persistent arthritis and chronic encephalitis. Treatment is with oral antibiotics, usually doxycycline.

The rash would not be in keeping with any of the other organisms listed. Herpes simplex (A) causes an acute viral disease. Type 1 is primarily responsible for oral–facial lesions, whereas Type 2 is responsible for genital disease – remember this as Type 2 requires 2 people to lead to the disease! Several anti-virals can be effective in treating the disease, particularly acyclovir.

The Epstein–Barr virus (B) is also one of the herpes viruses, and is responsible for causing infectious mononucleosis. A rash is not typically a feature of this disease, but sometimes the virus can cause erythema multiforme. This rash usually consists of itchy papules, which may evolve into target lesions.

Streptococcus pyogenes (C) is a Gram-positive bacterium responsible for many conditions, including impetigo and rheumatic fever. The rash in rheumatic fever is known as erythema marginatum, which can be easily confused with erythema chronicum migrans of Lyme disease. A good way to remember which is which is to picture a person sucking a Lyme and getting a 'chronic migraine' from doing so! In terms of appearance, erythema marginatum consists of pink ring lesions which usually occur on the trunk, arms and legs but with facial sparing.

Treponema pallidum (D) is another spirochaete, like *Borrelia burgdorferi*, but is the organism responsible for causing syphilis. The skin lesion with syphilis is called a chancre, and is classically a painless ulcer with sharp borders.

Swollen joint (1)

15   A   The patient in this question is presenting with septic arthritis. Other differentials might include gout or pseudogout, but it is paramount to consider septic arthritis as it is a rheumatalogical emergency! Typical features are like those described in the question: the patient is often pyrexial, the joint is swollen and painful with limited range of movement, and the skin overlying the joint is warm and erythematous.

Classically the patient will refuse to move the joint at all. The most important investigation is an aspirate of the joint: the fluid aspirated may appear purulent and have a high neutrophil count.

The most common cause of septic arthritis in young, sexually active adults is *Neisseria gonorrhoeae* (A). A Gram-stain of this aspirate would reveal Gram-negative diplococci. It is less likely for this organism to lead to joint destruction than a staphylococcal arthritis. The two forms of disseminated gonoccocal infection are the septic arthritis form (as described in this case), and the bacteraemic form. Other clinical features of the bacteraemic form might include a migratory polyarthralgia and a vesicular or papular rash.

Staphyloccocus aureus (B) is the most common causative organism in older patients. A Gram-stain of the joint aspirate would reveal Gram-positive cocci. It is thought that a septic arthritis infected with this organism is more likely to be destructive than a gonoccocal arthritis, and a joint can be destroyed within 24 hours if left untreated. *Haemophilus influenzae* (C) is a Gram-negative bacterium that used to be the most common cause of septic arthritis in children, but is not typically found in adults. *Streptococcus viridans* (D) is an alpha haemolytic, optochin resistant streptococcus that does not typically cause septic arthritis. It is, however, the most common cause of sub-acute bacterial endocarditis.

Swollen joint (2)

16 E   The patient in this question is presenting with septic arthritis, and the most likely cause given the joint aspiration findings of Gram-negative diplococci is *Neisseria gonorrhoeae*. The *British National Formulary* (BNF) advises the use of intravenous cefotaxime for 4–6 weeks (E) if gonococcal arthritis or a Gram-negative infection is suspected. The BNF is a good source of information for looking up the latest guidelines regarding antibiotic treatment regimens for common types of infection.

Cefotaxime is a third generation cephalosporin. Cephalosporins are part of the beta-lactam group of antibiotics which work by inhibiting cell wall synthesis. The penicillins are also part of this group. There are different generations of cephalosporins, with those of later generations having increasing Gram-negative but decreasing Gram-positive cover. Cefotaxime is also used to treat meningitis and gonorrhoea. Some of the other commonly used third generation cephalosporins are ceftizoxime and ceftriaxone – you can remember these because they all have a 't' in their names, just like in 'third' generation.

If a staphylococcal cause of septic arthritis is suspected, IV flucloxacillin for 4–6 weeks (B) would be the preferred regimen. Flucloxacillin is a narrow spectrum beta-lactam antibiotic, used to treat infections caused by Gram-positive organisms. Some bacteria, such as *Staphylococcus aureus*, produce an enzyme called beta-lactamase which renders this class of antibiotics ineffective. However, flucloxacillin is beta-lactamase stable, and so is used to treat staphylococcal infections. It is ineffective against MRSA, in which case vancomycin is preferred.

Oral flucloxacillin (A) or IV therapy of only 2–4 weeks' treatment (C) would not be sufficient to clear the infection in this case. IV flucloxacillin and vancomycin (D) together would not be needed.

Hepatitis B serology (1)

17 A   The HBsAg positive indicate that the patient has hepatitis B, and the HBeAg indicates that it is highly infectious (A). The anti-HBc IgG is also a marker that it is a chronic infection.

The different hepatitis B surface antigens and antibodies can become quite confusing, but are often asked about in exam questions. Here is a summary of what you should know:

- HBsAg – The 's' stands for surface, and refers to a protein on the surface of the virus. It is the first detectable antigen to appear after someone has been infected, and can be positive in acute or chronic disease. Patients who still carry this antigen after 6 months are termed hepatitis carriers. It is this antigen that is used to make the hepatitis B vaccine
- Anti-HBs – This is an IgG antibody that appears after the host has cleared the infection, and indicates recovery. It is also found in a person who has been vaccinated against hepatitis B (D)
- HBeAg – the 'e' antigen is often used as a marker of infectivity, as it is only found in the blood when the virus is actively replicating. If you find this hard to remember, think of the 'e' standing for 'eek! I'm infectious!' If the patient was not infectious (B), this would not be present
- Anti-HBc IgM – this indicates that the patient has recently been infected with hepatitis B, and is a marker of acute infection (C)
- Anti-HBc IgG – this is produced in response to the core antigen, and often persists for life. You can remember this as the 'c' standing for 'chronicity', as it is the difference between IgM and IgG antibodies which can tell you whether the infection is acute or chronic. And to remember which way round it is, think of 'My Gosh, he's chronic!' If the patient was immune from natural infection (E), HBsAg would not be positive, but anti-HBc IgG would be.

Hepatitis B serology (2)

18 D   Remember from the previous question that the anti-HBs antibody appears after the host has cleared the infection, and indicates recovery.

It is also found in a person who has been vaccinated against hepatitis B (D). If you get an exam question which only has the anti-HBs positive, think of vaccination! Levels of this antibody are measured to see if the patient has responded adequately to the vaccine.

The patient has not got hepatitis (E) nor is he highly infectious (A) given that HBsAg and HbeAg are negative. HBsAg can be negative in the case of a resolved infection (C), but you would expect to see some marker of previous infection such as anti-HBc IgG, which usually persists for life.

It is much more likely that the patient has been vaccinated than it is to be a false positive result (B)!

Treatment for diarrhoea (1)

19 B   Broad spectrum antibiotics, such as those used for pneumonia, can eradicate a patient's normal gut flora and therefore increase their susceptibility to *Clostridium difficile* infection. This is particularly true of penicillin derivatives (as was most likely used to treat her pneumonia), clindamycin, and third generation cephalosporins. It classically presents with profuse watery diarrhoea, usually of acute onset. The most common time for it to occur is 4–9 days after the antibiotics are started, but it can occur up to 2 months after discontinuing treatment. *Clostridium difficile* is a Gram-positive, anaerobic rod-shaped bacterium. The gold standard for diagnosis is detection of the *C. difficile* toxin in a stool sample.

The two most feared complications are pseudomembranous colitis and toxic megacolon. Pseudomembranous colitis is essentially an acute, severe colitis, which is named as such because of the formation of 'pseudomembranes' on the mucosa of the colon. These are thought to be composed of exudative material produced from the bacterium. Toxic megacolon can also be a complication of inflammatory bowel disease. The colon becomes severely distended, and clinical features include pyrexia, severe abdominal pain and bloating.

First line treatment for infection with *C. difficile* is oral metronidazole, with a suggested duration of treatment of 10–14 days (B). Metronidazole is classified as a nitroimidazole antibiotic, and is particularly useful for the treatment of anaerobic organisms and protozoa. You can remember three of the key organisms it is used to treat by remembering that 'Met is out to G.E.T you difficult bugs!' (Giardia, Entamoeba, Trichomonas and C. difficile). Patients are usually advised to avoid consuming alcohol whilst taking this antibiotic because of the potential reaction that can occur characterized by nausea, shortness of breath, flushing and vomiting.

The course of treatment should be at least 10–14 days, so 7 would not suffice (A). Whilst the patient must be isolated and rehydrated adequately, this alone would not be enough (C). IV metronidazole is not necessary in the first instance (D), unless the patient had a life-threatening infection. Co-amoxiclav (E), otherwise known as augmentin, is not used to treat *C. difficile* infections.

Treatment for diarrhoea (2)

20 **B** This patient's repeated diarrhoea may be caused by persistent infection with *Clostridium difficile* (spore germination), new infection or resistant bacteria. Current guidelines recommend the use of a repeat course of metronidazole for the treatment of recurrent *C. difficile* infection (B).

As explained previously, a 7-day course of metronidazole (A) is not considered a sufficient duration of treatment to eradicate the bacterium. Again, isolation and IV fluid resuscitation (C) is necessary but not adequate as a single measure in the management of this woman. Intravenous metronidazole (D) is only needed if a patient is not responding to vancomycin, the infection is life-threatening, or for patients with ileus.

Oral vancomycin for 10–14 days (E) is given for:

- Third or subsequent episodes
- Severe infection
- Infection not responding to metronidazole
- Patients who cannot tolerate metronidazole

Vancomycin is classified as a glycopeptide antibiotic. Its mechanism of action is to inhibit cell wall synthesis in Gram-positive bacteria, and it is not effective for Gram-negative bacteria. You can remember this if you picture an ambulance 'Van' with a big red cross (for Gram-positive) on the side! Because it cannot pass through the lining of the intestine, it is usually given intravenously. However, in the case of *Clostridium difficile* infection we give it orally, as this stays in the gut where it is needed.

One rare but important side effect you might hear about is 'red man syndrome', a reaction to the drug which consists of a sudden onset erythematous, pruritic rash over the face, neck and upper torso. To remember this fact, picture the driver of the red cross van emerging very angry, with a bright red face!

Confusion (1)

21 **B** The key here is the rapidly progressive nature of the condition in a relatively young patient. He shows the characteristic sudden decline in cognitive function, combined with the presence of myoclonic jerks and the

lack of positive investigation results so far. This is highly suggestive of sporadic Creutzfeldt–Jakob disease (CJD), the name given to a common group of prion diseases. The word prion is derived from the words 'protein' and 'infection', and it so follows that a prion is a highly infectious agent composed of protein.

There are essentially three different forms of CJD which you should be aware of:

1   Sporadic Creutzfeldt–Jakob Disease (80 per cent)

2   Acquired (<5 per cent): Kuru, variant CJD, iatrogenic CJD

3   Genetic (15 per cent): e.g. Gerstmann–Straussler–Sheinker syndrome, familial fatal insomnia

The key clinical features of sporadic CJD are **dementia** at a mean age of 65 years, and lower motor neuron signs, akinetic mutism (a clinical state of not speaking or moving), myoclonus, and cortical blindness. This can be remembered as the '**demented L.A.M.B**'. The most striking feature is the rapidity of the dementia, as in this case.

In terms of the pathology behind sporadic CJD, the characteristic feature found at autopsy in these patients is known as spongiform vacuolation (essentially the presence of many round vacuoles in the grey matter). This is not unique to sporadic CJD, but unlike in other forms of dementia, such as Alzheimer's disease, there is no associated brain atrophy. This may be because the disease progresses so rapidly.

The diagnostic test of choice here is the electroencephalogram (B), which is abnormal in two-thirds of patients and would classically demonstrate generalized triphasic sharp wave complexes. Do not confuse this with an electrocardiogram (ECG) (C), which would not be diagnostic in this case. An MRI brain (A) may show increased signal in the basal ganglia, but would not be the best investigation here. An ultrasound scan of both carotids (D) is a useful test if investigating a transient ischaemic attack (TIA) to look for carotid stenosis, but this is not relevant with this patient. Finally, a tonsillar biopsy (E), is a useful diagnostic test for variant CJD (for which it has 100 per cent sensitivity and specificity), but not for sporadic CJD.

Confusion (2)

22   B   The lumbar puncture in CJD is used to analyze the CSF for a protein named '14-3-3' (B). Note that routine analysis of the cerebrospinal fluid (CSF) is normal in CJD, therefore looking at levels of protein, glucose and polymorphs (A) would not be useful to distinguish between possible causative agents of the clinical features as it is in meningitis.

'14-3-3' is a term for a large group of proteins which have different functions in eukaryotic cells, such as in cell signalling. However, its measurement in CJD is a time consuming process, and as it is a normal neuronal protein it can be released into the CSF as a result of many other normal neuronal insults. It is therefore not a specific finding (C), and the test can be positive in other conditions such as a recent stroke, viral encephalitis or a subarachnoid haemorrhage. The 14-3-3 protein is present in both variant and sporadic CJD, therefore (D) is incorrect.

Variant CJD has several important differences from sporadic CJD:

1   It typically occurs in younger patients (median age of onset 26 years) than sporadic CJD

2   The median survival time is approximately 14 months, compared to 4 months for sporadic CJD

3   Psychiatric features may dominate in the initial stages, before neurological features such as ataxia, myoclonus, chorea, dementia and peripheral sensory symptoms appear

4   The MRI in variant CJD shows the 'positive pulvinar sign' (enhanced signal of nuclei in the thalamus)

5   The classical EEG findings are often absent in the variant form

6   A tonsillar biopsy is sensitive and specific in the variant form, but is not a useful test in the sporadic form (E).

Lumbar puncture

23   In this context, the two most immediately worrying diagnoses for the onset of an acute headache are a subarachnoid haemorrhage and bacterial meningitis as both of these may be fatal if rapid intervention does not occur.

A lumbar puncture can be used to differentiate between the different aetiological agents of meningitis as follows:

Cause	Appearance	Neutrophil count (x 10^6/L)	Lymphocyte count (x 10^6/L)	Protein (g/L)	Glucose (mmol/L)
Normal	Clear	0	<5	<0.4	2.2–3.3
Bacterial	Turbid	100–10 000	Usually <100	↑↑ 0.4–3	↓ 0.0–2.2
Viral	Clear/slight turbidity	Usually <100	10–1000	↑ 0.4–1	Normal
Tuberculous	Clear/slight turbidity	Usually <100	50–1000	↑↑↑ 1–5	↓ 0.0–2.2

Rather than trying to remember specific numbers, try to remember the normal features and then the main differentiating factors between each agent:

- Bacterial meningitis typically has a very high neutrophil count, with a high protein and low glucose
- Viral meningitis typically has a very high lymphocyte count
- Tuberculous meningitis has similar features to viral meningitis in terms of the cell types found in the CSF, but has a particularly high protein

Using this, the easiest way to tell what the cause of the patient's headache is in this scenario is the high lymphocyte count found on the lumbar puncture. This, combined with its clear appearance and slightly high protein content, indicates that the most likely cause is viral meningitis (D). A bacterial meningitis (C) is more likely to look turbid in appearance and would not have a predominant lymphocytosis, whilst a meningitis caused by TB (E) would usually have a higher protein content.

A lumbar puncture in a subarachnoid haemorrhage (A) may be normal, or may have an increased number of red blood cells. The CSF is also examined for the presence of xanthochromia – this is the term for the yellowish appearance seen when red blood cells enter the CSF and are broken down. The presence of pyrexia combined with lumbar puncture results clearly points towards excluding a simple tension headache (B).

Abdominal distension

24 E   This patient is presenting with features suggestive of spontaneous bacterial peritonitis (SBP), which is a form of peritonitis in the absence of a contiguous source of infection. This usually results from the development of portal hypertension in patients with chronic liver disease. This group of patients are particularly susceptible as they are often immunocompromised.

The pyrexia and tachycardia, in conjunction with the clinical features of abdominal tenderness and ascites, make this the most likely diagnosis in this patient. Other typical clinical features might include nausea, vomiting, confusion, general malaise or features of hepatic encephalopathy. In approximately 15 per cent of patients SPB can be asymptomatic.

A prompt diagnostic paracentesis is needed to make the diagnosis, and SPB is confirmed by the presence of:

1   Ascitic fluid WCC of 500 cells/mm^3

2   or Neutrophil count of >250 cells/mm^3

Do not confuse a diagnostic paracentesis with a therapeutic paracentesis (A): in the latter the purpose is to remove the fluid, for example to relieve abdominal pressure or in the case of respiratory compromise. This may be appropriate later, but only once SBP has been excluded from the results of a diagnostic paracentesis or treated.

The most common organisms isolated in patients with SBP include *E. coli*, Gram-positive cocci and enterococci. Although local antibiotic guidelines may differ, of the options listed cefotaxime (E) is one of the most extensively studied and has been proven to be effective. It is usually given for at least 5 days. Other third generation cephalosporins such as ceftriaxone can also be used. Amoxicillin (D) would not provide sufficient cover against Gram-negative organisms.

Whilst analgesia and close observation are also important measures (B), the high risk of mortality in SBP necessitates prompt antibiotic treatment. Spironolactone (C) is used for the treatment of uncomplicated ascites, but initial antibiotic treatment would take precedence in the case of SBP.

Hepatitis C (1)

25 D Hepatitis C is a single stranded RNA virus that is similar in structure to the 'flaviviruses'. It can cause a slowly progressive disease of the liver that is frequently asymptomatic and which cannot be vaccinated against. Routes of transmission include:

- blood products (before 1991, when screening of blood donors for the disease was introduced)
- intravenous drug use
- sexual transmission
- vertical transmission
- less commonly: needle-stick injuries, tattoos

Acute hepatitis occurs in approximately 20 per cent of patients following exposure to the virus. The symptoms are usually mild, such as malaise, arthralgia, jaundice and lethargy. Others may remain asymptomatic. Up to 85 per cent of patients this may persist and cause chronic infection, and approximately 20 per cent of these will develop liver cirrhosis in 20 years.

There are six different genotypes of the virus. The most common in the UK is genotype 1 (40–50 per cent), genotypes 2 and 3 are responsible for another 40–50 per cent, and the remainder is due to genotypes 4, 5 and 6. It has been found that genotype 1 is associated with a poorer response to anti-viral treatment (with interferon and ribavarin) than the other genotypes, so the answer here is (D). In fact, the recommended duration for combination therapy is 24 weeks for people with the 2nd and 3rd genotypes, but 48 weeks for genotypes 1, 4, 5, and 6.

Patients with hepatitis C who develop cirrhosis are estimated to have approximately a 1–2 per cent annual risk of developing hepatocellular carcinoma. Alpha-feto protein is the main tumour marker for this cancer, but its levels do not influence response to treatment (E). Similarly, the length of time between contracting the disease and being diagnosed (A), the route by which she contracted the disease (B), or her liver function test results (C) do not impact her response as significantly as the viral genotype does. A liver biopsy is also often performed and is thought to be the most accurate way to obtain information about the severity of the liver disease. It is thought that the severity of the fibrosis can also help to predict which patients are more likely to respond to antiviral treatment.

Hepatitis C (2)

26 D There are several different tests which are helpful in investigating the disease:

1 Hepatitis C RNA PCR (D) – This can be used to differentiate between a current and past infection. A quantitative test to detect the number of hepatitis C RNA particles (called the 'viral load') can also be performed. This can be very useful to detect a patient's response to the anti-viral treatment. Therefore, this is the best diagnostic test for hepatitis C

2 Anti-hepatitis C antibodies (B) – a positive test would indicate exposure to the disease, but results should be interpreted with caution because it cannot distinguish between current or past infection. In addition, it can take up to 3 months for these antibodies to appear after exposure, so an initial negative test can be misleading. It has also been suggested that a weakly positive test might actually be a false positive, so this is not the best diagnostic test. However, it may be performed initially, and if the patient has two positive results a hepatitis C RNA PCR is used to confirm the diagnosis

3 Viral genotyping (E) – this is used to determine the genotype of virus present. The most common, genotype 1, is less likely to respond to treatment than genotypes 2 or 3 and requires longer therapy

4 Liver biopsy (A) – this would be the most accurate means of determining the stage and severity of liver damage caused by the virus, and may be useful to assess the patient's likelihood to respond to treatment. However, it would be performed after the suspected diagnosis has been confirmed

5 Alanine aminotransferase levels (ALT) (C) – this is not a diagnostic test, but can be useful aid in the initial stages of confirming the diagnosis. The ~~ALT~~ to ~~AST~~ (aspartate aminotransferase) ratio is typically <1 in
AST to ALT

liver damage caused by hepatitis, whereas if it is >2 this is more suggestive of alcoholic liver disease. You can remember this because AST is indicative of Smirnoff drinking, whereas ALT is indicative of viraL aetiology!

Lethargy

27 C   Human African trypanosomiasis is also known as sleeping sickness, and is an infection transmitted by the tsetse fly in sub-Saharan Africa. There are two main types:

1   *Trypanosoma brucei gambiense* (B) is found in west and central Africa, is responsible for over 95 per cent of cases, and causes a chronic infection. It can take months or even years for symptoms to appear. You can remember this as gambiense causes a gradual infection

2   *Trypanosoma brucei rhodesiense* (C) is found in south and eastern Africa, accounts for under 5 per cent of cases, and causes an acute infection with symptoms appearing over a few weeks or months. You can remember this as rhodesiense causes a rapid infection. As this patient's symptoms appeared 3 months after returning from his travels, this is more likely to be the causative agent here

A subcutaneous chancre can develop at the site where the tsetse fly bites, and symptoms such as fevers, weakness, arthralgia and headache can then appear. Posterior cervical lymphadenopathy can also occur, especially with *T. brucei gambiense*. This is known as Winterbottom's sign. Later the parasite can cross the blood–brain barrier resulting in neurological features such as disturbance of the sleep cycle, ataxia, behavioural changes and psychiatric disturbance. Treatment is with drugs such as pentamidine and suramin in the early stages.

Plasmodium falciparum (A) is an organism responsible for causing malaria. Whilst it should be considered in all patients with a fever returning from an endemic area, the changes in behaviour and sleep disturbance described in this patient make this a less likely cause. *Trypanosoma cruzi* (D) causes Chagas disease which is carried by the reduviid bug. Chronic infection can appear weeks to years after the initial infection, affecting the cardiac and gastrointestinal systems. *Leishmania infantum* (E) is responsible for leishmaniasis, features of which can include fever, hepatosplenomegaly and lymphadenopathy. Again, it is less likely to cause behavioural changes and sleep is unlikely to be affected.

Difficulty swallowing

28 B   *Trypanosoma cruzi* is responsible for causing Chagas disease, a potentially life-threatening disease which is spread by reduviid bugs (B) in

Brazil. These are also known as 'kissing bugs'. A red nodule, called a chagoma, can appear at the site of the bite.

There are two forms of the disease: acute and chronic. In the acute phase, patients may experience non-specific symptoms such as fever, lethargy, diarrhoea, and vomiting. A characteristic feature, but one which occurs in less than 50 per cent of cases, is a purplish swelling of the eyelids (called Romana's sign). To put this all together, picture Tom Cruise (*Trypanosoma cruzi*) starring in a gladiator film as a Roman (Romana's sign) wearing purple sunglasses (swollen eyelids) and being kissed (kissing bugs) by lots of fans 'ready with their video cameras' (reduviid!)

The chronic phase can occur even years after the initial bite, and typically affects the heart and gastrointestinal tract. You can remember its effects by thinking of it causing both dilatation and dysfunction in three organs: in the heart (dilatation = dilated cardiomyopathy, dysfunction = arrhythmias), in the colon (dilatation = megacolon, dysfunction = constipation) and in the oesophagus (dilatation = mega oesophagus, dysfunction = dysphagia). Bennzimidazole or nifurtimox are effective medications used to treat this disease.

The tsetse fly (A) is responsible for causing human African trypano-somiasis, also known as sleeping sickness, in sub-Saharan Africa. The clinical features of this disease can include changes to the sleep–wake cycle and psychiatric disturbance. The sandfly (C) transmits *Leishmania* species in Africa, America and the Middle East. The *Aedes* mosquito (D) is a type of mosquito that causes Dengue fever. The *Ixodes* tick (E), also known as the 'deer tick', transmits the organism responsible for causing Lyme disease. None of these vectors would cause the spectrum of clinical features described in this patient.

Treatment for a cough (1)

29 A Current guidelines in the UK recommend the following antibiotic treatment for pulmonary tuberculosis:

- Isoniazid and rifampicin for 6 months
- Pyrazinamide and ethambutol for the first 2 months

The purpose of the initial phase where all four drugs are taken together is to rapidly reduce the number of bacteria and prevent drug resistant bacteria emerging. Culturing TB can take several weeks, so treatment is started without waiting for the culture results if clinical features or histopathology results are highly suggestive. Streptomycin (D) is an aminoglycoside that is rarely used in the UK, but may be used in the initial phase if it has been shown that the organism is resistant to isoniazid.

It is not usually necessary to continue all four drugs after 2 months (E). The continuation phase consists of rifampicin and isoniazid alone for

2 months. A good way to remember this is to think of the word **R.I...P.E** (rifampicin, isonizaid, pyrazinamide, ethambutol), with the first two letters given for 6 months, and the last two letters on the end of the word dropping off after 2 months! Answers (B) and (C) are therefore incorrect.

In the case of tuberculous meningitis, direct spinal cord involvement, and for resistant organisms a longer course of treatment may be necessary. A corticosteroid such as dexamethasone should be started at the same time as anti-tuberculosis therapy in meningeal or pericardial tuberculosis.

Treatment for a cough (2)

30 E Remember that treatment for pulmonary TB usually consists of two phases – an initial phase with rifampicin, isoniazid, pyrazinamide and ethambutol for 2 months, and then a continuation phase with rifampicin and isoniazid only for 4 months.

Streptomycin and ethambutol are two anti-tuberculous drugs which should preferably be avoided in patients with renal impairment (E). If they have to be used the dosage should be reduced and the plasma drug concentration closely monitored. A patient's renal function should be checked routinely before anti-tuberculous medication is started.

The side effect that is particularly worrying with the use of ethambutol is its ocular toxicity, and this is more likely in renal impairment as it is renally excreted. This can present with changes in visual acuity, colour blindness and restriction of visual fields. Therefore a patient's visual acuity should be assessed with a Snellen chart prior to starting treatment, and they should be strongly advised to stop the medication and seek advice if they become aware of any change in their vision. This side effect does not occur with rifampicin (D).

Liver function should be tested in everyone before starting antituberculous therapy, as isoniazid, rifampicin and pyrazinamide are all hepatotoxic (A). Further checks are not needed unless the patient has pre-existing liver disease, is alcohol dependent or develops symptoms of liver disease. Rifampicin can commonly cause a transient disturbance to liver function tests in the first 2 months, but this does not usually necessitate any changes to the treatment regimen.

The only common side effect of isoniazid is a peripheral neuropathy. This can be remembered by 'isoniazid causes a sensory neuropathy'. Pyridoxine (vitamin B_6) is not given routinely as a prophylactic measure in patients using isoniazid, but may be given in those with pre-existing risk factors such as diabetes, alcohol dependence and HIV (C). Ethambutol does not cause a peripheral neuropathy (B).

Muscle weakness

31   C   This scenario is characteristic of Guillan–Barrè syndrome. If you remember that this disease is also known as AIDP – acute inflammatory demyelinating polyradiculopathy – you can remember the underlying pathology more easily. It is usually triggered by an infection, and it is thought that a suppressed T-cell response results in an immunological reaction that targets the peripheral nerves.

The triggering infection is most commonly *Campylobacter jejuni* (as alluded to here), but other common causes can include *Mycoplasma pneumoniae* and viruses such as cytomegalovirus and influenza. The key clinical features that guide you to this diagnosis are:

1   An antecedent infection

2   Sudden progressive muscle weakness within approximately 3 weeks of the onset of the original infection

3   The muscle weakness evolving rapidly over 1–3 weeks

4   The weakness is often symmetrical, and usually begins distally and ascends over time

5   Cranial nerves can also be affected, most commonly presenting as a unilateral facial weakness

6   Reflexes are usually absent

7   Sensory abnormalities are not a common feature

The key worrying features of this disease are:

1   Autonomic involvement – with tachycardia, fluctuating blood pressure and arrhythmias

2   Respiratory involvement – which can lead to type 2 respiratory failure

Treatment is usually supportive, but intravenous immunoglobulin therapy for 5 days or plasma exchange has been shown to be effective.

Polio (A) would not characteristically have an antecedent diarrhoeal infection, and facial weakness is less likely. The paralytic phase would not typically have an ascending pattern of weakness, and fasciculations prior to paralysis are an important feature. Lyme disease (B) can cause facial weakness, but you would normally expect a question pointing you to this diagnosis to mention the characteristic target rash of erythema chronicum migrans. The somewhat unusual features of the second stage of Lyme disease can be remembered using the word PEACH: Peripheral neuropathy, Erythema chronicum migrans (persists in this stage), Arthritis, Cranial nerve palsies and Heart block. Haemolytic uraemic syndrome (D) is a triad remembered by the phrase

'He's (haemolytic) got **your** (ur-aemic) MAT (the triad of microangio-pathic haemolytic anaemia, acute renal failure and thrombocytopenia). Cases that feature diarrhoea often occur in children, and are usually caused by *E. coli* O157. The neurological features described here would not normally be associated with this syndrome. Influenza (E) is again not likely to manifest with this characteristic neurological pattern of symptoms.

Malaria (1)

32   D   Malaria should always be considered as a diagnosis in a patient pre-senting with a fever from an endemic country – mainly Africa, South and Central America, Asia and the Middle East. It is transmitted by the female *Anopheles* mosquito.

There are five different types as listed below. They can be differentiated clinically according to the pattern of the fever they cause. Each of the different members of the *Plasmodium* genus results in a different periodicity of fever. 'Tertian' malaria means that the fever occurs every 3 days (i.e. days 1, 3 and 5 and so on) and 'quartan' malaria means it occurs every fourth day (i.e. days 1, 4, 7 and so on), as in this case. *P. malariae* (D) causes quartan malaria, so is the correct answer here. This type of malaria is said to be benign, and is the least common form found in the UK.

The following table summarizes the features of the different types of malaria:

Plasmodium genus	Incubation period	Type of malaria	Comment
Plasmodium falciparum (A)	7–14 days	Malignant tertian	This is the most severe form
Plasmodium vivax (B)	12–17 days	Benign tertian	Relapse can occur with these forms because the parasite can lie dormant in the liver, and can produce symptoms months or years later
Plasmodium ovale (C)	15–18 days	Benign tertian	
Plasmodium malariae (D)	18–40 days	Benign quartan	Relapse can occur with this too, but this time the parasites lie dormant in the blood
Plasmodium knowlesi (E)	12 days	Quotidian (daily)	This form mainly occurs in southeast Asia (such as in Borneo), and not in Africa. It does not normally relapse

It is worth remembering that malaria does not usually cause a rash or lymphadenopathy, so think again if these are featured in a question on a fever in a returning traveller! Features of malaria on examination might include anaemia, jaundice and hepatosplenomegaly.

Malaria (2)

33 C Malaria has a complex life cycle, with two phases. The 'erthrocytic' phase involves red blood cells, whereas the 'exoerthryocytic phase' involves the liver. The basic stages are:

    1   An infected mosquito injects sporozites (A) from its saliva into a person's blood stream when it bites

    2   These enter the blood stream and are taken to the liver where they infect hepatocytes

    3   Here they multiply for a varying period of time, and then differentiate to form haploid merozites (C). These have a 'signet ring' appearance. Schizonts (B) are oval-shaped inclusions that contain the merozoites. Note that *P. vivax* and *P. ovale* sporozoites may not develop into merozites immediately, but can form hypnozoites (D) that remain dormant in the liver

    4   The merozites escape from the liver into the blood stream and infect red blood cells – the erythrocytic phase

    5   They multiply further in the erythrocytes, and will be released from them at intervals. The waves of fever the patient experiences correspond to when the merozites are released from the erythrocytes

    6   Some of the merozites develop into sexual forms of the parasite, called male and female gametocytes (E). When a mosquito bites an infected human, it ingests the gametocytes which form gametes inside the mosquito

    7   These then fuse to form oocytes and then sporozites – ready to inject into a person.

Malaria (3)

34 E All patients with falciparum malaria should be admitted to hospital initially, so answers (A) and (B) are automatically excluded. Children should be kept in for at least 24 hours, and infants, pregnant women and the elderly need to be closely monitored because they can deteriorate rapidly. The treatment options then depend on whether the malaria is uncomplicated or complicated.

Uncomplicated malaria can be treated with one of the following:

    1   Oral quinine plus doxycycline for 5–7 days (E)

    2   Co-artem (artemetherelumefantrine) for 3 days

    3   Atovaquone–proguanil (Malarone) for 3 days

Therefore the correct answer here is (E). Giving paracetamol without anti-malarials would not be adequate, so clearly (C) is not suitable. Chloroquine and mefloquine (B) are not recommended for the treatment of falciparum malaria in the UK.

Oral treatment would suffice in an uncomplicated case of falciparum malaria such as this, but in a severe case the first line anti-malarial used in the UK is IV quinine (D). IV artesunate may also be considered in the case of very severe disease instead of or in addition to quinine, but this is not always widely available.

The treatment for non-falciparum malaria is quite different. In uncomplicated infection, chloroquine is used initially followed by a 2-week course of primaquine. The choloroquine treats the parasites in the erythrocytes only, thus primaquine is still needed to kill the hypnozoites that remain latent in the liver.

Glucose-6-phosphate dehydrogenase deficiency is an X-linked recessive hereditary disease, and anti-malarial drugs can cause acute haemolysis in these patients. The drugs thought to be particularly troublesome are primaquine and choloroquine, but others may be dangerous at high doses. For this reason glucose-6-phosphate dehydrogenase levels are checked in patients before starting anti-malarial treatment.

Malaria (4)

35 A The most reliable way to diagnose malaria is via a blood film, and traditionally a thick and thin blood film are requested. Most people remember this fact, but not the reason behind it! Thick films are better than thin films at picking up lower levels of infection, but thin films allow the specific species to be identified. Both types of films are used together to make the diagnosis.

In the erythrocytic life cycle of the malarial parasite, disc-like granulations can be seen at the edge of the cell using an electron microscope. These are known as Maurer's clefts, and are found in falciparum malaria (A). They are thought to be used by the parasite for protein sorting and export. They are larger and coarser than the Schuffner's dots seen with *P. vivax* (B) and *P. ovale* (C). These are punctuate granulations again seen under the microscope in erythrocytes invaded by the tertian malaria parasite. These two structures are worth remembering for exam questions!

P. malariae (D) causes 'quartan' malaria, meaning the fever occurs every fourth day (i.e. days 1, 4, 7 and so on). *P. knowleski* (E) is much less common, and mainly occurs in southeast Asia (such as in Borneo). Maurer's clefts and Schuffner's dots would not typically be found in infection with these species.

SECTION 9:
HISTOPATHOLOGY EMQs

Questions

Answers

QUESTIONS

1. Cardiovascular pathology

A	Monckeberg arteriosclerosis	F	Left heart failure
B	Infective endocarditis	G	Hypertrophic obstructive cardio-
C	Dressler's syndrome		myopathy
D	Dilated cardiomyopathy	H	Aortic stenosis
E	Rheumatic heart disease	I	Carcinoid syndrome

For each scenario below, choose the most appropriate answer from the list above. Each option may be used once, more than once or not at all.

1 A 36-year-old man presents to accident and emergency with a 1-day history of a fever of 39.2°C and night sweats. A new heart murmur is detected by the on-call cardiologist. The patient admits to being an intravenous drug user.

2 A 64-year-old man presents to accident and emergency due to a collapse at home. An ejection systolic murmur is heard at the upper-left sternal edge.

3 A widowed 72-year-old woman who has passed away at home is sent for autopsy due to unknown cause of death. Post-mortem examination reveals a nutmeg liver and haemosiderin-laden macrophages in the lungs.

4 A 54-year-old man presents to accident and emergency with fever and pleuritic chest pain. It is noted that the patient suffered a myocardial infarction 4 weeks previously.

5 A 46-year-old man is referred to the cardiology outpatient clinic. On investigation he is found to have mitral regurgitation and has a past history of St Vitus Dance when he was in school and a mild pericarditis.

2. Respiratory pathology

A	Hyaline membrane disease	F	Chronic bronchitis
B	Small cell carcinoma	G	Pulmonary oedema
C	Extrinsic allergic alveolitis	H	Cystic fibrosis
D	Bronchiectasis	I	Sarcoidosis
E	Non-small cell carcinoma		

For each scenario below, choose the most appropriate answer from the list above. Each option may be used once, more than once or not at all.

1 A 40-year-old male presents to his GP with chronic cough with copious amounts of purulent mucus production. High resolution CT scans demonstrate dilated bronchi.

2   A 14-year-old girl is admitted to hospital after suffering her third bout of pneumonia caused by *Pseudomonas aeruginosa* infection. She also has a previous admission for pancreatitis.

3   A 58-year-old man presents to his GP with haemoptysis and weight loss. He has a 30 pack–year history of smoking. He is referred to the oncologist for a biopsy, who determines 'oat-shaped' cells on microscopy.

4   A 62-year-old man presents to his GP with shortness of breath, lethargy and weight loss. The patient's chest X-ray reveals a peripheral focal lesion in the left lung field.

5   A 53-year-old woman with a history of rheumatic fever presents to accident and emergency with severe shortness of breath, and has been coughing up pink frothy sputum for the past 2 days.

3. Connective tissue pathology

A	Systemic lupus erythematosus	F	Dermatomyositis
B	Sjögren's syndrome	G	CREST syndrome
C	Diffuse scleroderma	H	Polymyositis
D	Amyloidosis	I	Microscopic polyangitis
E	Takayasu arteritis		

For each scenario below, choose the most appropriate answer from the list above. Each option may be used once, more than once or not at all.

1   A 35-year-old woman is referred to the rheumatology clinic due to recent onset dysphagia. The patient also reports that her fingers have turned very pale and cold. One examination she is found to have tightening of the skin near her finger tips and small dilated vessels on her skin.

2   A 35-year-old woman with a history of recurrent miscarriages presents to her GP with joint pains. Blood tests reveal she is anti-double stranded DNA antibody positive.

3   A 68-year-old man presents to accident and emergency with symptoms suggestive of heart failure. All initial investigations do not determine an underlying cause. However, a tongue biopsy sample gains an apple-green birefringence under polarized light using Congo red stain.

4   A 45-year-old woman presents to accident and emergency with signs suggestive of renal failure. She is found to be p-ANCA positive.

5   A 52-year-old man presents to his GP with limb weakness and shortness of breath. A distinctive rash is noted around both eyes as well as plaques on the joints of his hands.

4. Cerebrovascular pathology

A   Subarachnoid haemorrhage
B   Parkinson's disease
C   Extradural haemorrhage
D   Vascular dementia
E   Subdural haemorrhage

F   Intracerebral haemorrhage
G   Multiple sclerosis
H   Duret haemorrhage
I   Alzheimer's disease

For each scenario below, choose the most appropriate answer from the list above. Each option may be used once, more than once or not at all.

1   A 54-year-old man is seen in the neurology clinic due to tremor and rigidity. A DAT scan reveals reduced uptake in the substantia nigra.

2   A 74-year-old man presents to accident and emergency with increasing head-ache and confusion. The man's wife suggests her husband may have tripped and fallen 3 days previously.

3   A 45-year-old woman presents to accident and emergency with the worst head-ache she has ever experienced. She is noted to have polycystic kidney disease.

4   A 35-year-old woman presents to the neurology clinic with weakness of her left side. On examination she is found to have nystagmus and an intention tremor. The patient complains of blurred vision for the past month.

5   A 42-year-old man who suffers from Down syndrome is brought to see his GP by his carer. The carer describes how the patient has been wandering out of the house with increased frequency as well as becoming uncharacteristically aggres-sive, especially in the evening.

5. Gastrointestinal pathology

A   Ulcerative colitis
B   Chronic gastritis
C   Oesophageal cancer
D   Coeliac disease
E   Gastric carcinoma

F   Barrett's oesophagus
G   Gardener's syndrome
H   Crohn's disease
I   Peptic ulcer disease

For each scenario below, choose the most appropriate answer from the list above. Each option may be used once, more than once or not at all.

1   A 35-year-old man has a 3-week history of bloody stools without mucus with associated weight loss. A biopsy of the gastrointestinal tract reveals non-caseating granulomas with transmural inflammation.

2   A 24-year-old woman presents to her GP with a 2-week history of diarrhoea, weight loss and fatigue. Biopsy of the gastrointestinal tract reveals villous atrophy with crypt hyperplasia.

3   A 54-year-old man presents to his GP with a 2-week history of worsening dysphagia. The patient's past medical history reveals severe gastro-oesophageal reflux disease. A duodenoscopy suggests metaplastic transformation of the lower oesophageal region.

4   A 45-year-old man is referred to the gastroenterology outpatient clinic due to severe epigastric pain and an episode of haematemesis. Further testing reveals he is *Helicobacter pylori* positive and has a 20 pack–year history of smoking.

5   A 56-year-old man presents to his GP with abdominal pain, weight loss and fatigue. A duodenoscopy allows a biopsy of a gastric lesion to be taken, which demonstrates signet ring cells and linitis plastica.

6. Liver pathology

A	Cholangiocarcinoma	F	Haemochromatosis
B	Cirrhosis	G	Hepatocellular carcinoma
C	α1-Antitrypsin deficiency	H	Primary sclerosing cholangitis
D	Haemosiderosis	I	Wilson's disease
E	Primary biliary cirrhosis		

For each scenario below, choose the most appropriate answer from the list above. Each option may be used once, more than once or not at all.

1   A 56-year-old man with previous history of hepatitis C infection presents to accident and emergency with jaundice. His wife notes that he has recently been bruising very easily. Ultrasound of the patient's liver reveals irregular echogenicity demonstrating nodules.

2   A 35-year-old man presents to his GP with his mother with signs of Parkinsonism (tremor, rigidity and slow movement) as well as recent changes in his behaviour.

3   A 56-year-old woman is investigated by the hepatology team for decompensated liver disease. A liver biopsy sample stains blue with Perl's Prussian blue stain.

4   A 53-year-old man who has recently emigrated from sub-Saharan Africa is referred to the hepatology department due to recent onset weight loss, jaundice and ascites. There is history of previous aflatoxin exposure.

5   A 45-year-old woman presents to accident and emergency with jaundice and pruritis. Xanthelasma are noted on examination. The patient is found to be anti-mitochondrial antibody positive.

7. Skin pathology

A	Pemphigoid	F	Psoriasis
B	Bowen's disease	G	Basal cell carcinoma
C	Pityriasis rosea	H	Erythema multiforme
D	Lichen planus	I	Malignant melanoma
E	Actinic keratosis	J	Pemphigus

For each scenario below, choose the most appropriate answer from the list above. Each option may be used once, more than once or not at all.

1   A 65-year-old man presents to his GP with blisters along his left arm that are about 1.0 cm in diameter. Gentle rubbing of the affected area does not lead to skin exfoliation.

2   A 38-year-old man on the respiratory ward has been diagnosed with *Mycoplasma pneumoniae* and develops a number of target shaped rashes on his body.

3   A 45-year-old woman presents to her GP with salmon-pink plaques with a silver–white scale on the extensor surfaces of her elbows.

4   A 54-year-old man is referred to the dermatologist with a brown warty lesion on his nose which has a rough consistency. Biopsy of the lesion reveals solar elastosis.

5   A 59-year-old woman presents to her dermatologist with a 3 cm black irregular lesion on her cheek. Over the next month the lesion spreads to cover 6 cm with new onset pain.

8. Renal pathology

A	Nephritic syndrome	F	Goodpasture's syndrome
B	Wegener's granulomatosis	G	IgA nephropathy
C	Membranous glomerulonephritis	H	Nephrotic syndrome
D	Acute tubular necrosis	I	Focal segmental glomerulo-nephritis
E	Minimal change glomerulo-nephritis		

For each scenario below, choose the most appropriate answer from the list above. Each option may be used once, more than once or not at all.

1   A 45-year-old man presents to accident and emergency with haematuria and admits to passing less urine than previously. He is found to be hypertensive. Microscopy of the patient's urine reveals red and white cell casts.

2 A 42-year-old man presents to accident and emergency with an episode of haemoptysis and haematuria. Blood tests reveal he is in acute renal failure. Once the patient is stable a renal biopsy demonstrates a crescent morphology on immunofluorescence.

3 A 64-year-old man on the Care of the Elderly ward is found to be in acute renal failure secondary to statin-related rhabdomyolysis. Urinalysis reveals the presence of 'muddy' casts.

4 An 8-year-old girl presents to accident and emergency with frank haematuria. Her parents state that she had just recovered from a throat infection 2 days previously.

5 A 62-year-old woman on the Care of the Elderly ward is found to have new onset ankle swelling. A urine dipstick demonstrates proteinuria and the only blood abnormality is a low albumin level.

9. Breast pathology

A	Mastitis	F	Gynaecomastia
B	Phylloides tumour	G	Fibrocystic disease
C	Fibroadenoma	H	Fat necrosis
D	Duct ectasia	I	Infiltrating ductal carcinoma
E	Ductal carcinoma *in situ*		

For each scenario below, choose the most appropriate answer from the list above. Each option may be used once, more than once or not at all.

1 A 55-year-old parous woman presents to her GP with a 2-week history of green discharge from her right nipple.

2 A 35-year-old woman presents to her GP with a soft 3 cm mobile mass in her left breast. The patient suggests the size of the lump fluctuates with her menstrual cycle.

3 A 54-year-old woman presents to her GP with a single lump in her left breast. A mammogram reveals a focal area of calcification.

4 A 60-year-old woman presents to her GP with a 5.5 cm mobile lump in her right breast. Biopsy reveals an 'artichoke-like' appearance.

5 A 58-year-old woman presents to her GP with a painful lump in her right breast. On examination there is also evidence of *peau d'orange*.

10. Bone pathology

A   Osteoporosis
B   Fibrous dysplasia
C   Paget's disease
D   Osteomalacia
E   Osteochondroma

F   Osteoid osteoma
G   Renal osteodytrophy
H   Enchondroma
I   Giant cell tumour

For each scenario below, choose the most appropriate answer from the list above. Each option may be used once, more than once or not at all.

1   A 35-year-old man with pain and difficulty bending his left knee. X-ray reveals many lytic lesions in the epiphysis of the patient's left knee.

2   A 38-year-old woman presents to her GP with generalized bone pain. X-ray reveals areas of pseudofracture, especially in the ribs.

3   A 65-year-old woman is referred to the rheumatologist after suffering recurrent falls. Blood tests are all unremarkable but a DEXA scan reveals a T-score of 2.8.

4   An 8-year-old boy has been diagnosed with precocious puberty. A routine examination by the paediatrician reveals café-au-lait spots on the child's back. The boy has had numerous fractures of his femur and tibia bilaterally after falls.

5   A 50-year-old man presents to his GP with pain in his arms and legs. The patient also complains of shooting pains down his left leg as well as worsening shortness of breath.

ANSWERS

1. Cardiovascular pathology

ANSWERS: 1) B 2) H 3) F 4) C 5) E

Infective endocarditis (IE; B) results from bacterial-vegetation of heart valves. Acute IE has a time course of days and is usually caused by *Staphylococcus aureus* in intravenous drug users; both sides of the heart can be affected, but the right heart is most commonly affected, because the lungs filter out many organisms, so that the left side of the heart gets less exposure to organisms. Subacute IE has a time course of weeks/months and is generally secondary to *Streptococcus viridans* infection after dental procedures; only abnormal valves are affected and hence these are more likely to be on the left side of the heart because those valves are more commonly damaged as they are on the high pressure side of the heart. Perforation of the valve leaflets and rupture of papillary muscles may lead to aortic or mitral regurgitation.

Aortic stenosis (H) occurs when there is an opening defect in the aortic valve. Causes include age-related degenerative calcification, rheumatic heart disease and congenital malformations (bicuspid valve). Calcification is confined to the cusps. Clinical presentation includes syncope, angina and dyspnoea. On examination an ejection systolic murmur, narrow pulse pressure and/or slow rising pulse may be detected. If due to a bicuspid valve an ejection systolic click may be heard. Left ventricular hypertrophy may develop as a consequence of chronic pressure overload.

Left heart failure (F) results in the inability of the heart to meet the demands of the body. It is either due to increased demand (high output failure) or reduced supply (low output failure) of blood. Causes of high output failure include severe anaemia and hyperthyroidism, while low output failure occurs due to ischaemic heart disease, hypertension and aortic/mitral valve defects. Clinical features include dyspnoea, orthopnoea and paroxysmal nocturnal dyspnoea. Histological findings include dilated ventricles, thin walls, nutmeg liver and haemosiderin macrophages in the lungs.

Dressler's syndrome (C) is an autoimmune complication of myocardial infarction (MI) that occurs approximately 4 weeks after the episode. It is characterized by chest pain, fever and a pericardial rub. The complications of MI can be classified according to how they present temporally. Complications of MI that may occur within 1 week include arrhythmias (most commonly ventricular fibrillation and ventricular tachycardia), myocardial rupture, valve incompetence (causing regurgitation) and cardiogenic shock. Later developments include ventricular aneurysm, pericarditis and the aforementioned Dressler's syndrome.

Rheumatic heart disease (E) is an inflammatory condition most commonly affecting the connective tissue of the heart (but also joints and central nervous system). It occurs several weeks after throat infection with group A β-haemolytic streptococci usually under the age of 10 years. Cardiac complications include endocarditis (causing verroucous lesions of the heart valves); myocarditis (containing Aschkoff-bodies and Anitschow cells causing dilatation of the mitral ring, hence mitral regurgitation); pericarditis (fibrous exudate causing friction rub). Any layer of the heart can be affected, potentially leading to pancarditis. Many years after recovery from acute rheumatic fever, chronic rheumatic heart disease occurs, with fibrosis of the mitral and aortic valves that can occur. The history of St Vitus Dance Suggests Sydenham's chorea, a well known feature of acute rheumatic fever.

Monckeberg arteriosclerosis (A) involves focal calcification of the media of small medium-sized arteries. It usually presents in patients over 50 years of age and unlike atherosclerosis, there is no associated inflammation in the pathogenesis.

Dilated cardiomyopathy (D) occurs due to a progressive loss of myocytes resulting in a left ventricular ejection fraction of less than 40 per cent. Causes include alcohol, chemotherapy (e.g. doxorubicin) and viral myocarditis.

Hypertrophic obstructive cardiomyopathy (G) is an autosomal dominant condition caused by a mutation in the β-myosin heavy chain. Histological features include myocyte hypertrophy and disarray.

Carcinoid syndrome (I) occurs due to 5-hydroxyindoleacetic acid producing tumours and is characterized by episodic flushing, abdominal cramps and diarrhoea. Right sided valve abnormalities may also result.

2. Respiratory pathology

ANSWERS: 1) D 2) H 3) B 4) E 5) G

Bronchiectasis (D) is defined as the permanent dilatation of bronchi and bronchioles secondary to chronic inflammation. Causes are numerous, and include chronic pneumonia, for example due to *Staphylococcus aureus* or *Haemophilus influenzae* infection, obstructing tumours and cystic fibrosis. Histopathological findings include bronchial wall destruction and transmural inflammation. High-resolution computed tomography (CT) is the diagnostic modality of choice. Abscess formation, haemoptysis and pulmonary hypertension are complications that may arise as a result of bronchiectasis.

Cystic fibrosis (CF; H) is an autosomal recessive condition caused by a mutation in the cystic fibrosis transmembrane conductance regulator (CFTR) protein that primarily affects the exocrine glands. There are several mutations responsible for CF, the most common being ΔF508 mutation. Defective CFTR causes reduced secretion of chloride ions across epithelial cell membranes, resulting in increased sodium and hence water reabsorption into these cells. The result is viscous secretions from exocrine glands affecting multiple organs including the lungs (recurrent infections and bronchiectasis), gastrointestinal tract (distal intestinal obstruction syndrome) and pancreas (pancreatitis).

Small cell carcinoma (B) is also known as 'oat-cell' carcinoma due to the appearance of the malignant cells under the microscope. They appear as nests of small round hyper-chromatic cells that are fragile (chromatin smudging) and possess nuclear moulding. Small cell carcinomas are very aggressive with approximately 80 per cent of cases having metastasized at the time of diagnosis. Small cell carcinomas also express neuroendocrine markers and can cause paraneoplastic syndromes such as Lambert–Eaton myasthenic syndrome. On chest X-rays, the cancer may be seen arising centrally.

Non-small cell carcinomas (E) comprise adenocarcinoma, squamous cell carcinoma and large cell carcinoma. Adenocarcinomas are gland forming and therefore will have mucin vacuoles within. This sub-type of non-small cell carcinoma may lead to atypical adenohyperplasia whereby atypical cells are seen to line the alveolar walls; hence adenocarcinoma is usually a peripheral lung cancer. Squamous cell carcinomas are histologically characterized by keratinization and intracellular 'prickle' desmosomes. Large cell carcinomas are undifferentiated forms of adenocarcinoma or squamous cell carcinoma.

Pulmonary oedema (G) is defined as fluid collections in the alveoli which impairs gas exchange that can potentially lead to respiratory failure. Increased hydrostatic pressure causes of pulmonary oedema include heart failure, mitral stenosis, fluid overload and renal failure. Increased capillary permeability can also cause pulmonary oedema, for example due to pneumonia. Chest X-rays can distinguish between cardiac and non-cardiac causes of pulmonary oedema; the former will demonstrate alveolar oedema (bat's wing appearance), Kerley B-lines, cardiomegaly, upper lobe diversion of blood vessels and effusions.

Hyaline membrane disease (A) is also known as respiratory distress syndrome. It occurs in premature neonates due to surfactant deficiency leading to hyaline deposition and hypoxia.

Extrinsic allergic alveolitis (C) occurs secondary to a type III hypersensitivity reaction. Long-term exposure to an inhaled allergen leads to pulmonary fibrosis.

Chronic bronchitis (F) is one end of the chronic obstructive pulmonary disease spectrum. Histological features include mucus gland hypertrophy, goblet cell hyperplasia/metaplasia and mucosal oedema.

Sarcoidosis (I) is a multisystem, non-caseating granulomatous disease. Inflammatory markers such as TNF-α, IFN-γ and IL-12 play an important role in the inflammatory process.

3. Connective tissue pathology

ANSWERS: 1) G 2) A 3) D 4) I 5) F

CREST syndrome (G), also known as limited scleroderma, represents a combination of conditions: calcinosis (calcium deposition in the skin), Raynaud's disease (vasospasm of blood vessels in response to triggers such as cold), oesophageal dysmotility, sclerodactyly (thickening and tightening of skin surrounding fingers/hands) and telangiectasia (dilation of blood capillaries causing red marks on the surface of the skin). The pathogenesis relates to excessive release of PDGF causing widespread fibroblast activation and multi-organ fibrosis. Chronic fibrosis leads to initimal thickening of the microvasculature known as 'onion skinning.'

Systemic lupus erythematosus (SLE; A) is a multi-system connective tissue disease that is antinuclear antibody (ANA) positive. The underlying pathology of SLE relates to failure in the regulatory mechanisms of self-tolerance. Autoantibodies form against nuclear components such as DNA, RNA and histones. This leads to complement activation and complex formation, which are deposited in organs. Cytology of tissues reveals haematoxylin bodies which are denatured nuclei that are produced when ANA bind to exposed nuclei. LE cells are also visible on microscopy; these are macrophages that have phagocytosed a haematoxylin body.

Amyloidosis (D) occurs due to the extracellular deposition of fibrillar proteins that accumulate in tissues and organs. Amyloid proteins arise due to dysfunctional folding resulting in non-branching fibrils. Proteins aggregate into insoluble crossed beta-pleated sheet tertiary conformation. Amyloid proteins contain P-component which causes biopsy samples to characteristically gain an apple-green birefringence using polarized light and Congo red stain. Four major amyloid proteins exist: AA, derived from serum amyloid assisted protein and associated with inflammation; AL, derived from IgG light chains and associated with myeloma; $\alpha\beta_2$, linked with Alzheimer's disease; β_2 microglobulin, associated with patients undergoing dialysis treatment.

Microscopic polyangitis (I) is a small vessel vasculitis affecting the arterioles, venules and capillaries. The pathology involves a trigger factor such as microorganisms and drugs causing immune complex formation in a previously sensitized host. These immune complexes deposit in small vessels leading to neutrophil-related inflammation. Microscopic polyangitis affects the skin, heart, brain and kidneys. Histopathological features of affected vessels include fibrinoid necrosis that leads to fragmented neutrophilic nuclei within vessel walls. Microscopic polyangitis is associated with p-ANCA.

Dermatomyositis (F) is an inflammatory myopathy that involves skeletal and thoracic muscles. Skeletal muscle involvement will lead to proximal muscle fatigue, especially in the hips and shoulders. Thoracic muscle involvement can affect the lungs (dyspnoea), heart (arrhythmia) and oesophagus (dysmotility). There is, however, sparing of the ocular muscles which differentiates dermatomyositis from myasthenia gravis. Dermatomyositis is also defined by a heliotrope rash (violet erythema around the periorbital region) and Gottron papules (violet scaly plaques over hand joints). Muscle inflammation will also cause an increased blood creatine kinase level.

Sjögren's syndrome (B) is defined by the immune mediated destruction of the lacrimal and salivary glands that causes dry eyes and dry mouth.

In diffuse scleroderma (C), in contrast to limited scleroderma (CREST), there are extensive skin lesions, with an early visceral involvement and rapidly progressive course.

Takayasu arteritis (E) results in a thickened section of the aorta (usually the aortic arch). Features include no pulses and low blood pressure in the arms and cold hands.

Polymyositis (H) is part of the inflammatory myopathy spectrum. Similar to dermatomyositis there is proximal muscle weakness as well as heart and lung involvement, however with no dermatological lesions.

4. Cerebrovascular pathology

ANSWERS: 1) B 2) E 3) A 4) G 5) I

Parkinson's disease (B) is a degenerative disorder associated with basal ganglia dysfunction. Clinical features can be remembered by the mnemonic SMART: shuffling gait, mask-like-face, akinesia, rigidity and tremor. Degeneration of the substantia nigra and locus coeruleus of the basal ganglia leads to reduced production of dopamine. At the microscopic level, inclusion bodies known as Lewy bodies are deposited in the cytoplasm of neurons that are made up of α-synuclein. Parkinson's disease may be associated with Lewy body dementia.

Subdural haemorrhage (E) occurs between the dura and arachnoid due to an acute tear in bridging veins. This tends to occur after a clear history of trauma. Bleeding results in features of raised intracranial pressure. As the bleeding is venous in nature, haematoma development is slow (usually taking 48 hours) and as a result raised intracranial pressure takes time to become apparent. Chronic subdural haemorrhage refers to a re-bleed of a previous bridging vein subdural haemorrhage. Patients will usually present with an altered mental state.

Subarachnoid haemorrhage (A) occurs in the subarachnoid space. Potential causes include a saccular 'berry' aneurysm (most commonly occurring at artery bifurcations of the anterior circulation), hypertension, trauma, arteriovenous malformations and coagulation disorders. Clinical features include a severe 'thunder clap' headache radiating to the occiput; this may be preceded by a warning bleed causing a sentinel bleed. Subarachnoid haemorrhages are more commonly associated with polycystic kidney disease, coarctation of the aorta and fibromuscular dysplasia.

Multiple sclerosis (MS; G) is a demyelinating disease of the upper motor system which follows a relapsing and remitting course. Histological features along the central nervous system include active (contain lymphocytes and macrophages) and inactive plaques (reduced nuclei and myelin). Clinical features include optic neuritis, intranuclear opthalmoplegia (disruption of medial longitudinal fasciculus) and cerebellar signs, as well as spasticity and weakness of limbs. Variants of MS include Devic disease (a more aggressive form) and Marburg MS (a fulminant form).

Alzheimer's disease (I) is a progressive degenerative disease which mainly occurs in patients over the age of 50 years and the condition is most commonly sporadic. In some instances, there may be a genetic component such as the amyloid precursor protein as well as presenelins 1 and 2 mutations associated with Down syndrome. Inheritance of the ε4 allele of apolipoprotein E increases risk of developing Alzheimer's disease. Histological features include vascular wall deposition of β-amyloid (amyloid angiopathy), neurofibrillary tangles and neuritic plaques.

Extradural haemorrhage (C) is a bleed above the dura due to damage to the middle meningeal artery. It is usually associated with severe trauma and fracture to the pterion and a subsequent lucid interval.

Vascular dementia (D) often progresses in a step-wise manner. It is associated with cardiovascular risk factors such as hypertension, smoking and diabetes mellitus.

Intracerebral haemorrhage (F) cause approximately 20 per cent of strokes and is perpetuated by hypertension and arteriovenous malformations. Hypertension may lead to either hyaline arteriosclerosis or Charcot–Bouchard aneurysms.

Duret haemorrhage (H) is associated with tentorial (medial temporal lobe) and tonsillar (cerebellar tonsil) herniation, due to tearing of vessels. Herniation may occur due to raised intracranial pressure.

5. Gastrointestinal pathology

ANSWERS: 1) H 2) D 3) F 4) I 5) E

Crohn's disease (H) is an inflammatory bowel disease which can affect any section of the gastrointestinal system. Characteristics include transmural inflammation (full intestinal wall thickness), skip lesions and fistulae. Biospy of the gastrointestinal wall will reveal non-caseating granulomas in approximately 60 per cent of cases. Complications include thickening of the bowel wall (also known as a 'rubber hose wall') which can lead to bowel obstruction. Extra-intestinal manifestations of Crohn's disease include arthritis, ankylosing spondylosis, stomatitis and uveitis, as well as dermatological lesions (pyoderma gangrenosum and erythema nodosum).

Coeliac disease (D) is an autoimmune disease that occurs due to gluten sensitivity, specifically gliadin found in wheat, barley and rye. It affects primarily the duodenum and jejunum. CD8+ cells are sensitized to gliadin; they accumulate in the gut and attack enterocytes and as a result villi disappear. As a compensatory mechanism immature enterocytes in the crypts proliferate causing deeper crypts. Therefore, features of gut biopsy samples include intraepithelial lymphocytes, villous atrophy and crypt hyperplasia. Clinical features include steatorrhoea, bloating, weight loss and fatigue (anaemia secondary to malabsorption).

Barrett's oesophagus (F) occurs as a result of chronic gastro-oesophageal reflux disease. At the squamo-columnar junction between the lower oesophagus and stomach, squamous epithelial cells usually exist. Acidity causes transformation of squamous epithelial cells to columnar epithelial cells, a metaplastic change. The metaplastic columnar epithelial cells include goblet cells that produce intestinal mucin; hence the process is termed intestinal metaplasia. The major complication of Barrett's oesophagus is an increased risk of adenocarcinoma of the oesophagus.

Peptic ulcer disease (I) can either be duodenal or gastric. Ulcers differ from erosions as they extend to the submucosa (sometimes to the muscularis mucosa) and take weeks to heal, whereas erosions breach the mucosa only and take days to heal. The main causes of peptic ulcers are *Helicobacter pylori*, NSAIDs, Zollinger–Ellison syndrome and smoking. These factors disrupt the balance between protective (mucus layer and bicarbonate secretion) and damaging (acid and enzymes) elements leading to ulceration.

Gastric carcinoma (E) is usually a consequence of chronic gastritis and hence *Helicobacter pylori* is implicated in the pathogenesis. *H. pylori* causes intestinal metaplasia leading to gastric atrophy which becomes dysplasia and eventually carcinoma. On histology the carcinoma can be ulcer-like, but differs from peptic ulcers as they have irregular borders and raised edges. Features of gastric carcinoma are the presence of signet ring cells (cells with compressed nuclei) and linitis plastica (the stomach becomes thick and rigid resembling a leather bottle).

Ulcerative colitis (A) is an inflammatory bowel disease, which differs from Crohn's disease as inflammation is confined to the colon, superficial and continuous.

Chronic gastritis (B) may be caused by *Helicobacter pylori* or autoimmune disease. Histological features include lymphocyte infiltrate and intestinal metaplasia. There is a long-term risk of carcinoma or MALT lymphoma.

Oesophageal cancer (C) exists as squamous cell carcinoma (90 per cent) primarily caused by smoking or alcohol, and adenocarcinoma (10 per cent) caused by Barrett's oesophagus.

Gardener's syndrome (G) is similar to familial adenomatous polyposis (presence of adenomas in the gastrointestinal tract caused by a defect in the *APC* gene), with the addition of extra-intestinal growths (osteomas, epidermoid cysts and desmoid tumours).

6. Liver pathology

ANSWERS: 1) B 2) I 3) F 4) G 5) E

Cirrhosis (B) is defined as the diffuse fibrosis of the liver with abnormal architecture characterized by nodules secondary to chronic hepatic disease. This can be sub-classified as micronodular (<3 mm; usually alcoholic aetiology) or macronodular (>3 mm; usually viral aetiology). Fibrosis results from stellate cell activation, which deposit collagen. Nodules represent proliferating hepatocytes that lack normal acinar structure and hence have a haphazard blood supply; this leads to shunt formation and portal hypertension. Causes of cirrhosis include alcohol, hepatitis B and C, primary biliary cirrhosis, haemochromatosis, Wilson's disease and α1-antitrypsin deficiency.

Wilson's disease (I) is an autosomal recessive condition that results from a mutation in the ATP7B gene leading to multi-organ copper accumulation. ATP7B is a protein that facilitates the transport of copper across cell membranes. Liver involvement will lead to cirrhosis, most commonly in children, whilst accumulation in the brain can lead to Parkinsonism, seizures and dementia. Psychological features include behavioural changes, depression and psychosis. Other organs affected include the eyes (Kayser–Fleischer rings), kidneys (renal tubular acidosis) and heart (cardiomyopathy).

Haemochromatosis (F) is an autosomal recessive condition that is due to a mutation in the HFE gene. The HFE protein regulates iron absorption that is stored as haemosiderin. Histological features of haemochromatosis include a golden-brown haemosiderin deposition in the parenchyma of many organs. Haemosiderin eventually leads to inflammation and subsequent fibrosis. Histological samples of affected tissue will stain blue with Perl's Prussian blue. Organs affected include the liver (cirrhosis), pancreas (diabetes), skin (bronzed pigmentation), heart (cardiomyopathy) and gonads (atrophy and impotence).

Hepatocellular carcinoma (HCC; G) is the most prevalent primary liver malignancy. Most commonly HCC occurs secondary to cirrhosis. The risk factors for HCC are therefore the numerous causes of cirrhosis. However, carcinogens such as aflatoxin, produced by the fungal genus *Aspergillus* can directly cause HCC; aflatoxin contaminates many crops in the developing world, notably cereals and nuts. α-Fetoprotein is a marker that may suggest the presence of HCC. There is also evidence that the metabolic syndrome contributes to risk of developing HCC.

Primary biliary cirrhosis (PBC; E) is an autoimmune disease of the liver, affecting the small and medium-sized intra-hepatic ducts. The primary histological feature is the dense accumulation of lymphocytes around bile ducts creating granulomas and total destruction of the ducts. This results in an obstructive cholestasis causing the triad of jaundice, xanthelasma (cholesterol is normally excreted in bile) and pruritis. Biochemically PBC is linked with anti-mitochondrial antibodies, as well as raised ALP, GGT, IgM and cholesterol. PBC is also strongly associated with Sjögren's syndrome.

Cholangiocarcinoma (A) is an adenocarcinoma of the bile ducts. Risk factors for the development of cholangiocarcinoma include primary sclerosing cholangitis, parasitic liver fluke infection and exposure to medical imaging contrast media.

α1-Antitrypsin deficiency (C) results in destruction of tissues due to the lack of inhibition of neutrophil proteases, resulting in emphysema in the lungs and cirrhosis.

Haemosiderosis (D) is defined as excess haemosiderin deposition due to an acquired cause (alcohol and blood transfusions). Unless severe, there is no architectural change and therefore no development of cirrhosis.

Primary sclerosing cholangitis (H) affects the large intra- and extra-hepatic ducts. Histological features include periductal fibrosis that eventually invades the lumen causing concentric onion-ring fibrosis.

7. Skin pathology

ANSWERS: 1) A 2) H 3) F 4) E 5) I

Pemphigoid (A) is an autoimmune deep bullous (blisters >0.5 cm) condition that occurs in the elderly. Bullae are fluid filled and therefore do not rupture easily; pemphigoid is Nikolsky sign negative. The underlying pathology involves IgG binding to hemi-desmosomes. This causes activation of eosinophils that are recruited to the area. Pemphigoid should not be confused with pemphigus (option J), also an autoimmune bullous disease that affects middle-aged patients, causing superficial bullae on the skin (Nikolsky positive). IgG bind to desmosomes in the intra-epidermal region resulting in acantholysis.

Erythema multiforme (H) is a hypersensitivity reaction secondary to infections (herpes simplex, mycoplasmas and fungi) and drugs (penicillin, phenytoin and barbiturates). The pathogenesis is unclear but is thought to be due to immune-complex deposition in the microvasculature of the skin and oral mucous membranes. Most commonly the rash is self-limiting and target shaped as well as being maculo-papular with sub-epidermal bullae in the centre. In severe cases, the rash may involve mucosal surfaces leading to Steven–Johnson's syndrome, characterized by epidermal necrosis with minimal inflammatory cell infiltrate.

Psoriasis (F) is an autoimmune condition primarily affecting the extensor surfaces of the skin. Histological features include parakeratosis (corneum nuclei mixed with keratin to form a thick keratin layer creating 'silvery scales'); Munro-abscesses (white blood cells entering the corneum); loss of the granular layer leading to pin-point bleeding (Auspitz sign); clubbing of the rete ridges, whereby they grow downwards leading to a 'test-tubes in a rack' appearance. Clinical features include salmon-pink plaques with a silver–white scale on the skin and onycholysis.

Actinic keratosis (solar keratosis; E) is defined as epidermal dysplasia that occurs secondary to sunlight and presents as a brown–red warty lesion with a sandpaper-like consistency. Histological features include solar elastosis, focal parakeratosis, atypical cells and inflammatory cell infiltrates. Actinic keratosis does not affect the full thickness of the epidermis. It is a premalignant condition that may progress to squamous cell carcinoma in approximately 20 per cent of cases.

Malignant melanoma (I) is a malignant tumour of melanocytes. The characteristic features can be remembered by the mnemonic ABCDE: asymmetry, border irregularity, colour (usually black; sometimes demonstrate colours of the French flag), diameter >5 cm and evolution (change in size, colour and/or new onset itchiness/pain). Malignant melanomas initially grow radially *in situ* within the epidermis; over time there is growth vertically into the dermis, eventually leading to metastases. Sub-types include lentigomaligna (LM), acrallentigious (AL), superficial spreading (SS) and nodular (N).

Bowen's disease (B) is also called squamous carcinoma *in situ*. Histological features include atypical cells involving the full thickness of the epidermis but not invading the basement membrane.

Pityriasis rosea (C) begins as a single scaly macule that is salmon-pink, <5 cm and known as a 'herald patch'. After several days multiple small pink rashes appear posteriorly creating a fir-tree pattern.

Lichen planus (D) histologically appears as inflammation at the epidermal-dermal junction. The lymphocytic infiltrate creates a saw-tooth pattern. The 7 Ps reflect the features of lichen planus: pruritic, purple, polygonal, planar, popular, plaques and pearl sheen.

Basal cell carcinomas (G) occur secondary to sun exposure. They are very invasive locally and are hence termed 'rodent ulcers.' On examination they are pearly, raised, irregular, ulcerated and have telangiectasia.

8. Renal pathology

ANSWERS: 1) A 2) F 3) D 4) G 5) H

Nephritic syndrome (A) involves the following: haematuria, red cell and white cell casts, dysmorphic red cells, oliguria and hypertension. The pathogenesis begins with inflammation of glomerular vessels allowing red blood cells to enter the renal tubule; as they enter they are damaged. The body compensates for the inflammation by slowing renal blood flow causing oliguria, which leads to water retention and hence hypertension. Cellular casts form as a result of Tamm–Horsefall secretions in the distal collecting duct and collecting duct that 'glue' cells together, hence forming a cast.

Goodpasture's syndrome (F) is an anti-glomerular basement membrane disease that causes rapidly progressive glomerulonephritis (RPGN). RPGN all demonstrate a crescent sign on biopsy, which represents the proliferation of macrophages and parietal cells in the Bowman's space. There are numerous causes of RPGN; these can be differentiated by looking at the IgG and C3 deposition pattern on immunofluorescence. Goodpasture's syndrome occurs due to IgG against the A3 chain of type-4 collagen, creating a linear pattern on immunofluorescence.

Acute tubular necrosis (D) is defined as damage to the tubular epithelium leading to acute renal failure. Ischaemic or toxic injury reduces GFR in three ways: 1) Loss of polarity (loss of membrane channels reduces sodium reabsorption; more sodium reaches macula densa constricting afferent arteriole, hence reducing GFR); 2) Glomerular back-pressure (formation of casts in distal convoluted tubule creates back-pressure reducing GFR); and 3) Interstitial leakage (back-pressure forces fluid into interstitium causing swelling and compression of tubules).

IgA nephropathy (Berger's disease; G) usually occurs 1–4 days after a respiratory or gastrointestinal infection (mucosal defence is primarily IgA). IgA is deposited in the mesangium which may lead to RPGN. On immunofluorescence a granular staining of IgG and C3 will demonstrate IgA nephropathy (other conditions causing this pattern are SLE, Henoch–Schlönein purpura, post-streptococcal infection and Alport's syndrome). There is frank haematuria in 50 per cent of cases and microscopic haematuria in 50 per cent of patients.

Nephrotic syndrome (H) is the combination of proteinuria, hypoalbuminaemia and oedema (with associated hyperlipidaemia and lipiduria). Primary causes such as IgA nephropathy are most common in children, whereas systemic causes such as diabetes and SLE are more common in adults. Damage to the glomerulus causes increased permeability and hence proteins pass into the tubules leading to proteinuria and hypoalbuminaemia. A reduced oncotic pressure therefore causes oedema. The liver compensates by producing increased amounts of lipids which are then excreted via the damaged kidneys causing lipiduria.

Wegener's granulamatosis (B) is a c-ANCA mediated pauci-immune RPGN, creating an absent/scant pattern on IgG and C3 immunofluorescence staining.

Membranous glomerulonephritis (C) is defined on histological investigation as a thickened glomerular basement membrane, spike/dome protrusions, sub-epithelial immunoglobulin and a granular staining pattern.

Minimal change glomerulonephritis (E) appears normal with light microscopy but podocyte effacement is visible on electron microscopy. Most cases will respond to steroid treatment.

Focal segmental glomerulonephritis (I) appears with obliterated lumen and podocyte effacement on histological examination. Focal segmental glomerulonephritis is not responsive to steroids.

9. Breast pathology

ANSWERS: 1) D 2) C 3) E 4) B 5) I

Duct ectasia (D) is defined as the chronic ductal inflammation due to acini secretions that become clogged in the ducts causing them to dilate and rupture. This leads to a green/white discharge being produced. Duct ectasia occurs in women older than 40 who have had children. It is an important diagnosis to make as it mimics breast cancer; the presentation may be nipple retraction due to fibrosis and bloody discharge secondary to rupture of the ducts.

Fibroadenoma (C) is the most common benign breast tumour. Fibroadenomas arise from stroma as well as lobules and hence are mixed tumours. They characteristically grow rapidly in pregnancy and during the menstrual cycle as lobules are oestrogen driven; conversely, fibroadenomas regress at menopause due to the lack of oestrogen. On examination, fibroadenomas are very mobile (sometimes known as a breast mouse), well circumscribed, discrete and usually less than 5 cm. They tend to be soft in a young female and firm in elderly women (as stroma becomes more fibrous).

Ductal carcinomas *in situ* (DCIS; E) occur in pre- or post-menopausal women. They are usually unilateral and unifocal. On mammogram, microcalcification may be visible secondary to central necrosis.

Microscopic features include the presence of central necrosis and pleomorphic nuclei. In contrast, lobular carcinoma *in situ* (LCIS) usually occurs mainly in pre-menopausal women and is bilateral and multifocal. No calcification occurs and hence there is no detection on mammogram. Histologically there is no necrosis and uniform nuclei are present.

Phylloides tumours (B) are similar to fibroadenomas as they are mixed; they arise from stroma and duct epithelium. They are also similar to fibroadenomas as they are discrete, well-circumscribed and mobile. They differ in that they are usually greater than 5 cm, occur in women over the age of 40 years and can be malignant. Histological investigation reveals an 'artichoke-like' appearance as the stroma pushes up on the epithelium to form clubs.

Infiltrating ductal carcinoma (IDC; I) is an invasive cancer and therefore penetrates the basement membrane. IDC is also called no special type and usually results from DCIS. Macroscopically IDC has a scirrhous look whereby the centre is very fibrous giving a dense white appearance. IDC has the worst prognosis compared to all other invasive carcinomas (medullary, mucinous, tubular and papillary carcinoma). Features of invasive carcinoma also include peau d'orange, Paget's disease of the breast, tethering, nipple retraction, lymphadenopathy, ulceration of the mass and pain.

Mastitis (A) occurs in breast-feeding mothers. As a result of cracked nipples, bacteria such as *Staphylococcus aureus* are able to enter. On examination, the area is tender to touch, erythematous and oedematous.

Gynaecomastia (F) is defined as enlargement of male breasts due to epithelial hyperplasia. Causes include: malnutrition, spironolactone, ketoconazole and cirrhosis.

Fibrocystic disease (G) is usually a peri-menopausal disease that regresses after menopause. It occurs due to irregular menstrual cycles that result in unbalanced oestrogen.

Fat necrosis (H) occurs after trauma to the breast resulting in a tender lump consisting of necrosed fat surrounded by macrophages.

10. Bone pathology

ANSWERS: 1) I 2) D 3) A 4) B 5) C

Giant cell tumour (GCT; I) is a borderline malignant tumour of giant osteoclast cells. The cells are similar to those found in Paget's disease as they have multiple nuclei (>20). The osteoclastic cells cause lytic lesions in the epiphyses (especially around the knee) that are visible on X-ray and may give a characteristic 'soap bubble' appearance. Histological features include multinucleated giant osteoclasts with surrounding ovoid and spindle cells.

Osteomalacia (D) is defined as the insufficient mineralization of bone due to vitamin D deficiency. Reduced intake, malabsorptive conditions, phenytoin and chronic liver disease can cause vitamin D deficiency. A low vitamin D level causes hypocalcaemia resulting in increased PTH release (normalizing calcium). PTH stimulates osteoclastic activity causing bones to be soft and epiphyses to widen. Clinical features include craniotabes, bone pain, proximal weakness and pseudo-fractures (looser zones). Craniotabes is the descriptive term for the soft and elastic occipito-parietal bones causing an elastic recoil sensation when pushed.

Osteoporosis (A) is defined by reduced bone density (reduced quantity) but normal quality. Reduced circulating oestrogen concentration causes IL-1 and IL-6 levels to rise causing osteoclastic activity. Osteoporosis primarily affects the vertebrae and hips. Primary osteoporosis occurs in post-menopausal women. Secondary causes include lifestyle choices (smoking, alcohol, inactivity), drugs (steroid, goserelin), low BMI as well as thyroid and parathyroid disease. Diagnosis is made using a DEXA scan; a T-score of <1 reflects osteopenia and a score of <2.5 suggests osteoporosis. All blood markers of metabolic bone disease are normal.

Fibrous dysplasia (B) occurs due to the developmental arrest of normal bone structures secondary to an osteoblast maturation defect. The most common sites affected are the proximal femur and ribs. On X-ray, fibrous dysplasia may cause a ground-glass or soap bubble appearance. Histological investigation reveals trabeculae that lack osteoblastic rimming. Two possible syndromes can arise: 1) Mono-ostotic (70 per cent) affecting femurs more than ribs occurring in patients under 30 years of age, and 2) McCune–Albright syndrome (30 per cent) that is poly-ostotic and causes café-au-lait spots and precocious puberty.

Paget's disease (C) is a disease of bone remodelling whereby new bone is larger but weaker and prone to fracture. During the initial lytic phase giant osteoclasts with multiple nuclei rapidly resorb bone. In the mixed phase, osteoblast activity leads to increased bone mass. In the final osteosclerotic phase, bone formation continues but is woven and weak, with collagen arranged haphazardly resulting in a mosaic pattern. Complications can arise from deformities that cause impingement of nerves. Bone marrow infiltration of weak woven bone can lead to high output heart failure.

Osteochondroma (E) is a bone neoplasm affecting those aged between 10 and 30 years. It targets the large joints and is a low malignancy risk.

Osteoid osteoma (F) is a painful bone neoplasm. X-ray investigation reveals central nidus (luscent) with sclerotic rim (opaque) pattern.

Renal osteodystrophy (G) is also known as secondary hyperparathyroidism. It occurs in patients with renal failure due to build-up of phosphate, damage to 1α-hydroxylase, osteosclerosis and aluminium toxicity.

Enchondroma (H) is a bone neoplasm most prevalent in patients aged between 10 and 40 years. It affects the small joints and has a high risk of malignant transformation.

SECTION 10:
HISTOPATHOLOGY SBAs

Answers

QUESTIONS

1. Mitral valve vegetation

A 65-year-old patient with advanced breast malignancy and a history of multiple systemic emboli suffers a stroke. On examination, there are no cardiac murmurs but an echocardiogram reveals small bland vegetations on the mitral valve. Blood cultures are negative. What is the most likely diagnosis?

A   Infective endocarditis
B   Acute rheumatic fever
C   Non-bacterial thrombotic endocarditis
D   Chronic rheumatic valvular disease
E   Libman–Sacks endocarditis

2. Congenital causes of cardiovascular disease

A 41-year-old man presents with severe central chest pain which he describes as 'tearing' in nature and radiating to the back. He is tall, with long limbs and long thin fingers. He also has an aortic regurgitation murmur. Histologically there is cystic medial necrosis in the aortic wall. In which syndrome are these findings most likely?

A   Ortner's syndrome
B   Ehlers–Danlos syndrome
C   Down syndrome
D   Turner syndrome
E   Marfan syndrome

3. Acute myocardial infarction

A 57-year-old overweight patient suffers an acute myocardial infarction and subsequently dies. A post-morterm examination of the infarcted area shows extensive cell infiltration including polymorphs and macrophages. There is also extensive debris post necrosis and the cytoplasm is homogeneous making it difficult to see the outlines of the myocardial fibres. There is no evidence of collagenization or a scar. How long after the initial attack did the patient die?

A   At the time of the attack (0–6 hours)
B   Hours after the attack (6–24 hours)
C   Days after the attack (1–4 days)
D   Within the first 2 weeks of the attack (4–14 days)
E   Weeks and months after (14 days +)

4. Anti-topoisomerase antibodies

A 35-year-old woman presents to accident and emergency with nausea, severe malaise, swelling and stiffness of the fingers. On examination, her blood pressure is 155/95 mmHg and she has Raynaud's phenomenon. Blood tests reveal positive anti-topoisomerase antibodies and deranged serum creatinine and urea. A biopsy result of her small arteries reveals an onion skin appearance. What is the most likely diagnosis?

A   Systemic lupus erythematosus
B   Diffuse scleroderma
C   Kawasaki's disease
D   Polyarteritis nodosa
E   Limited scleroderma/CREST

5. Muscle weakness

A 46-year-old woman presents with gradual muscle weakness in her neck and upper arms over the past 3 weeks. She is also said to have a purple 'heliotrope' rash on her upper eyelids, an erythematous scaling rash on her face and red patches on the knees. She has also experienced some weight loss. Blood tests reveal elevated skeletal muscle enzymes but electromyogram results were negative. What is the most likely diagnosis?

A   Polymyositis
B   Henoch–Schönlein purpura
C   Dermatomyositis
D   Kawasaki disease
E   Sarcoidosis

6. Lewy bodies

A 43-year-old man presents with a rest tremor, slowness of voluntary movement and rigidity. It is reported that he has a mutation of the alpha-synuclein protein and he is free of Lewy bodies on histological examination. What is the most likely diagnosis?

A   Familial Parkinson's disease
B   Alzheimer's disease
C   Multiple system atrophy
D   Multiple sclerosis
E   Idiopathic Parkinson's disease

7. Plaques of multiple sclerosis

The activity of the plaques in a 25-year-old multiple sclerosis patient is described with the presence of oedema and macrophages, and some myelin breakdown. Which ICDNS (International Classification of Diseases of the Nervous System) plaque type classification best fits the description?

A   Acute plaque
B   Early chronic active plaque
C   Late chronic active plaque
D   Chronic inactive plaque
E   Shadow plaque

8. Causes of dementia

A 72-year-old woman is diagnosed with a disease that accounts for 50–75 per cent of all cases of dementia. The four characteristic pathological features for her diagnosis are severe brain atrophy, loss of neurons, senile plaques and neuro-fibllirary tangles. What is the most likely diagnosis?

A   Huntington's disease
B   Alzheimer's disease
C   Multiple system atrophy
D   Dementia with Lewy bodies
E   Parkinson's disease

9. Cell changes

A 32-year-old man has a past medical history of severe gastro-oesophageal reflux disease. His most recent oesophageal biopsy shows a columnar epithelium with goblet cells suggestive of a diagnosis of Barrett's oesophagus. What form of cell change is this also known as?

A   Anaplasia
B   Hyperplasia
C   Metaplasia
D   Dysplasia
E   Neoplasia

10. Gastritis

A 38-year-old man is a known gastritis patient. The most recent endoscopy and biopsy has detected that the area most severely affected is the pyloric antrum. He also has susceptibility for developing a gastric MALT lymphoma in the future. What is the most likely diagnosis?

A   Menetrier's disease (hyperplastic hypersecretory gastropathy)
B   Acute gastritis
C   *Helicobacter*-associated chronic gastritis
D   Autoimmune chronic gastritis
E   Reactive/reflux chronic gastritis

11. Diseases of the exocrine pancreas

A 50-year-old known alcoholic man has persistent severe epigastric pain radiating to the back and has experienced weight loss of 5 kg in 2 months. On initial presentation, the patient is not jaundiced. On contrast enhanced CT scan there are multiple calcific densities along the line of the main pancreatic duct. On histological examination, there is evidence of parenchymal fibrosis and large ducts containing insipissated secretions. What is the most likely diagnosis?

A   Chronic pancreatitis
B   Carcinoma in the head of the pancreas
C   Diabetes mellitus type 2
D   Acute pancreatitis
E   Pseudocysts

12. Diseases of the endocrine pancreas

A 22-year-old man presents with polyuria and polydipsia. His fasting plasma glucose is 7.3 mmol/L. He is Glutamic Acid Decarboxylase (GAD) antibody positive. What is the most likely diagnosis?

A   Diabetes mellitus type 1
B   Diabetes insipidus
C   Psychogenic polydipsia
D   Diabetes mellitus type 2
E   Zollinger–Ellison syndrome

13. Viral hepatitis

A 37-year-old man, while abroad, was involved in a road traffic accident and required a blood transfusion. He had an episode of acute hepatitis with the contraction of a DNA virus of the Hepadna group. There is a small chance this may progress to chronic hepatitis. What is the most likely viral hepatitis type?

A   Hepatitis A
B   Hepatitis B
C   Hepatitis C
D   Hepatitis D
E   Hepatitis E

14. Anti-mitochondrial antibodies

A 42-year-old woman, who has a history of joint and skin symptoms, presents with jaundice. Anti-mitochondrial antibodies are present and histologically there is evidence of a progressive, chronic granulomatous inflammation of the bile duct. What is the most likely diagnosis?

A   Primary sclerosing cholangitis
B   Autoimmune hepatitis
C   Primary biliary cirrhosis
D   α-1 Antitrypsin deficiency
E   Alcoholic liver disease

15. Congenital metabolic disorders

A 23-year-old patient has an autosomal recessive disorder. The patient has demonstrated parkinsonian symptoms such as a hand tremor and has developed chronic hepatitis. On examination, he is found to have Kayser–Fleischer rings. Blood levels of serum ceruloplasmin are low. What is the most likely diagnosis?

A   Wilson's disease
B   Genetic haemochromatosis
C   α-1 Antitrypsin deficiency
D   Reye's syndrome
E   Budd–Chiari syndrome

16. Gastrointestinal diseases in children

An 8-year-old Down syndrome boy presents with constipation, distended abdomen, vomiting and overflow diarrhoea. The cause is believed to be absence of ganglion cells in the myenteric plexus causing the failure of the dilation of the distal colon. What is the most likely diagnosis?

A   Stenosis
B   Hirschsprung's disease
C   Atresia
D   Intussusception
E   Volvulus

17. Colitis

A 25-year-old white man is experiencing bloody diarrhoea and mucous discharge. Macroscopic analysis shows abnormality in the colon and rectum only and is continuous with a normal bowel wall thickness. The pattern of inflammation is confined to the mucosa of the bowel wall and no evidence of granulomas exists. What is the most likely diagnosis?

A Crohn's disease
B Ulcerative colitis
C Ischaemic colitis
D Pseudomembranous colitis
E Viral gastroenteritis

18. Neoplastic disease of the intestine

A 39-year-old man is diagnosed with a colon cancer proximal to the splenic flexure that is poorly differentiated and highly aggressive. There are no associated adenomata. It is an autosomal dominant condition that involves gene mutations of DNA mismatch repair genes. What is the most likely diagnosis?

A Familial adenomatous polyposis
B Gardner's syndrome
C Colorectal carcinoma
D Hereditary non-polyposis colorectal cancer
E Hamartomatous polyps

19. Hydrosalpinx

A 25-year-old woman presents to clinic with an inability to conceive and a past history of *Chlamydia trachomatis* infection. On ultrasonography, she is diagnosed with hydrosalpinx. Hydrosalpinx is the most likely complication of which of the below options?

A Endometriosis
B Adenomyosis
C Cervical intraepithelial neoplasia
D Salpingitis
E Human papillomavirus

20. Gynaecological tumours

A 42-year-old Afro-Caribbean woman is nulliparous and trying to conceive. She has been experiencing dysmenorrhoea. Ultrasound scan shows multiple rounded nodules within the myometrium. What is the most likely diagnosis?

A Cervical intraepithelial neoplasia
B Vulval carcinoma
C Leiomyoma
D Endometrial carcinoma
E CGIN (endocervical glandular dysplasia)

21. Ovarian tumours

A 20-year-old woman presents to accident and emergency with a distended abdomen resembling a pregnancy. She later develops acute onset of severe abdominal pain. An ultrasound identified a mass in her right ovary. Her abdomen is rigid and she is admitted for emergency surgery. It is believed that three embryonic germ cell layers are present. What is the most likely diagnosis?

A   Teratoma of the ovary
B   Serous tumour of the ovary
C   Mucinous tumour of the ovary
D   Endometrioid tumour of the ovary
E   Clear cell carcinoma

22. Peripheral blood film

A 32-year-old woman presents with generalized fatigue. Full blood count shows a reduced haemoglobin level and reduced mean corpuscular volume. A peripheral blood film has revealed iron deficiency anaemia. What features are most likely to be seen on her peripheral blood film?

A   Hypochromic and microcytic red blood cells with anisopoikilocytosis and acanthocytes
B   Hypochromic and microcytic red blood cells with hypersegmented neutrophils
C   Hypochromic and microcytic red blood cells with anisopoikilocytosis and no evidence of basophilic stippling
D   Hypochromic and microcytic red blood cells with Howell–Jolly bodies and basophilic stippling
E   Hypochromic and macrocytic red blood cells with target cells, acanthocytes and Howell–Jolly bodies

23. Coeliac disease

A 26-year-old woman presents with fatigue 'all the time'. She has a family history of coeliac disease and blood tests reveal hypochromic, microcytic anaemia. She is referred to the gastroenterology clinic for tests. The gold standard investigation is the duodenal biopsy, which is carried out after positive serological testing. Which current serological testing and histopathology findings in the options below are most consistent with a coeliac disease diagnosis?

A   Anti-reticulin antibodies only/villous atrophy, crypt hyperplasia, increased intraepithelial lymphocytes
B   Anti-gliadin antibodies only/no villous atrophy, crypt hyperplasia, decreased intraepithelial lymphocytes
C   Anti-endomysial antibodies only/villous atrophy, crypt hyperplasia, increased intraepithelial lymphocytes
D   Anti-endomysial antibodies and anti-tissue transglutaminase antibodies/ villous atrophy, crypt hyperplasia, increased intraepithelial lymphocytes
E   Anti-endomysial antibodies and anti-tissue transglutaminase antibodies/villous atrophy, no evidence of crypt hyperplasia, increased intraepithelial lymphocytes

24. Non-neoplastic bone tumours

A 27-year-old woman has developed pain in her right proximal femur. She has a history of intermittent hip pain since childhood. An X-ray has demonstrated a 'soap bubble' appearance indicative of osteolysis and a characteristic shepherd's crook deformity. The biopsy would show irregular trabeculae of woven bone said to resemble Chinese letters. What is the most likely diagnosis?

A   Non-ossifying fibroma
B   Fibrous dysplasia
C   Giant cell reparative granuloma
D   Ossifying fibroma
E   Simple bone cyst

25. Benign bone tumours

A 36-year-old man presents with swelling of his middle finger and subsequently a fracture. His X-ray shows cotton wool calcification and histopathology shows evidence of a tumour composed of benign hyaline cartilage. It is believed that he has only a very slight risk of malignant transformation. What is the most likely diagnosis?

A   Osteochondroma
B   Multiple myeloma
C   Osteoid osteoma
D   Giant cell tumour
E   Enchondroma

26. Malignant bone tumours

An 18-year-old man presents with pain and a mass in his right knee. His X-ray shows an ill defined mass in the metaphyseal region of the distal femur that is sclerotic and lytic. There is also an elevated periosteum (known as a Codman's triangle). Prognosis is said to be poor and the treatment required is multi-disciplinary involving intensive chemotherapy and surgery. In cytology, these tumour cells will be positive for alkaline phosphatase. What is the most likely diagnosis?

A   Osteosarcoma
B   Chondrosarcoma
C   Fibrosarcoma
D   Malignant fibrous histiocytoma
E   Ewing's sarcoma

27. NHS cervical screening programme

A 25-year-old woman is due for her cervical smear test. Which method of cyto-pathology is going to be used?

A   FNA
B   Ultrasound guided FNA
C   Washings
D   Brushings
E   Liquid based cytology

28. Obstructive lung disease

A 57-year-old man who is a heavy smoker presents to his GP with gradually worsening dyspnoea and cough productive of green sputum. On examination, he is cyanosed, tachypnoeic and wheezing. What is the most likely diagnosis?

A   Chronic bronchitis
B   Pulmonary embolus
C   Asthma
D   Bronchiolitis
E   Emphysema

29. Pneumonia

A 57-year-old man presents to accident and emergency with dyspnoea, fever, cough and purulent sputum. Histopathology confirms widespread fibrinosup-purative consolidation on the left lower lobe and the top differential diagnosis is lobar pneumonia. Which organism is the most likely cause?

A   *Streptococcus pneumoniae*
B   *Staphylococcus aureus*
C   *Haemophilus influenzae*
D   *Streptococcus pyogenes*
E   *Mycobacterium tuberculosis*

30. Diffuse alveolar damage

A 27-year-old man with severe second degree burns is admitted to the ITU and develops severe shortness of breath and tachypnoea the next day. Diffuse alveolar damage is indicated in the histopathology report. What is the most likely diagnosis?

A   Pulmonary oedema
B   Acute respiratory distress syndrome
C   Cryptogenic fibrosing alveolitis
D   Bronchiectasis
E   Chronic bronchitis

31. Respiratory disease (1)

A 47-year-old construction worker presents with a 6-month history of cough, haemoptysis and 5 kg weight loss. He is a heavy smoker and a centrally located lesion is found on his chest X-ray. Histology showed keratinization and intercellular 'prickles'. What is the most likely diagnosis?

A   Tuberculosis
B   Squamous cell carcinoma
C   Mesothelioma
D   Emphysema
E   Large cell carcinoma

32. Respiratory disease (2)

A 55-year-old non-smoking woman presents to her GP with a 6-month history of cough, haemoptysis and 5 kg weight loss. A chest X-ray showed the lesion is in the periphery and histopathology showed evidence of glandular differentiation and cytology showed mucin vacuoles. Mode of treatment most suitable is surgical. What is the most likely diagnosis?

A   Small cell carcinoma
B   Adenocarcinoma
C   Large cell carcinoma
D   Sarcoidosis
E   Pneuomoconiosis

33. Erythema multiforme

A 27-year-old man presents with fever, fatigue and a rash. He has also noted a few painful ulcers in his mouth. The rash is described as numerous round lesions about an inch in diameter on the face, trunk, arms and legs, diagnosed as erythema multiforme. What is the most likely diagnosis for this patient?

A   Systemic lupus erythematosus
B   Stevens–Johnson syndrome
C   Pemphigoid
D   Pityriasis rosea
E   Contact dermatitis

34. Skin tumours

A 55-year-old Australian man presents with a flat black lesion on his back that appears asymmetrical with an irregular border and 6 mm in diameter. Breslow's depth is 0.4 mm. What is the most likely diagnosis?

A   Malignant melanoma
B   Basal cell carcinoma
C   Squamous cell carcinoma
D   Keratoacanthoma
E   Bowen's disease

35. Inflammatory conditions

A 23-year-old Irish man presents with an itchy blistering eruption on his buttocks and elbows. He also has diarrhoea and abdominal pain. Histopathology reveals papillary microabscesses and a neutrophilic infiltrate. He has a family history of gluten sensitivity. Which rash is most often associated with his presentation?

A   Psoriasis
B   Atopic eczema
C   Dermatitis herpetiformis
D   Lichen planus
E   Seborrhoeic dermatitis

36. Types of fractures

A 26-year-old man presents to accident and emergency having fallen off his skateboard and landed with a big impact on his right side. His X-ray shows a fracture in the midshaft of his right humerus that appears splintered although the soft tissue is intact. What type of fracture is this?

A   Greenstick fracture
B   Transverse fracture
C   Compound fracture
D   Impacted fracture
E   Comminuted fracture

37. Non-neoplastic bone disease

An 80-year-old woman presents complaining of pain on movement and stiffness after inactivity in her legs, most notably in her hips and knees. She also complains of pain in her hands and marked symmetrical swelling is noted in her distal interphalangeal joints. The X-ray of her right knee shows subchondral sclerosis, subchondral cyst formation, joint space narrowing and osteophytes. What is the most likely diagnosis?

A   Osteoarthritis
B   Rheumatoid arthritis
C   Ankylosing spondylitis
D   Psoriatic arthritis
E   Osteoporosis

38. Painful joint

A 59-year-old man presents to accident and emergency with a painful, swollen and hot big toe. The joint aspirate shows negatively birefringent crystals under polarized red light. The crystals are needle shaped. What is the most likely diagnosis?

A   Pseudogout
B   Lyme disease
C   Reiter's sydrome
D   Gout
E   Osteomyelitis

39. Renal disease

A 23-year-old man presents to accident and emergency with a 2-day history of left-sided loin pain, fever, rigors and vomiting. Urine analysis reveals microscopic haematuria and white cell casts. What is the most likely diagnosis?

A   Cystitis
B   Prostatitis
C   Urolithiasis
D   Acute pyelonephritis
E   Hydronephrosis

40. Urological neoplasia

A 4-year-old boy presents with a large abdominal mass and haematuria. His blood pressure is 165/120 mmHg. The mass has a large necrotic solid tumour with extrarenal invasion. Microscopically, there are immature-looking glomerular structures. Aggressive therapy with surgery, chemotherapy and radiotherapy is indicated. What is the most likely diagnosis?

A   Teratoma
B   Wilm's tumour
C   Oncocytoma
D   Spermatocytic seminoma
E   Bowen's disease

41. Gleason's grading system

A 79-year-old man has hesitancy and terminal dribbling urinary symptoms secondary to a tumour growth. No other symptoms are present. On rectal examination, the prostate is reported as hard and craggy. The patient has been given a Gleason's score of 8; a primary grade of 3, describing that the tissue has recognizable glands and these cells are beginning to invade the surrounding tissue. There is also a secondary grade of pattern 5 suggesting poorly differentiated cells. What is the most likely diagnosis?

A   Prostatic adenocarcinoma
B   Seminoma
C   Prostatic intraepithelial neoplasia
D   Benign prostatic hyperplasia
E   Transitional cell carcinoma

42. Non-neoplastic disorders of the breast

A 27-year-old lactating mother presents with a painful red left breast. On closer examination, there are cracks and fissures on the left nipple. What is the most likely diagnosis?

A   Fat necrosis
B   Acute mastitis
C   Duct ectasia
D   Simple fibrocystic change
E   Epithelial hyperplasia

43. Neoplasms of the breast (1)

A 56-year-old woman presents with blood stained nipple discharge and a solitary mass located just superior to the nipple in her left breast. A histopathology analysis shows that a papillary mass is lined by epithelium and myoepithelium. It is believed that there is no increased risk of malignancy. What is the most likely diagnosis?

A   Intraductal papilloma
B   Phylloides tumour
C   Fibroadenoma
D   Radial scar
E   Ductal carcinoma *in situ*

44. Neoplasms of the breast (2)

A 53-year-old overweight woman with a positive family history of breast cancer attends her appointment for the NHS Breast Screening Programme. She is one of the 5 per cent of women who have an abnormal mammogram and are called for a core biopsy. She has been given a B code of B5b. What is the most likely diagnosis?

A   Benign abnormality
B   Lesion of uncertain malignant potential
C   Ductal carcinoma *in situ*
D   Invasive carcinoma
E   Suspicious of malignancy

45. Cystic diseases of the kidneys

A 44-year-old man has developed end stage renal failure over the past 5 years with numerous episodes of macroscopic haematuria. He was asymptomatic previously. Ultrasound scan has shown numerous asymmetrical large cysts bilaterally. The patient's mother had a similar condition. What is the most likely diagnosis?

A   Acquired cystic disease
B   Medullary sponge disease
C   Adult polycystic kidney disease
D   Cystic renal dysplasia
E   Simple renal cysts

46. Glomerular disease

A 48-year-old man presents with oliguria and a vasculitic rash on his legs. Investigations indicate that he has a reduced glomerular filtration rate and urinalysis finds urine casts containing red and white blood cells. Histopathology shows scanty deposits of immunoglobulins and complement present with associated anti-neutrophil cytoplasm antibodies (ANCA). What is the most likely diagnosis?

A   IgA nephropathy
B   Thrombotic microangiopathy
C   Anti-GBM crescentic glomerulonephritis disease
D   Pauci-immune crescentic glomerulonephritis disease
E   Amyloidosis

47. Clinical manifestations of glomerular disease

A 35-year-old oedematous woman is found to have urinary protein loss of 5.1 g daily. Further tests show a low albumin level and significant interference with podocyte function. No glomerular crescents were detected. What is the most likely diagnosis?

A   Acute glomerulonephritis
B   Nephritic syndrome
C   Nephrotic syndrome
D   Acute tubular necrosis
E   Acquired cystic disease

48. Cerebrovascular aneurysm

A 58-year-old woman is known to have a Berry aneurysm in the basilar artery. She develops sudden onset severe headache, nausea and loss of consciousness. There was evidence of a 'warning bleed' but no history of brain trauma. What is the most likely fatal diagnosis caused by the ruptured Berry aneurysm?

A   Intracerebral haemorrhage
B   Subarachnoid haemorrhage
C   'Watershed' strokes
D   Transient ischaemic attack
E   Tonsillar brain herniation

49. Cerebral infections

A 9-year-old boy presents with fever, headache, stiff neck and altered mental state. His cerebrospinal fluid is turbid and contains mostly neutrophils. The meninges appear congested and there is purulent material in the subarachnoid space. What is the most likely causative organism?

A   Coxsackie virus
B   *Treponema pallidum*
C   *Staphylococcus aureus*
D   *Streptococcus pneumoniae*
E   *Haemophilus influenzae*

50. HIV in children

A 22-year-old HIV-infected woman is pregnant with her second child. HIV has been transmitted perinatally to her first child. One of the most successful interventions to reduce vertical transmission of HIV during pregnancy to less than 1 per cent is the use of combination anti-retroviral treatment, which ideally should reduce the viral load to?

A   50 copies/mL
B   800 copies/mL
C   1000 copies/mL
D   5000 copies/mL
E   10000 copies/mL

ANSWERS

Mitral valve vegetation

1 C   Non-bacterial thrombotic endocarditis (NBTE; C) commonly affects
        patients over 40 years of age and is often characterized by the absence
        of inflammation or bacteria. Sterile fibrin and platelet vegetations are
        present on cardiac valves, more commonly affecting left-sided heart
        valves (mitral > aortic) and are also associated with numerous diseases,
        especially advanced stage malignancy. NBTE is a source of thrombo-
        embolism to the brain, heart, kidneys, and recurrent emboli are a hallmark
        feature. Infective endocarditis (A) is unlikely in this case because of the
        absence of a persistent fever, no new or changing murmur and negative
        blood cultures. Other absent features of infective endocarditis include
        Roth's spots, Janeway lesions and Osler's nodes. Acute rheumatic fever
        (B), mainly affecting children, commonly involves the endocardium and
        typically results in verruca formation on the left-sided heart valves.
        Vegetations are small as described, but they are much more likely to
        cause stenosis and are therefore inconsistent with this patient. Chronic
        rheumatic valvular disease (D), mainly affecting adults, is a sequela of
        earlier rheumatic fever and causes thickening of valve leaflets, especially
        along lines of closure, and thickening, shortening and fusion of the
        chordate tendineae. Libman–Sacks endocarditis (E) is very commonly
        associated with systemic lupus erythematosus and rarely causes emboli.

Congenital causes of cardiovascular disease

2 E   Cystic medial necrosis is a disorder particularly affecting the aorta,
        causing focal degeneration of the elastic tissue and muscle fibres in the
        media, with accumulation of basophilic ground substance. This leads
        to cyst-like pools between the fibres disrupting the normally paral-
        lel arrays. Clinically, aneurysm formation becomes more likely. It is
        more frequent after 40 years of age and is twice as common in males.
        There is evidence that links cystic medial necrosis to aortic dissection
        in patients with a variety of syndromes, the most common of which is
        Marfan's syndrome (E). These patients are characteristically tall with
        long limbs and long thin fingers. All other syndromes are inconsistent
        with this patient. The most common murmur in Ortner's syndrome (A)
        is mitral stenosis, associated with an enlarged left atrium and recurrent
        laryngeal nerve palsy. Turner's syndrome (D) is only present in females.
        Congenital heart defects include: aortic coarctation, aortic stenosis,
        ventricular septal defect and atrial septal defect, but aortic dissection is
        uncommon. In Ehlers–Danlos syndrome (B), cystic medial necrosis can
        cause fragile blood vessels but aortic regurgitation is not commonly

present. Down syndrome (C) patients may have congenital atrioventricular septal canal defects. Other causes of cystic medial necrosis in patients without Marfan's syndrome are advanced age and chronic hypertension.

Acute myocardial infarction

3 C   In the first 6 hours (A) in the evolution of an acute myocardial infarction (MI), the histology is normal. Necrotic cell death takes place between 6 and 24 hours (B). Pathologically, there is contraction band necrosis (dark red/pink wavy lines extending across the myocardial fibres), loss of nuclei in the myocardial cells and the start of a homogeneous appearing cytoplasm. At 1–4 days (C) following an acute MI, the start of an extensive acute inflammatory response takes place with cell infiltration. Debris is left by the necrosis in the previous stage and the cytoplasm is homogeneous so that it is difficult to see the outlines of the myocardial fibres. Infiltration of polymorphs, and later macrophages, takes place. Removal of the debris takes place at about 5–10 days. At approximately 2 weeks (D), the area undergoes repair and a classic young scar with new capillaries is seen with early collagenization. Macrophages and myofibroblasts are present in large numbers. Some granulation tissue and collagen synthesis will continue on to the next stage. In the months (E) following an acute MI, the area starts to strengthen with the formation of a decellularizing scar. This established scar will be seen as a pale white collagenized area within the interstitium between myocardial fibres.

Anti-topoisomerase antibodies

4 B   Scleroderma exists as limited and diffuse forms. This patient has internal involvement with the evidence of renal failure, which is consistent with diffuse scleroderma (B), which is a rapidly progressing condition that affects a large area of skin and one or more internal organs such as the kidneys, oesophagus and heart. In limited scleroderma (E) there are predominantly cutaneous manifestations affecting the hands, arms and face associated with Calcinosis, Raynaud's phenomenon, Esophaegeal dysfunction, Sclerodactyly and Telangiectasias, i.e. CREST syndrome. The immune system abnormalities in scleroderma are: decreased CD8 cells, antibodies to DNA topoisomerase (in the diffuse form only) and anti-centromere antibody (in limited form). The pathology underlying scleroderma is fibrosis with the unique 'onion skin' intimal thickening of small arteries, which is due to arteriolosclerosis. The remaining three options are unlikely for the following reasons: systemic lupus erythematosus (A) often presents with the characteristic photosensitive butterfly malar rash on the face and antibodies to double-stranded DNA. Polyarteritis nodosa (D) is the inflammatory necrosis of the walls of small and medium-sized arteries. It is usually associated with chronic hepatitis B infection and the presence of

anti-neutrophil cytoplasmic antibodies (ANCA). Kawasaki disease (C) is an autoimmune condition that largely affects children under 5 years of age.

Muscle weakness

5   C   Dermatomyositis (C) has the muscle components involved in polymyositis but in addition it is accompanied by periorbital oedema and a characteristic purple 'heliotrope' rash on the upper eyelids. Heliotrope is a pink/purple colour that one only hears about in reference to dermatomyositis, but is actually the colour of the heliotrope flaver. It is also commonly present with an erythematous, scaling rash on the face, shoulders, upper arms and chest, with red patches over the knuckles, elbows and knees. Weight loss and arthralgia may also present. Polymyositis (A) is characterized by weakness, pain and swelling of proximal limb muscles and facial muscles, often with ptosis and dysphagia. It is not associated with any skin presentations and often there are positive electromyogram results. Kawasaki disease (D) is a paediatric condition that does not cause any muscle weakness. Henoch–Schönlein purpura (B) is a systemic vasculitic condition that typically presents with symptoms including palpable purpura, joint pains and abdominal pains. Impaired renal function is a fairly common complication of Henoch–Schönlein purpura, which this patient does not have. Sarcoidosis (E) is common in the age and gender of this patient but primarily affects the lungs and lymph nodes. The key presenting complaint here is the muscle weakness and this would exclude sarcoidosis: http://emedicine.medscape.com/article/1170205-diagnosis

Lewy bodies

6   A   The alpha-synuclein protein is a major component of Lewy bodies. Its true function is unknown but its accumulation has a toxic effect on plasma membranes. In the rare cases of familial forms of Parkinson's disease (A), there is a mutation in the gene coding for alpha-synuclein and this condition is free of Lewy bodies. Patients with these mutations have a worse prognosis with earlier onset and non-responsiveness to levodopa. The alpha-synuclein protein can aggregate to form insoluble fibrils in pathological conditions characterized by Lewy bodies, such as idiopathic Parkinson's disease (E), Alzheimer's disease (B) and multiple system atrophy (C) (ruling them all out for being inconsistent with the case). Idiopathic Parkinson's disease is a degenerative disease with cell death of the dopamine-producing neurons of the substantia nigra, resulting in depigmentation. Furthermore, patients with this condition are alpha-synuclein and ubiquitin positive. Multiple sclerosis (D) often presents between the ages of 20 and 40 and is pathologically characterized by demyelinating plaques. It is also more common in females. The remaining diseases often present in an older patient.

Plaques of multiple sclerosis

7 B   Multiple sclerosis (MS) is the leading cause of disability in Western
        countries among young individuals between 20 and 40 years of age.
        The pathological hallmark of MS is the presence of demyelinating
        plaques on MRI scanning of the central nerves (spinal cord and brain).
        Particular things to look for are myelin loss, destruction of oligodendro-
        cytes, and reactive astrogliosis, often with relative sparing of the axon
        cylinder until later stages. The number of plaques, which range from a
        few to several hundreds, is indicative of the severity of the disease.

        According to the activity, the International Classification of Diseases
        classifies plaques as follows;

        Acute plaque (A): Minor changes (e.g. oedema) and often difficult to
        recognize
        Early chronic active plaque (B): Oedema and macrophages, indicative of
        an inflammatory disorder of the central nervous system, with some myelin
        breakdown. Reactive astrocytosis is present
        Late chronic active plaque (C): Complete loss of myelin. Some macrophages
        will contain myelin debris and there will be often very mild perivascular
        inflammation at this stage with enlarged perivascular spaces
        Chronic inactive plaque (D): Complete loss of myelin with the absence of
        macrophages
        Shadow plaque (E): Nearly complete remyelination as a thin myelin with some
        scattered macrophages and a mild microglial up-regulation.

Causes of dementia

8 B   Alzheimer's disease (AD) (B) accounts for 50–75 per cent of all cases
        of dementia in Western countries. Dementia is the progressive loss of
        cognitive function due to degeneration of the cerebral cortex. There is
        severe brain atrophy particularly prominent in the hippocampus and
        the frontal lobes and the brain weight is reduced to 1000 grams or
        less (normal average being 1400 grams). Histological hallmarks of the
        disease include senile plaques, which are complex spherical structures
        involving the grey matter and the aggregation of beta-amyloid appears
        to play a central role in developing the senile plaques. Neurofibrillary
        tangles are abnormal tangles in neuronal cell bodies of insoluble
        cytoskeletal-like tau protein. It is believed that the major antigenic com-
        ponent is the phosphorylated tau.

        Dementia with Lewy bodies (D) is another likely possibility for this
        patient and even though it can only be diagnosed at autopsy, cortical
        Lewy bodies will be prominent. This condition is believed to account for
        25 per cent of all dementias. The remaining three diseases (A, C, E) are

not often associated with dementia. Huntington's disease characteristically shows cerebral atrophy in the caudate nucleus and putamen and several changes in neurotransmitters. Multiple system atrophy is associated with glial cytoplasmic inclusion bodies (i.e. Papp–Lantos bodies). Parkinson's disease is characteristically associated with depigmentation of the substantia nigra.

Cell changes

9   C   The normal oesophagus is lined by stratified squamous epithelium and the squamo-columnar junction lies 2 cm above the gastro-oesophageal junction and is recognized by an irregular white line known as the Z line. Barrett's oesophagus occurs due to long standing reflux, and is the re-epithelialization by metaplastic columnar epithelium with goblet cells replacing normal squamous epithelium. This is known as metaplasia (C), which is the conversion from one type of differentiated tissue to another. It is reversible and often represents an adaptive response to environmental stress. Surveillance is crucial with repeated biopsy to detect a potential adenocarcinoma early, which is becoming more common than squamous cell carcinomas. Metaplasia can lead to dysplasia (D), which is an abnormal pre-malignant disordered pattern of growth. The cells are altered in size, shape and organization. If it leads to neoplasia (E), histologically there will be an abnormal proliferation and the process of tumour growth is detected.

Anaplasia (A) is defined as dedifferentiation or the reversion of differentiated cells and is characteristic of malignant neoplasms, implying loss of structure or function, which is not the case here. Hyperplasia (B) is a physiological proliferation and increase in the number of cells in a tissue or organ, which is not consistent with Barrett's oesophagus.

Gastritis

10   C   *Helicobacter pylori*-associated gastritis (C) is the most common form of chronic gastritis, accounting for 90 per cent of cases, and it is known that the pyloric antrum is the most severely affected area. An immune response is established and the infection may potentially persist for years. Around three-quarters of MALT (mucosa-associated lymphoid tissue) lymphoma or MALToma cases are associated with *H. pylori* infection. MALT is a system of small lymphoid tissue that regulates mucosal immunity and is present in a variety of organs in the body.

In addition to the infectious cause of chronic gastritis, there are two other forms. The autoimmune chronic gastritis (D) is associated with pernicious anaemia in the elderly and typically affects the body of the stomach. In reactive gastritis (E) the dominant feature is the epithelial change with minimal inflammation that can be idiopathic or due to reflux of bile-containing duodenal fluid or drugs. Acute gastritis (B) is often a superficial form resulting from ingested chemicals and hypotension, unlikely in this patient who appears to have a more chronic presentation. Menetrier's disease (A) is a rare disease characterized by gross hyperplasia of gastric pits and a marked increase in mucosal thickness and typically affects the fundus and body of the stomach.

Diseases of the exocrine pancreas

11   A   Chronic pancreatitis (A) causes irreversible loss of function. Histology shows chronic inflammation with parenchymal fibrosis, loss of pancreatic parenchymal elements and duct strictures with formation of intrapancreatic calculi. Jaundice may occur; it is a presenting feature in only a small proportion of patients and would be secondary to common bile duct obstruction during its course through the fibrosed head of the pancreas. Grossly, the pancreas is replaced by firm fibrous tissue within which are dilated ducts and areas of calcification. The pathogenesis of acute pancreatitis (D) is similar but with a lack of permanent impairment and often resolves with supportive therapy. Histologically it would only show acute inflammation and necrotic changes.

Carcinoma in the head of the pancreas (B) presents early with obstructive jaundice, which this patient does not have, despite the history of weight loss and epigastric pain. Diabetes mellitus type 2 (C) is a metabolic disorder, where patients may present with polyuria and polydipsia due to the chronic hyperglycaemia and not with severe epigastric pain. Pseudocysts (E) are collections of fluid and necrotic inflammatory debris in the pancreas that may be associated with acute or chronic pancreatitis but often resolve spontaneously.

Diseases of the endocrine pancreas

12   A   Diabetes mellitus type (1) (A) is an autoimmune disorder of childhood/ adolescent onset that is characterized by antibody-mediated destruction of beta-cells of the islets of Langerhans. Ninety to ninety-five per cent of patients are HLA DR3 and HLA DR4 positive. Type 1 diabetes can present with polyuria as in this case, or, if the polyuria is ignored, with diabetic ketoacidosis. The peak incidence of type 1 diabetes is 12–14 years, so the patient being young also makes this type 1 diabetes. Diabetes mellitus type 2 (D) is not an autoimmune disorder and has no HLA associations and the patient usually is a bit older. Type 2 diabetes used to be called "maturity asset diabetes", as it commonly affected people over the age of 50 years, although with the increase in obesity recently, patients are beginning to present with type 2 diabetes at a younger age, and in some patients, further tests are required before one can easily distinguish type 1 from type 2 diabetes. Patients with type 1 diabetes are GAD (glutamic Acid Decarboxylase Autoantibodies test) antibody positive, and this test

has superceded the HLA tissue type, which is not diagnostic. The diagnosis of diabetes mellitus is on the finding of hyperglycaemia. Diagnosis of diabetes mellitus is made with fasting venous plasma glucose levels of >7.0 mmol/L or a random venous plasma glucose level of >11.1 mmol/L.

Diabetes insipidus (B) is a disorder of the pituitary where there is either a failure of ADH production (cranial DI) or the renal distal tubules are refractory to the water reabsorptiveaction of ADH (nephrogenic DI). While both present with polyuria and polydipsia, DI is not related to plasma glucose levels. Psychogenic polydipsia (C) is excessive fluid intake with no organic pathology. It has been described in schizophrenics and young children with emotional difficulties. Zollinger–Ellison syndrome (E) is where there is gastric hypersecretion, multiple peptic ulcers and diarrhoea caused by gastric-secreting tumour of the pancreatic G cells. This may be part of MEN1 syndrome, with adenomas present in other endocrine glands.

Viral hepatitis

13   B   Hepatitis B (B) is a DNA virus of the Hepadna group. Transmission is commonly blood-borne but these can also be sexual and vertical transmission from mother to child. Most commonly, the infection can be asymptomatic with complete recovery, but also patients can develop acute or chronic hepatitis B infection. These patients always have a risk of developing chronic hepatitis. Hepatitis A (A) infection never causes chronic hepatitis.

Hepatitis C (C) is an RNA flavivirus that also shows predominantly blood-borne spread and is very common among intravenous drug abusers. A high percentage (70 per cent) will develop chronic hepatitis, increasing the life-long risk of cirrhosis and hepatocellular carcinoma. Hepatitis D (D) is an RNA virus that is incomplete and can only cause infection in the presence of hepatitis B virus. Hepatitis E (E) is an RNA virus that behaves in a similar fashion in terms of transmission and clinical features to hepatitis A virus.

Anti-mitochondrial antibodies

14   C   Primary biliary cirrhosis (C) is the destruction of the intrahepatic bile duct, often associated with an immune component, with anti-mitochondrial antibodies present in 90 per cent of cases and associations with other autoimmune diseases such as rheumatoid arthritis or scleroderma. Primary sclerosing cholangitis (A) also presents with obstructive jaundice and probably has an autoimmune element to it, but is very unlikely to show any autoantibodies. Sixty per cent of cases are associated with ulcerative colitis. Autoimmune hepatitis (B) is similar histologically to chronic viral hepatitis, and is associated with hyperglobulinaemia and anti-smooth muscle antibodies. Alpha-1 antitrypsin deficiency (D) is an inherited condition, where individuals fail to produce protease inhibitor alpha-1

antitrypsin. This can cause hepatitis in adults due to the accumulation of abnormal alpha-1 antitrypsin globules in the liver. Alcoholic liver disease (E) requires a history of alcohol abuse and the ethanol toxicity damages hepatocytes leading to fatty liver, acute hepatitis and cirrhosis.

Congenital metabolic disorders

15   A   Wilson's disease (A) is an autosomal recessive metabolic disorder that is caused by a mutation in the copper transport ATPase gene on chromosome 13. It results in failure of the liver to secrete the copper–ceruloplasmin complex into the plasma. This creates an overspill of copper into the blood that typically causes liver disease, central nervous system disease resembling Parkinson's disease and the characteristic development of brown discolouration around the cornea (Kayser–Fleischer rings). Genetic haemochromatosis (B) is excessive deposition of iron in tissues due to increased absorption of iron from the gut. Iron accumulates as haemosiderin in various organs giving them a rusty brown appearance, including hyperpigmentation of the skin. The diagnosis is based on the high saturation of transferrin in the blood, high serum iron and ferritin levels. Alpha-1 antitrypsin deficiency (C) is not known to affect the central nervous system, but may cause chronic hepatitis and cirrhosis due to accumulation of the abnormal alpha-1 antitrypsin globules in the liver. Reye's syndrome (D) often occurs following an upper respiratory tract infection and was thought to occur in children exposed to aspirin. It is rare and presents with acute encephalopathy secondary to severe impairment of liver function. Budd–Chiari syndrome (E) is the rare condition that is characterized by the occlusion of the main hepatic vein due to either local compression or thrombosis, or is idiopathic.

Gastrointestinal diseases in children

16   B   Congenital aganglionic megacolon, also known as Hirschsprung's disease (B), is believed to be due to the absence of ganglion cells in the myenteric plexus causing the failure of the dilation of the distal colon. Macroscopically, there is narrowing of an abnormally innervated bowel segment yet dilation and muscular hypertrophy of the bowel segment proximal to this. Microscopically, there is an absence of normal myenteric and submucosal plexus ganglion cells. The condition often presents in early childhood with symptoms of colonic obstruction. There has been a reported association of this condition with Down syndrome.

Stenosis (A) implies incomplete obstruction, while atresia (C) implies complete obstruction. Both are rare in the colon but more commonly found in the duodenum and small intestine. Intussusception (D) occurs when one portion of the bowel invaginates into the adjoining segment, most commonly at the ileoceacal valve. Bleeding takes place due to the venous congestion of the invaginated portion, which this patient does not have signs of. Volvulus (E) is a type of mechanical disorder, where there is complete twisting of a loop of bowel at the mesenteric base causing obstruction and infarction and severe pain on presentation.

Colitis

17 B   Ulcerative colitis (B) is inflammation affecting the rectum and colon only in a contiguous fashion. There are many extra-intestinal manifestations including arthritis, myositis, uveitis/iritis, erythema nodosum, pyoderma gangrenosum and primary sclerosing cholangitis. Crohn's disease (A), on the other hand, can affect any region of the gastrointestinal tract with 'skip lesions'. It is also associated with transmural inflammation and non-caseating granulomas, which this patient does not have evidence of. Wall is thickened and described as 'rubber-hose' and 'cobblestone mucosa'. Ulcers tend to be linear and the lumen is narrowed. Extra-intestinal manifestations are also common in Crohn's disease.

Ischaemic colitis (C) is the most common vascular disorder of the intestinal tract and usually occurs in segments in 'watershed zones' such as the splenic flexure or the rectosigmoid flexure. It may be transmural and may lead to perforation. Pseudomembranous colitis (D) is a type of bacterial enterocolitis caused by the protein exotoxins of *Clostridium difficile*. The necrosis of the colonic mucosa characteristically causes the formation of a pseudomembrane. Patients develop fever, abdominal pain and diarrhoea. Viral gastroenteritis (E) is the most common in children and infants and typically presents with cramps, vomiting and fever but no blood in stools.

Neoplastic disease of the intestine

18 D   Hereditary non-polyposis colorectal cancer (HNPCC) (D) is an uncommon autosomal dominant disease but the cancers are poorly differentiated and highly aggressive, therefore screening for identification of carriers for surveillance is necessary. Familial adenomatous polyposis (FAP) (A) is also a rare autosomal dominant condition that is caused by a mutation in the *FAP* gene on chromosome 5. It is characterized by the presence of adenomata in the large bowel, which this patient did not have, yet also carries a 90 per cent risk of developing into carcinoma by the age of 45. Gardner's syndrome (B) is similar clinically, pathologically and aetiologically to FAP and also carries a high carcinoma risk. However, there are very distinct extra-intestinal manifestations of Gardner's syndrome, including multiple osteomas of the skull and mandible, epidermoid cysts and desmoid tumours. Colorectal carcinoma (C) of the sporadic type is inconsistent with the history and age of the patient, as it is more commonly present in patients over the age of 60. Hamartomatous polyps (E) often present in childhood or adolescence as part of Peutz–Jeghers syndrome and these carry a small risk of carcinomas. Patients also tend to have pigmented lesions around the mouth that are characteristic of this condition.

Hydrosalpinx

19 D   Salpingitis (pelvic inflammatory disease; D) is inflammation of the fallopian tubes that is almost always caused by infection, in particular
sexually transmitted infections including chlamydia, mycoplasma and
gonococcus. Other related infections, such as an actinomyces infection,
are associated with intrauterine contraceptive device use. Hydrosalpinx,
a complication of salpingitis, is the dilation of the fallopian tube that is
thin-walled and contains clear fluid. This is believed to be a sequel to
previous inflammatory damage to the tube. The scarring sequelae are
believed to include plical fusion, adhesions to the ovary, tubo-ovarian
abscess, peritonitis, hydrosalpinx, infertility and ectopic pregnancy.

Endometriosis (A) occurs when endometrial glands develop outside
the uterus and is associated with development of fibrous adhesions. It
may develop in the fallopian tube but will not cause a hydrosalpinx
and is not often associated with a history of an infectious episode.
Adenomyosis (B) is a disorder of the uterus whereby the endometrium
grows to develop deep within the myometrium. Cervical intraepithelial
neoplasia (C) is a pre-neoplastic (dysplastic) proliferation of epithelium
of the transformation zone of the cervix. This is strongly associated
with human papillomavirus (E) infection, particularly serotypes 16
and 18.

Gynaecological tumours

20 C   Leiomyoma (C), also called fibroids, is a benign smooth muscle tumour
arising in the myometrium. They are the most common of all pelvic
tumours, presenting often in women over 30 years of age and are more
common in nulliparous and Afro-Caribbean women. The presentation
often involves multiple large rounded nodules. They are well circumscribed with a pseudocapsule that may become pedunculated forming
polyps.

Cervical intraepithelial neoplasia (A) is a dysplastic transformation
at the cervix; it is associated with HPV infection and does not present as nodules in the myometrium, nor with dysmenorrhoea. Vulval
carcinoma (B) is often squamous and associated with HPV 16 infection and does not present with internal symptoms such as dysmenorrhoea. Endometrial carcinoma (D) is malignant and more common
in postmenopausal women. There is a hyperoestrogenic form and a
non-hyperoestrogenic form, with superficial invasion of the myometrium and deep invasion respectively. The condition classically presents
with postmenopausal bleeding and not dysmenorrhoea. CGIN (E) is
a rare disorder of the cervix that is difficult to diagnose and manage
and may compromise fertility of the patient but does not involve the
myometrium.

Ovarian tumours

21 A Teratoma (A) is a common benign cyst that contains all three embryonic germ cell layers and this is a torsion presentation which is the most common complication of teratomas. In mature cases there have been reports of teratomas containing features such as hair, teeth, bone and eyes. As they are encapsulated, teratomas are usually benign but may rarely undergo malignant change in postmenopausal women. Serous, mucinous and endometrioid tumours (B, C, D) are epithelial ovarian tumours where serous tumours differentiate to mimic tubal epithelium, mucinous tumours differentiate to mimic endocervical or intestinal wall and endometrioid tumours mimic the endometrium. Pseudomyxoma peritonei, metastases from the appendix, are sometimes a characteristic feature of mucinous tumours. Clear cell carcinomas (E) are uncommon and tend to be malignant with a poor prognosis. As the name suggest, they have a clear cytoplasm and are often associated with endometriosis.

Peripheral blood film

22 C Features of iron deficiency anaemia are hypochromic (pale) and microcytic (small) red blood cells. Poikilocytes are red blood cells that are abnormally shaped. When there are variations in shape and size, it is known as anisopoikilocytosis. Basophilic stippling (aggregation of ribosomal material) is absent in iron deficiency and present in β-thalassaemia trait and lead poisoning.

In megaloblastic anaemia, there is impaired DNA synthesis and this can be caused by B_{12} deficiency, folate deficiency and drugs. Here the features are the characteristic hypersegmented neutrophils and macrocytic red blood cells.

In hyposplenism, there is presence of target cells known as codocytes (red blood cells that have a high surface area:volume ratio). Acanthocytes (spiculated blood cells/spur cells) and Howell–Jolly bodies (nuclear remnants visible in red cells) are also present in the hyposplenism picture.

Coeliac disease

23 D The following investigations are key in diagnosing coeliac disease: inflammatory markers (CRP and ESR), current serological tests (anti-endomysial antibodies and anti-tissue transglutaminase antibodies), and upper GI endoscopy and distal duodenal biopsies.

There are four serological investigations for coeliac disease; two are out-dated because of non-specificity and unreliability (anti-reticulin antibodies and anti-gliadin antibodies) and two are currently used (anti-endomysial antibodies and anti-tissue transglutaminase antibodies). The IgA autoantibody to endomysial cells is both specific and sensitive, however interpretation requires considerable operator expertise. The most sensitive (at 90–94 per cent) and specific (~95 per cent) for coeliac disease is said to be the IgA anti-tissue transglutaminase (anti-TTG) antibody.

The endoscopy, if positive, will show mucosal folds and lack of villi. Histopathology will show villous atrophy, crypt hyperplasia, and increased intraepithelial lymphocytes. Normally, enterocytes are constantly shed from the tips of the villi and replenished by migration of cells up the villi from the proliferative compartment in the crypts. With higher rates of cell loss, a stage is soon reached when the increased proliferative compartment (evidenced by elongation, hypercellularity and high mitotic activity of the crypts) cannot maintain a normal number of maturing and functioning 'end cells', the size of this compartment diminishes and villous atrophy results. This degenerate epithelial surface is infiltrated by large numbers of T lymphocytes, which are further enhanced by the local production of TNF-alpha.

Non-neoplastic bone tumours

24 B Fibrous dysplasia (B) is a benign disorder of children and young adults, whereby lesions composed of fibrous and bony tissue develop usually in the ribs, femur, tibia or skull. It mostly presents as bone pain and weakness in female patients under 30 years of age and results from congenital dysplasia of bone, consistent with the patient's history. There are three forms: the more common monostotic form (lesions localized to only one bone), polyostotic (multiple lesions) and McCune–Albright syndrome, which also has endocrine manifestations. Shepherd's crook deformity refers to a varus angulation of the proximal femur commonly seen in the femoral involvement of polyostotic fibrous dysplasia. Histologically, it is characterized by loose fibrous tissue with metaplastic immature or woven bone trabeculae arranged in a 'Chinese letters' formation.

Non-ossifying fibroma (A) is often asymptomatic and merely an incidental finding on X-ray and occurs in an even younger group of patients. Ossifying fibroma (D) is a benign, fibrous tumour with reactive bone formation that shows local aggressive behaviour. Lesions are found in the mandible for adults, and the tibia for children. Giant-cell reparative granuloma (C) is an uncommon benign reactive intraosseous lesion and can occur in the skull, jaw, hand and foot. The histology resembles giant cell tumour of bone (see below). A simple bone cyst (E) is common in the proximal metaphysis of the humerus and asymptomatic unless there has been a fracture.

Benign bone tumours

25 E Enchondroma (E) is a benign intramedullary cartilage tumour usually
found in the central mature hyaline cartilage of the short tubular bones
of the hands and feet. It may present at any age (average is 40 years)
and is often asymptomatic, but some patients present with pain, fracture
or swelling of the affected area. There are lytic lesions on X-rays that
usually contain variably calcified chondriod matrix and histopathological findings showing bluish-grey lobules of hyaline cartilege. There may
be a thin layer of lamellar bone surrounding the cartilage nodules but
no permeation of pre-existing host bone which is a positive sign that the
lesion is benign. Each potential enchondroma needs to be evaluated on
imaging and histology to distinguish it from low-grade chondrosarcoma.

Osteochondroma (A) is the most common skeletal neoplasm, often affecting boys in their teens and often found in the long bones. When the
growth plates close in late adolescence, there is usually no further growth
of the osteochondroma. There is a low risk of malignancy in osteochon-
dromas associated with syndromes that involve multiple lesions such as
Ollier's disease or Maffucci's syndrome. Osteoid osteoma (C) is a small,
benign lesion surrounded by a zone of reactive bone. It mostly occurs in
the long bones, with a very distinct clinical picture in that pain is dull,
worse at night and relieved by aspirin. Similar radiology and histology
are seen in osteoblastomatomours that are larger than 1 cm diameter and
that commonly affect the vertebrae. Pathological fracture is a common
presentation of giant cell tumour (D), which is more common in females,
is locally aggressive and can metastasize. It does not occur in the immature skeleton. It is more common in the metaphysics of the long bones,
especially the distal femur and proximal tibia. There is no calcification
on X-ray and, histologically, there would be numerous multinucleated
giant cells. The mono-nuclear cell population is the neoplastic cells.
Multiple myeloma (B) is highly unlikely as it is a different classification
of bone tumours altogether and is considered as a blood cell malignancy
rather than a primary bone tumour. It is a malignant tumour of plasma
cells that causes widespread osteolytic bone damage. It may be in are
bone only when it is known as plasmacytoma rather than myeloma.

Malignant bone tumours

26 A Osteosarcoma (A) is the most common primary bone malignancy that is
aggressive with poor prognosis (60 per cent of patients with 5-year survival). The vast majority of these tumours occur in teenagers and young
adults. The most common presentation is pain and a mass, which occurs
near a joint such as the knee, with the distal femur and proximal tibia
being the most common sites. X-rays show a mixed sclerotic and lytic
lesion in the metaphysis that may permeate the bone causing a soft tissue

mass and a periosteal reaction. Bone formation within the tumour is characteristic of osteosarcoma and is usually visible on X-rays. Bone alkaline phosphatase has significant value in diagnosing osteosarcoma, also indicating chemotherapy effectiveness and prognosis.

Chondrosarcomas (B) usually affect older patients. The prognosis is variable depending on the grade of tumour. They usually grow slowly and not only affect long bones but also the ribs, spine and pelvis. The only treatment is surgical excision as both chemotherapy and radiotherapy are ineffective. Fibrosarcomas (C) and malignant fibrous histiocytomas (D) are both spindle cell malignant tumours, arising from stromal cells and collectively they make up the majority of soft tissue sarcomas. Ewing's sarcoma (E) is one of the family of malignant small round cell tumours. It affects children and teenagers and has a characteristic chromosomal translocation (t11;22)(q24;q12). It is negative for alkaline phosphatase and positive for CD99 (MIC2) immunostain. It is more commonly found in the pelvis and diaphysis/metaphysis of long bones than around the knee. Widespread metastases and bone marrow involvement are frequent.

NHS cervical screening programme

27 E   Liquid based cytology (E) is an important method of preparing cervical samples for examination under the microscope. The sample is collected in the standard brushings method using a spatula but rather than smearing the sample onto a microscope slide as before, the head of the spatula is broken off into a small glass vial containing preservative fluid. This is then sent to the laboratory and obscuring material, e.g. mucus and pus, is removed and a representative sample of cells is deposited onto a slide for examination. The vial can also be tested for the human papillomavirus and other sexually transmitted diseases. Fine needle aspiration with or without ultrasound (A, B) is only suitable for lesions that are easily palpable by hand or easily detected via imaging; common sites include breast, thyroid and lymph nodes. They are not suitable for cervical samples. Washings (C) and brushings (D) are types of exfoliative cytology. This is used when cells are dislodged or spontaneously shed such as bronchial washings. The use of the spatula in the smear test is a form of brushing but liquid based cytology involves a crucial additional component that brings many benefits to patients and staff, including quicker results and fewer inadequate tests.

Obstructive lung disease

28 A   Obstructive lung disease is characterized by airway obstruction and a decreased FEV1/FVC ratio. Chronic obstructive pulmonary disease (COPD) includes chronic bronchitis (A) and emphysema (E). While the two often coexist, a predominantly chronic bronchitis cough produces

copious amounts of sputum, and infection is consistent with this patient, while sputum and infection are only occasional in emphysema. Chronic bronchitis is the damage caused to the airways/bronchi and the clinical definition is productive cough for at least 3 months per year for 2 consecutive years. Histopathology shows hypertrophy of mucous glands and goblet cell hyperplasia. Emphysema is alveolar parenchymal damage by activation of proteases (elastase) that are in turn activated by neutrophil/macrophage action secondary to cigarette smoking. Emphysema patients only have dyspnoea and no associated cough with no mucus excess. COPD is characteristically poorly reversible and gets progressively worse over time, consistent with this patient's presentation. In contrast, asthma (C) causes episodic wheezing, cough and dyspnoea. There is excessive mucus secretion in asthma, which poses a risk of mucus plug formation that can be fatal. Charcot–Leyden crystals indicative of eosinophilic inflammation would be found in these patients as the condition is under the allergic/immunological diseases umbrella. Pulmonary embolus (B) is not an obstructive lung disorder but vascular. Its presentation is acute with pleuritic chest pain and progressive dyspnoea. Bronchiolitis (D) is a paediatric presentation and the inflammation is often caused by a virus, e.g. respiratory syncytial virus.

Pneumonia

29 A Lobar pneumonia is one of two anatomical classifications of pneumonia, the other being bronchopneumonia. In up to 95 per cent of cases, the causative organism for lobar pneumonia is *Streptococcus pneumoniae* (A) type 1, 2, 3, and 7. The stages of pneumonia start with congestion in the first 24 hours; lobes are heavy, red and boggy due to hyperaemia, intra-alveolar fluid with scattered neutrophils and many bacteria. The second stage is red hepatization, with the lobe's transformation to a liver-like mass, characteristic of lobar pneumonia. The red hepatization is blood-stained pulmonary exudate with many intra-alveolar neutrophils. Grey hepatization is when the lung is dry and firm because the red cells disintegrate and fibrinosuppurative exudates persist within the alveoli. Finally, the resolution stage involves the enzymatic digestion of the exudates in the alveoli and normal architecture remerges. Pneumococcial infection can also cause bronchopneumonia, along with other low virulence organisms: *Staphylococcus aureus* (B), *Haemophilus influenzae* (C), *Streptococcus pyogenes* (D). Bronchopneumonia is more likely in patients with a compromised host defence system (e.g. elderly) and the pathology demonstrates a patchy bronchial and peribronchial distribution in the lower lobes. *Mycobacterium tuberculosis* (E) is the cause of tuberculosis, which is an infectious granulomatous disease. A granuloma is a collection of histiocytes and macrophages with or without multinucleate giant cells.

Diffuse alveolar damage

30 B Acute respiratory distress syndrome (ARDS) (B) is a severe lung disease often developing with 24–48 hours post trauma, burns or sepsis. It is characterized by inflammation in the lung parenchyma impairing gas exchange and is therefore responsible for this patient's symptoms. A less severe form is acute lung injury. Diffuse alveolar damage (DAD) is most commonly associated with ARDS. Pulmonary oedema (A) is fluid accumulation within the alveolar spaces and interstitium but no damage is caused. These patients also present with shortness of breath. Crytogenic fibrosing alveolitis (C) is a form of fibrosing lung disease that is chronic and progressive. It presents with shortness of breath and cough and is more likely to be seen in males over the age of 50. On histopathology, fibrosis and cyst formation are seen. Bronchiectasis (D) is the permanent abnormal dilatation of bronchi and is very common in children in a post-infectious episode. The complications associated with it include recurrent infections, haemoptysis and pulmonary hypertension. Chronic bronchitis (E) is defined as a chronic cough productive of sputum, for at least 3 months during a 2-year period. On histopathology, there is dilatation of airways and goblet cell hyperplasia.

Respiratory disease (1)

31 B Squamous cell carcinoma (B) is one type of lung cancer within the non-small cell lung carcinoma (NSCLC) group. This type of cancer is most closely associated with a history of tobacco smoking and is more common in men. These tumours, if well-differentiated, show keratin pearls and cell junctions (or desmosomes), which form the characteristic intercellular 'prickles'. TB (A) is a granulomatous disease, whereby the histopathology shows a granuloma consisting of a collection of histiocytes/macrophages and/or multinucleate giant cells. Mesothelioma (C) is a malignant tumour of the pleura and is associated with asbestos exposure decades earlier. Emphysema (D) is unlikely in this case as it does not cause haemoptysis and weight loss. Histopathology shows permanent loss of the alveolar parenchyma distal to the terminal bronchiole and two key causes are cigarette smoking and alpha-1 antitrypsin deficiency. Large cell carcinoma (E) is another type of NSCLC that is undifferentiated and diagnosis is made by exclusion of other tumour cells as there is no characteristic histological evidence.

Respiratory disease (2)

32 B Adenocarcinoma (B) is the most common type of lung cancer in non-smokers and is usually seen in the periphery in the lungs, as opposed to small cell lung carcinoma (A) and squamous cell lung cancer, which both tend to be more centrally located. Adenocarcinomas often metastasize and are not as responsive to chemotherapy as small cell lung carcinomas.

The precursor of adenocarcinomas is termed atypical adenomatous hyperplasia (AAH) and this involves the proliferation of atypical cells lining the alveolar walls. Later they increase in size and become invasive. Small cell carcinoma has a very close association with smoking and paraneoplastic syndromes and is very chemo-sensitive. They are poorly differentiated and the mutations commonly involved are p53 and RB1. Large cell carcinoma (C) is unlikely in this patient as histopathology would not show any characteristics or evidence of glandular differentiation. Sarcoidosis (D) is a granulomatous multi-organ disease and surgery is not the mode of treatment. Pneumoconiosis (E) is a type of fibrosing lung disease or 'dusty lung' caused by inorganic dust inhalation. It commonly affects the upper lobes, while asbestosis affects the lower lobes more severely. It is an alteration of the lung structure rather than neoplastic differentiation of cells and is therefore unlikely to be the diagnosis for this patient.

Erythema multiforme

33   B   Erythema multiforme is a pleomorphic skin eruption, with macules, papules, urticarial weals, vesicles and bullae. Its severest life-threatening form is related to Stevens–Johnson syndrome (B), believed to be mediated by the deposition of immune complexes in the microvasculature of the skin and oral mucous membranes following certain drugs, foods or infections. Systemic lupus erythematosus (A) is much more common in females (ratio of 9:1) and patients develop the characteristic butterfly rash on the face. The systemic form affects the skin and internal organs, but discoid lupus erythematosus is a skin condition that presents with red, inflamed patches with scaling and a crusty appearance on the face, ears and scalp. Pemphigoid (C) tends to present in the elderly with large tense bullae on flexor aspects of the forearms, groin and axillae, and histopathology reveals numerous eosinophils. IgG binds to basement membranes in pemphigoid (subepidermal bullae) but to desmosomes in pemphigus (intra-epidermal bullae). Pityriasis rosea (D) is a salmon-pink scaly eruption on the trunk with the characteristic herald patch (a larger start lesion) and may be associated with a viral infection. Contact dermatitis (E) is a localized skin reaction resulting from exposure and contact with an allergen/irritant, which this patient's presentation lacks. The rash varies in severity from a red rash to blisters/weals to itchy burning skins.

Skin tumours

34   A   Malignant melanoma (A) is the most life-threatening and aggressive form of skin tumour and must be monitored closely and treated assertively. It is key to examine for the 'ABCDE': asymmetry, border irregularity, colour, diameter and environment. The BRESLOW scale is used to quantify the tumour thickness and determine prognosis. Basal cell carcinoma (B) often presents as a 'rodent ulcer' on the face

that is locally destructive and is described to have a pearly edge with telangiectasia and central ulceration. Bowen's disease (E) is a sunlight-induced skin disease that is considered to be a predisposing factor for squamous cell carcinoma (C). Squamous cell carcinoma (SCC) of the skin begins as a small nodule that may become ulcerated and necrotic. Bleeding is quite common and the clinical presentation is highly variable. Keratoacanthoma (D) is a benign lesion that is rapidly growing and dome-shaped. It arises from the pilosebaceous glands and often resembles SCC. However, the growth of a keratoacanthoma retains its smooth surface, unlike an SCC and a malignant melanoma. Bowen's disease presents as an enlarging well-demarcated erythematous plaque with an irregular border but non-elevated. It is essentially an SCC *in situ*.

Inflammatory conditions

35 C Dermatitis herpetiformis (C) is a chronic blistering skin condition associated with gluten intolerance or coeliac disease. The itchy papulovesicular eruptions are distributed symmetrically on extensor surfaces. Gluten intake will exacerbate the symptoms. Psoriasis (A) affects 2 per cent of the UK population and also presents on the extensor aspects of limbs, and on nails and scalp. The most common form is psoriasis vulgaris, presenting with macules and papules covered with silvery scales (characteristic parakeratosis) and pinpoint bleeding. It is associated with arthritis. There is also a loss of granular layer, clubbing of rete ridges and Munro's microabscesses. Ezcema's histopathology is spongiosis of epidermis and perivascular chronic inflammatory infiltrate in the dermis. Acanthosis (epidermal thickening) would develop if eczema becomes chronic. Atopic eczema (B) has a strong family history and association with asthma and not gluten sensitivity. Seborrhoeic dermatitis (E) is a type of eczema that affects the apocrine areas of the face; sometimes known as the cradle cap in infants in severe forms (with lack of biotin causing a thick yellow crusty scalp rash). Lichen planus (D) is the eruption of purple flat-topped papules affecting the skin, tongue and oral mucosa. There is characteristic hyperkeratosis with saw toothing of rete ridges and basal cell degeneration with a lichenoid chronic inflammatory infiltrate.

Types of fractures

36 E Comminuted fractures (E) are also known as segmental fractures whereby the bone is splintered and a number of pieces are visible but with intact soft tissue. A greenstick fracture (A) is specifically a paediatric problem where the fracture is transverse, but only partially, and therefore the bone bends away from the long axis but remains attached. A transverse fracture (B) is a fracture that is at right angles to the bone's long axis and may be partial or complete (cortex to cortex). It is often a simple clean break with intact soft tissue. A compound fracture (C) is

when the fracture penetrates the skin surface and it is also known as an open fracture. These pose a very serious risk of infection due to contamination of the wound and exposed fracture. Impacted fracture (D) is when the fracture site is 'crushed' inwards.

Non-neoplastic bone disease

37 A Osteoathritis (A) affects mainly the vertebrae, hips, knees, distal interphalangeal joints, carpometacarpal and metatarsophalangeal joints. The presentation of this patient is typical of osteoarthritis. Rheumatoid arthritis (B) is severe chronic relapsing synovitis that often presents in a younger population than this patient (30–40 years of age). Eighty per cent of patients are rheumatoid factor positive and characteristic deformities include ulnar deviation of the fingers, swan-neck and Boutonniere deformity of the fingers and a 'Z'-shaped thumb. It characteristically spares the distal interphalangeal joint and affects symmetrically the small joints in the hands and feet, wrists, elbows, ankles and knees. Histopathology shows proliferative synovitis with thickening of the synovial membranes, hyperplasia of surface synoviocytes, intense inflammatory cell infiltrate and fibrin deposition and necrosis. Ankylosing spondylitis (C) is a chronic inflammatory arthritis with strong HLA B27 association affecting the spine and sacroilium that can cause eventual fusion of the spine (bamboo spine). It commonly presents in a male aged 20–40 with stiffness of the spine. In addition to joint involvement, psoriatic arthritis (D) will commonly present with psoriatic nail lesions (pitting, onycholysis), dactylitis and tendinitis. X-rays will show 'new fluffy' bone. Osteoporosis (E) would show osteopenia, cortical thinning and increased radiolucency in the X-rays.

Painful joint

38 D Only two conditions out of the five cause crystal-induced arthritis: gout and pseudogout. Gout (D) affects the big toe in 90 per cent of cases and needle-shaped crystals occur in the joint causing very severe pain. One might also see tophi, which are of monosodium glutamate precipitate in pathognoic for gout where monosodium urate crystals are deposited under the skin. Monosodium urate crystals are negatively bi-refringent when viewed using a polarising microscope. Pseudogout (A) is the calcium crystal deposition disease, either calcium pyrophosphate or calcium phosphate (hydroxyapatite). Chondrocalcinosis is seen on X-rays and the most commonly affected joint is the knee. On microscopic investigation with crossed polarizing filters of joint fluid obtained by aspiration, rhombus-shaped, positively birefringent crystals are seen.

Lyme disease (B) is an inflammatory arthropathy resulting from a tick bite, caused by *Borrelia burgdorferi*. The associated skin rash is erythema chronicum migrans and arthritis develops only in advanced disease.

Reiter's syndrome (C) characteristically presents following an infectious episode with the triad reactive arthritis, uveitis and urethritis. Reactive arthritis is a rheumatoid factor-seronegative, HLA B27-linked spondyloarthopathy commonly affecting the larger joints (e.g. sacroiliac and knee joints). Patients also sometimes develop circinate balanitis, keratoderma blenorrhagica and enthesitis of the Achilles tendon (causing heel pain). Osteomyelitis (E) in the big toe in adults is often secondary to diabetic skin ulcer, which this patient does not have.

Renal disease

39 D Acute pyelonephritis (D) is strongly indicated if white cell casts are present. Red cell casts are strongly suggestive of glomerulonephritis. Eosinophiluria is strongly suggestive of tubulointerstitial nephritis.

Most cases of pyelonephritis begin as lower urinary tract infections, including cystitis (A) and prostatitis (B), but given the pain distribution and presentation of this patient, it is much more likely to be infection of the left kidney (pyelonephritis). Urolithiasis (C) can cause the pain and haematuria present in this patient but it does not explain the fever and rigors as this condition is not caused by infection but by four types of calculi: calcium, triple phosphate/struvite, uric acid and cystine. However, these are likely to predispose to infection. Hydronephrosis (E) can present acutely with sudden onset severe pain or a more chronic presentation as episodes of dull discomfort. Nausea and vomiting may occur but it is unlikely to cause fever or rigors unless the blocking of urine flow results in a urinary tract infection.

Urological neoplasia

40 B Wilm's tumour (B) (nephroblastoma) is a malignant embryonic tumour derived from the primitive metanephros. It is the most common childhood urological malignancy and involves mutations of the tumour suppressor gene *WT1* located on chromosome 11. Macroscopically, the kidney is replaced by rounded masses of solid, fleshy, white lesions with vast amounts of necrosis. Microscopically, it is composed of four elements: immature-looking glomerular structures, primitive small cell blastaematous tissue, epithelial tubules and stroma composed of spindle cells and striated muscle.

Teratoma (A) is a tumour of germ cell origin involving the endoderm, ectoderm and mesoderm, with a peak age of onset of 20–30 years. Oncocytoma (C) is a benign epithelial tumour composed of large cells with granular, eosinophilic cytoplasm filled with mitochondria. It has little necrosis or haemorrhage. It is a variant of renal adenoma and is often confused with renal cell carcinoma. Spermatocytic seminoma (D) is a germ cell malignant tumour of the testes, with a peak age between 30 and 40 years of age. Histopathology shows large tumour cells with small cells resembling spermatocytes. Bowen's disease (E) is one of two types of penile carcinoma *in situ*, often associated with human papillomavirus infection and clinically appears as opaque plaques with shallow ulcerations.

Gleason's grading system

41 A Prostatic adenocarcinoma (A) is rare in men under 50 years of age. The gross histopathology involves the peripheral portion of prostate, posteriorly. It is poorly demarcated, firm and yellow and there may be urinary bladder, seminal vesicle and rectal invasion. The Gleason's scoring system is used to help evaluate the prognosis of men with prostate cancer. The pathologist assigns a grade to the most common tumour pattern and a second grade to the worst pattern, then the two grades are added together to get the Gleason score.

Seminoma (B) is the most common malignant testicular tumour and often presents as a painless swelling. Prostatic intraepithelial neoplasia (C) is a common finding in younger men and poses an increased risk for developing carcinoma. Benign prostatic hyperplasia (D) is a non-neoplastic enlargement of the prostate, which is very common and affects almost all men over 70 years of age. The treatment for benign prostatic hyperthrophy is different to malignant disease, and includes alpha blockers, and drugs to reduce intra-prostatic dihydrotestosterone. Less radical surgery such as TURP is commonly used. Transitional cell carcinoma (E) can arise anywhere in the bladder, with a significant association to smoking and chemical exposure. Clinically, there should be evidence of haematuria, previous cystitis and obstruction.

Non-neoplastic disorders of the breast

42 B Acute mastitis (B) is the acute inflammation of the breast that often affects lactating women. The usual causative organism is *Staphylococcus aureus*. An abscess may develop and drainage and antibiotics are curative. Fat necrosis (A) is an inflammatory reaction to trauma of the adipose tissue in the breast and histopathology shows necrosis with multinucleated giant cells and later fibrosis. It may present as a discrete firm lump mimicking a carcinoma. Duct ectasia (C) usually presents with nipple discharge and is due to inflammation and dilation of the large breast ducts. There may also be a breast mass and nipple retraction. Simple fibrocystic change (D) is not an inflammatory disorder but a fibrocystic disorder. It is very common and presents with breast lumpiness and nodularity which may be cyclical, representing exaggerated hormonal responses. Epithelial hyperplasia (E) is also a fibrocystic disorder that describes epithelial cell proliferation within the ducts or lobules in the breast, which increases risk of developing malignancy. It can only be diagnosed by histopathology.

Neoplasms of the breast (1)

43   A   Intraductal papilloma (A) is a benign papillary tumour arising within the duct system of the breast. The two forms are peripheral (arise within small terminal ductules) and central (arise in larger lactiferous ducts). Only central papillomas can present with nipple discharge that is blood stained, while peripheral papillomas can remain clinically silent.

A fibroadenoma (C) is a benign fibroepithelial neoplasm of the breast that is common and presents as a circumscribed mobile breast lump in younger women (aged 20–30). Phylloides tumours (B) are a group of potentially aggressive fibroepithelial neoplasms of the breast, they are uncommon and present as enlarging masses in women aged over 50. Some could have been pre-existing fibroadenomas. A radial scar (D) is a benign sclerosing lesion characterized by a central zone of scarring surrounded by a radiating zone of proliferating glandular tissue. They are common and usually present as stellate masses on screening mammograms. Ductal carcinoma *in situ* (E) has an inherent risk of progression to invasive breast carcinoma. Only 10 per cent produce clinical features such as a lump, nipple discharge or an eczematous change of the nipple (Paget's disease of the nipple).

Neoplasms of the breast (2)

44   D   Invasive breast carcinomas (D) are a group of malignant epithelial tumours which infiltrate within the breast and have capacity to spread to distant sites. The risk factors include: early menarche, late menopause, increased weight, high alcohol consumption, oral contraceptive use and a positive family history. *BRCA* mutations are known to cause a lifetime risk of invasive breast carcinoma of up to 85 per cent. The types of invasive carcinomas include: invasive ductal carcinoma, invasive lobular carcinoma, mucinous, tubular, medullary and papillary. Ductal carcinoma *in situ* (DCIS) is a form of non-invasive breast carcinoma.

The screening programme in the UK is a 3-yearly mammography for all women between 50 and 70 years of age. Those with an abnormal mammogram (5 per cent) are recalled for further investigation, which may include more mammograms or an ultrasound followed by sampling of the abnormal area, usually by core biopsy. The histology core biopsy codes are:

- B1 = normal breast tissue.
- B2 = benign abnormality (A)
- B3 = lesion of uncertain malignant potential (B)
- B4 = suspicious of malignancy (E)
- B5 = malignant
- B5a = ductal carcinoma *in situ* (C)
- B5b = invasive carcinoma

Cystic diseases of the kidneys

45 C Adult polycystic kidney disease (C) is an autosomal dominant condition, believed to involve two genes: PKD1 and PKD2. Both kidneys are replaced by fluid-filled cysts. It is asymptomatic initially, but in the fourth decade or later, the patient presents with a large lobulated abdominal mass, pain or haematuria. It is managed by blood pressure control and eventually dialysis or transplantation.

Acquired cystic disease (A) occurs in patients who are an dialysis and therefore inconsistent with this clinical picture. That does not mean that dialysis causes cysts. The cause is, in fact, not clear, but it seems that dialysis does not clear a circulating factor that causes such cysts. Without dialysis, these individuals would not survive, which is why patients on dialysis for long periods are those who have such cysts. Medullary sponge disease (B) is occasionally a familial condition that does not impair renal function and presents with renal stones predisposing to renal colic and infections. Cystic renal dysplasia (D) is a failure of differentiation of metanephric tissues, it is typically asymptomatic and it is not hereditary in nature but developmental, therefore often presenting in childhood. Simple renal cysts (E) are lesions in otherwise normal kidneys that can be solitary or occasionally multiple. They are typically asymptomatic and are acquired.

Glomerular disease

46 D Pauci-immune crescent glomerulonephritis (D) is associated with antineutrophil cytoplasm antibodies (ANCA) and vasculitis in other systems such as the skin and lungs. This patient has glomerulonephritis that is sufficient to cause acute renal failure and therefore is almost certain to be associated with glomerular crescents.

IgA nephropathy (A) is a cause of immune-complex crescentic glomerulonephritis, the key feature being immune complexes detected by immunohistochemistry and electron microscopy. IgA nephropathy is the most common form of glomerulonephritis worldwide, where there is a predominant IgA deposition in glomeruli, often present with microscopic or macroscopic haematuria. The anti-GBM form (C) is characterized by linear localization of IgG on GBM by immunofluorescence and because antibodies bind to alveolar basement membranes, it often leads to lung haemorrhage. Thrombotic microangiopathy (B) is where red blood cells may become damaged by fibrin leading to haemolysis (microangiopathic haemolytic anaemia). There are two forms: diarrhoea associated and non-diarrhoeal. Amyloidosis (E) is a systemic disease that can cause glomerular lesions, where the amyloid, an extracellular fibrillar protein can deposit. It can cause proteinuria, nephritic syndrome and chronic renal failure.

Clinical manifestations of glomerular disease

47   C   Nephrotic syndrome (C) is the breakdown of selectivity of the glomerular filtration barrier leading to massive protein leak. There is proteinuria at least of 3.5 g/day, hypoalbuminaemia, oedema and hyperlipidaemia. There are systemic and primary glomerular diseases. The latter interferes with podocyte function and can be one of three types: minimal change disease, focal segmental glomerulosclerosis (FSGS) and membranous glomerulonephritis.

Acute glomerulonephritis (A) is the acute inflammation of glomeruli leading to reduction in glomerular filtration rate. Characteristic presentation is with oliguria and urine casts containing red and white blood cells. A severe form can cause renal failure and is almost always associated with glomerular crescents. Crescents are accumulations of proliferating epithelial cells in Bowman's space and indicate destroyed glomeruli from which there can be no recovery. Nephritic syndrome (B) is characterized by haematuria, oedema, oliguria resulting in severe glomerular damage and red blood cell leakage. Acute tubular necrosis (D) is an acute, reversible renal failure caused by necrosis of renal tubular epithelial cells and therefore is a disease of the tubules and interstitium and not glomerular disease. Acquired cystic disease (E) is not glomerular disease and also commonly arises in kidneys *in situ* when the patient is on dialysis for chronic renal failure.

Cerebrovascular aneurysm

48   B   Subarachnoid haemorrhage (B) is usually non-traumatic and due to rupture of a Berry aneurysm, which are present in 1 per cent of the general population. They occur on the circle of Willis, mostly at the arterial bifurcations of the internal carotid artery and within the vertebrobasilar circulation. The Berry aneurysms enlarge with time and pose the greatest risk of rupture when at 6–10 mm diameter. They are more common in females than males and in 20 per cent of cases the patients have a 'warning bleed', which will lead to a rupture and poses a much worse prognosis than without a 'warning bleed'.

The basilar artery is an extracerebral artery and this rules out an intracerebral haemorrhage (A). 'Watershed' strokes (C) are infarctions caused by hypoperfusion at the periphery of a blood supply. There does not have to be an occlusion. Transient ischaemic attacks (D) often precede the main event, lasting several minutes to 24 h and caused by self-limiting vascular obstruction due to atheromatous emboli and/ or platelet–fibrin aggregates. One third of patients with a TIA get significant infarct within five years. Tonsillar brain herniation (E) is when cerebellar tonsils move downwards through the foramen magnum, this causes brainstem compression and is life threatening and often associated with secondary 'Duret' haemorrhage.

Cerebral infections

49   D   The diagnosis is acute purulent meningitis. It is a major cause of morbidity and mortality in all ages, but in children older than 6 years, *Streptococcus pneumoniae* (D) is the most common cause. It used to be *Haemophilus influenzae* (E) but incidence is falling due to vaccination. In neonates, the cause is usually the flora of the maternal genital tract, and the most likely organism would be group B *Streptococcus* and *Escherichia coli*. *Neisseria meningitidis* is the major cause of epidemics of meningitis in older children, adolescents and young adults and can present without a rash, although the presence of a non-blanching rash makes *Neisseria* a likely diagnosis, and this form of meningitis is rapidly fatal. *Staphylococcus aureus* (C) and Gram-negative rods are common causes in people with surgical shunts. Meninges appear congested and purulent material is present in the subarachnoid space. Prognosis depends on speedy accurate treatment.

If the organism is viral, the diagnosis will be acute lymphocytic meningitis. This can be caused by the Coxsackie's virus (A), echovirus, HIV and the mumps virus. The cerebrospinal fluid would contain mostly lymphocytes. Clinical features would often be less severe despite similar symptoms and signs to acute purulent meningitis. *Treponema pallidum* (B) is a cause of chronic meningitis and the infiltrate would characteristically contain lymphocytes, plasma cells and epithelioid macrophages.

HIV in children

50   A   Almost all new childhood HIV infections are due to mother-to-child (vertical) transmission; before (*in utero*), during childbirth (*intra partum*) or through breastfeeding. HIV viral load tests are reported as the number of HIV copies in a millilitre (copies/mL) of blood. A high viral load can be anywhere from 5000 to 10 000 copies/mL. Initial, untreated and uncontrolled HIV viral loads can range as high as one million or more copies/mL. A low viral load is usually between 40 and 500 copies/mL and this result indicates that HIV is not actively reproducing and that the risk of disease progression is low.

The clinical features of HIV infection include: suppurative ear infections, enlarged lymph nodes, hepatomegaly, splenomegaly, easy bruising, enlarged parotids, oral thrush, herpes zoster infection, clubbing, anaemia, progressive encephalopathy, frequent nose bleeds, failure to thrive, severe pneumonia (TB, LIP, PCC), severe nappy rash, recurrent or persistent diarrhoea. Classes of anti-retrovirals currently used for children in Africa are: non-nucleoside reverse transcriptase inhibitors, nucleoside reverse transcriptase inhibitors, nucleotide reverse transcriptase inhibitors and protease inhibitors.

The comprehensive approach to preventing HIV infection in infants is:

- Prevention of HIV in parents
- Prevention of unintended pregnancies among HIV-infected women
- Prevention of transmission from an HIV-infected woman to her infant
- Care and support for HIV-infected women, their infants and their families

Index